Update on the Shoulder

Guest Editor

JENNY T. BENCARDINO, MD

MAGNETIC RESONANCE IMAGING CLINICS OF NORTH AMERICA

www.mri.theclinics.com

Consulting Editors
VIVIAN S. LEE, MD, PhD, MBA
LYNNE STEINBACH, MD
SURESH MUKHERJI, MD

May 2012 • Volume 20 • Number 2

SAUNDERS an imprint of ELSEVIER, Inc.

W.B. SAUNDERS COMPANY
A Division of Elsevier Inc.

1600 John F. Kennedy Boulevard • Suite 1800 • Philadelphia, Pennsylvania 19103-2899

http://www.theclinics.com

MRI CLINICS OF NORTH AMERICA Volume 20, Number 2
May 2012 ISSN 1064-9689, ISBN 13: 978-1-4557-3888-5

Editor: Sarah Barth
Developmental Editor: Donald Mumford

Magnetic Resonance Imaging Clinics of North America (ISSN 1064-9689) is published quarterly by Elsevier Inc., 360 Park Avenue South, New York, NY 10010-1710. Months of issue are February, May, August, and November. Business and Editorial Offices: 1600 John F. Kennedy Blvd., Ste. 1800, Philadelphia, PA 19103-2899. Customer Service Office: 3251 Riverport Lane, Maryland Heights, MO 63043. Periodicals postage paid at New York, NY and additional mailing offices. Subscription prices are $337.00 per year (domestic individuals), $541.00 per year (domestic institutions), $172.00 per year (domestic students/residents), $376.00 per year (Canadian individuals), $678.00 per year (Canadian institutions), $488.00 per year (international individuals), $678.00 per year (international institutions), and $249.00 per year (international and Canadian students/residents). International air speed delivery is included in all *Clinics* subscription prices. All prices are subject to change without notice. **POSTMASTER:** Send address changes to *Magnetic Resonance Imaging Clinics*, Elsevier Health Sciences Division, Subscription Customer Service, 3251 Riverport Lane, Maryland Heights, MO 63043. Customer Service (orders, claims, online, change of address): Elsevier Health Sciences Division, Subscription Customer Service, 3251 Riverport Lane, Maryland Heights, MO 63043. Tel:1-800-654-2452 (U.S. and Canada); 314-447-8871 (outside U.S. and Canada). Fax: 314-447-8029. E-mail: journalscustomerservice-usa@elsevier.com (for print support); journalsonlinesupport-usa@elsevier.com (for online support).

Reprints. For copies of 100 or more of articles in this publication, please contact the Commercial Reprints Department, Elsevier Inc., 360 Park Avenue South, New York, NY 10010-1710. Tel.: 212-633-3812; Fax: 212-462-1935; E-mail: reprints@elsevier.com.

Magnetic Resonance Imaging Clinics of North America is covered in the *RSNA Index of Imaging Literature, MEDLINE/PubMed (Index Medicus),* and *EMBASE/Excerpta Medica.*

Printed in the United States of America.

GOAL STATEMENT

The goal of *Magnetic Resonance Imaging Clinics of North America* is to keep practicing physicians up to date with current clinical practice by providing timely articles reviewing the state of the art in patient care.

ACCREDITATION

The *Magnetic Resonance Imaging Clinics of North America* is planned and implemented in accordance with the Essential Areas and Policies of the Accreditation Council for Continuing Medical Education (ACCME) through the joint sponsorship of the University of Virginia School of Medicine and Elsevier. The University of Virginia School of Medicine is accredited by the ACCME to provide continuing medical education for physicians.

The University of Virginia School of Medicine designates this enduring material activity for a maximum of 15 *AMA PRA Category 1 Credit*(s)™ for each issue, 60 credits per year. Physicians should claim only the credit commensurate with the extent of their participation in the activity.

The American Medical Association has determined that physicians not licensed in the US who participate in this CME enduring material activity are eligible for a maximum of *15 AMA PRA Category 1 Credit*(s)™ for each issue, 60 credits per year.

Credit can be earned by reading the text material, taking the CME examination online at http://www.theclinics.com/home/cme, and completing the evaluation. After taking the test, you will be required to review any and all incorrect answers. Following completion of the test and evaluation, your credit will be awarded and you may print your certificate.

FACULTY DISCLOSURE/CONFLICT OF INTEREST

The University of Virginia School of Medicine, as an ACCME accredited provider, endorses and strives to comply with the Accreditation Council for Continuing Medical Education (ACCME) Standards of Commercial Support, Commonwealth of Virginia statutes, University of Virginia policies and procedures, and associated federal and private regulations and guidelines on the need for disclosure and monitoring of proprietary and financial interests that may affect the scientific integrity and balance of content delivered in continuing medical education activities under our auspices.

The University of Virginia School of Medicine requires that all CME activities accredited through this institution be developed independently and be scientifically rigorous, balanced and objective in the presentation/discussion of its content, theories and practices.

All authors/editors participating in an accredited CME activity are expected to disclose to the readers relevant financial relationships with commercial entities occurring within the past 12 months (such as grants or research support, employee, consultant, stock holder, member of speakers bureau, etc.). The University of Virginia School of Medicine will employ appropriate mechanisms to resolve potential conflicts of interest to maintain the standards of fair and balanced education to the reader. Questions about specific strategies can be directed to the Office of Continuing Medical Education, University of Virginia School of Medicine, Charlottesville, Virginia.

The faculty and staff of the University of Virginia Office of Continuing Medical Education have no financial affiliations to disclose.

The authors/editors listed below have identified no professional or financial affiliations for themselves or their spouse/partner:

Sarah Barth, (Acquisitions Editor); Asheesh Bedi, MD; Luis S. Beltran, MD; Javier Beltran, MD; Jenny T. Bencardino, MD (Guest Editor); Jean-François Budzik, MD, MSc; Eric Y. Chang, MD; Nancy A. Chauvin, MD; Jodi Cohen, MD; Randy M. Cohen, MD; Anne Cotten, MD, PhD; Eduard de Lange, MD (Test Author); Xavier Demondion, MD, PhD; Kevin S. Dunham, MD; Timothy Farley, MD; Evelyne Fliszar, MD; Soterios Gyftopoulos, MD; Brady K. Huang, MD; Igor Immerman, MD; Camilo Jaimes, MD; David A. Jamadar, MB, BS, FRCS, FRCR, DMRD; Diego Jaramillo, MD, MPH; Renata La Rocca Vieira, MD; Tal Laor, MD; Vivian S. Lee, MD, PhD, MBA (Consulting Editor); Peter J. MacMahon, MD; Yoav Morag, MD; Antoine Moraux, MD; Violeta Nikac, MD; George C. Nomikos, MD; William E. Palmer, MD; Vittorio Pansini, MD; Christopher Pettis, MD; Michael Recht, MD; Donald Resnick, MD; Leon D. Rybak, MD; A. Ross Sussmann, MD; Michael J. Tuite, MD; Christopher Wasyliw, MD; Guillaume Wavreille, MD, MSc.

The authors/editors listed below identified the following professional or financial affiliations for themselves or their spouse/partner:

Laura W. Bancroff, MD is on the Speakers' Bureau for IICME, and has book royalties with Lippincott.
Christine B. Chung, MD is an industry funded research/investigator for GE Healthcare.
Laith M. Jazrawi, MD is a consultant for Depuy Mitek, Knee Creations, Core Essence, Ferring Pharmaceuticals, and ConMed Linvatec.
Suresh Mukherji, MD (Consulting Editor) is a consultant for Philips Medical Systems.
Andrew S. Rokito, MD is on the Advisory Board for Core Essence Orthopaedics.
Mark E. Schweitzer, MD is on the Advisory Board for Pfizer, Inc. and Paradigm spine.
Lynne Steinbach, MD (Consulting Editor) is a consultant for Pfizer, Inc.
Joseph D. Zuckerman, MD receives royalties from Exactech, Inc.

Disclosure of Discussion of non-FDA approved uses for pharmaceutical products and/or medical devices:

The University of Virginia School of Medicine, as an ACCME provider, requires that all faculty presenters identify and disclose any "off label" uses for pharmaceutical and medical device products. The University of Virginia School of Medicine recommends that each physician fully review all the available data on new products or procedures prior to instituting them with patients.

TO ENROLL

To enroll in the Magnetic Resonance Imaging Clinics of North America Continuing Medical Education program, call customer service at 1-800-654-2452 or visit us online at www.theclinics.com/home/cme. The CME program is available to subscribers for an additional fee of $196.00.

Contributors

CONSULTING EDITORS

VIVIAN S. LEE, MD, PhD, MBA
Professor of Radiology; Vice President for Health Sciences, University of Utah, Salt Lake City, Utah

LYNNE STEINBACH, MD
Professor of Clinical Radiology and Orthopaedic Surgery, University of California, San Francisco, San Francisco, California

SURESH MUKHERJI, MD
Professor and Chief of Neuroradiology and Head and Neck Radiology; Professor of Radiology, Otolaryngology Head and Neck Surgery, Radiation Oncology, Periodontics and Oral Medicine, University of Michigan Health System, Ann Arbor, Michigan

GUEST EDITOR

JENNY T. BENCARDINO, MD
Associate Professor of Radiology, Department of Radiology, New York University Hospital for Joint Diseases, New York University Langone Medical Center, New York, New York

AUTHORS

LAURA W. BANCROFT, MD
Adjunct Professor, Department of Radiology, University of Central Florida School of Medicine; Clinical Professor, Florida State University School of Medicine, Florida Hospital, Orlando, Florida

ASHEESH BEDI, MD
Clinical Assistant Professor, Department of Orthopedic Surgery, University of Michigan Hospitals, Ann Arbor, Michigan

JAVIER BELTRAN, MD
Chairman of Radiology, Department of Radiology, Maimonides Medical Center, Brooklyn, New York

LUIS S. BELTRAN, MD
Assistant Professor of Radiology, Department of Radiology, New York University Langone Medical Center, New York, New York

JENNY T. BENCARDINO, MD
Associate Professor of Radiology, Department of Radiology, New York University Hospital for Joint Diseases, New York University Langone Medical Center, New York, New York

JEAN-FRANÇOIS BUDZIK, MD, MSc
Service d'Imagerie Médicale, Hôpital St Vincent de Paul, Lille, France

ERIC Y. CHANG, MD
Assistant Professor of Radiology, Department of Radiology, VA San Diego Healthcare System; Assistant Professor of Radiology, University of California San Diego Medical Center, San Diego, California

NANCY A. CHAUVIN, MD
Assistant Professor of Radiology, Department of Radiology, The Children's Hospital of Philadelphia, Perelman School of Medicine at the University of Pennsylvania, Philadelphia, Pennsylvania

CHRISTINE B. CHUNG, MD
Professor of Radiology, Department of
Radiology, University of California San Diego
Medical Center; Professor of Radiology,
Department of Radiology, VA San Diego
Healthcare System, San Diego, California

JODI COHEN, MD
Assistant Professor, Radiology, Hospital
for Joint Diseases/Orthopedic Institute,
New York, New York

RANDY M. COHN, MD
Resident, Orthopaedic Surgery, New York
University Hospital for Joint Diseases,
New York, New York

ANNE COTTEN, MD, PhD
Professeur, Service de Radiologie et Imagerie
Musculosquelettique, Centre de Consultation
et d'Imagerie de l'Appareil Locomoteur,
Lille, France

XAVIER DEMONDION, MD, PhD
Professeur, Service de Radiologie et Imagerie
Musculosquelettique, Centre de Consultation
et d'Imagerie de l'Appareil Locomoteur,
Lille, France

KEVIN S. DUNHAM, MD
Assistant Professor, Department of Radiology,
New York University Langone Medical Center,
New York, New York

TIMOTHY FARLEY, MD
Adjunct Assistant Professor, Department of
Radiology, University of Central Florida School
of Medicine, Florida Hospital, Orlando, Florida

EVELYNE FLISZAR, MD
Associate Professor of Radiology, Department
of Radiology, University of California San Diego
Medical Center, San Diego, California

SOTERIOS GYFTOPOULOS, MD
Assistant Professor, Department of Radiology,
New York University Hospital for Joint
Diseases, New York, New York

BRADY K. HUANG, MD
Assistant Clinical Professor of Radiology,
Division of Musculoskeletal Imaging,
San Diego School of Medicine, University of
California; University of California San Diego
Teleradiology and Education Center, San
Diego, California

IGOR IMMERMAN, MD
Resident, Department of Orthopaedic Surgery,
New York University Hospital for Joint
Diseases, New York, New York

CAMILO JAIMES, MD
Research Assistant, Department of Radiology,
The Children's Hospital of Philadelphia,
Perelman School of Medicine at the University
of Pennsylvania, Philadelphia, Pennsylvania

**DAVID A. JAMADAR, MB,BS, FRCS,
FRCR, DMRD**
Clinical Professor, Department of Radiology,
University of Michigan Hospitals, Ann Arbor,
Michigan

DIEGO JARAMILLO, MD, MPH
Radiologist-in-Chief, Professor of Radiology,
Department of Radiology, The Children's
Hospital of Philadelphia, Perelman School
of Medicine at the University of Pennsylvania,
Philadelphia, Pennsylvania

LAITH M. JAZRAWI, MD
Chief of the Division of Sports Medicine,
Associate Professor of Orthopaedic Surgery,
New York University Hospital for Joint
Diseases, New York, New York

RENATA LA ROCCA VIEIRA, MD
Assistant Professor, Department of Radiology,
New York University School of Medicine,
New York, New York

TAL LAOR, MD
Professor of Radiology and Pediatrics, Division
Co-Chief, Musculoskeletal Imaging,
Department of Radiology, Cincinnati Children's
Hospital Medical Center; Professor of
Radiology, University of Cincinnati College
of Medicine, Cincinnati, Ohio

PETER J. MACMAHON, MD
Clinical Fellow, Harvard Medical School;
Department of Musculoskeletal Imaging and
Intervention, Massachusetts General Hospital,
Boston, Massachusetts

YOAV MORAG, MD
Clinical Assistant Professor, Department of
Radiology, University of Michigan Hospitals,
Ann Arbor, Michigan

ANTOINE MORAUX, MD
Service de Radiologie et Imagerie
Musculosquelettique, Centre de Consultation
et d'Imagerie de l'Appareil Locomoteur,
Lille, France

VIOLETA NIKAC, MD
Department of Radiology, Maimonides Medical
Center, Brooklyn, New York

†GEORGE C. NOMIKOS, MD
Associate Professor, Department of Radiology,
Georgetown University Medical Center,
Washington, DC

WILLIAM E. PALMER, MD
Assistant Professor, Harvard Medical School;
Department of Musculoskeletal Imaging and
Intervention, Massachusetts General Hospital,
Boston, Massachusetts

VITTORIO PANSINI, MD
Service de Radiologie et Imagerie
Musculosquelettique, Centre de Consultation
et d'Imagerie de l'Appareil Locomoteur,
Lille, France

CHRISTOPHER PETTIS, MD
Adjunct Assistant Professor, Department
of Radiology, University of Central Florida
School of Medicine, Florida Hospital,
Orlando, Florida

MICHAEL RECHT, MD
Professor of Radiology and Chairman,
Department of Radiology, New York University
School of Medicine, New York, New York

DONALD RESNICK, MD
Professor of Radiology, Chief, Division of
Musculoskeletal Imaging, San Diego School
of Medicine, University of California; University
of California San Diego Teleradiology and
Education Center, San Diego, California

ANDREW S. ROKITO, MD
Associate Professor, Chief, Division of
Shoulder and Elbow Surgery, Department of
Orthopaedic Surgery and Hospital for Joint
Diseases, New York University Medical Center,
New York, New York

LEON D. RYBAK, MD
Assistant Professor, Acting Section Chief,
Department of Radiology, New York University
School of Medicine, New York, New York

MARK E. SCHWEITZER, MD
Professor and Chair of Radiology, Department
of Diagnostic Imaging, The Ottawa Hospital,
University of Ottawa, Ottawa, Ontario, Canada

A. ROSS SUSSMANN, MD
Radiology, Hospital for Joint Diseases/
Orthopedic Institute, New York, New York

MICHAEL J. TUITE, MD
Professor of Radiology, Head, Division of
Musculoskeletal Imaging and Intervention,
University of Wisconsin School of Medicine
and Public Health, Madison, Wisconsin

CHRISTOPHER WASYLIW, MD
Adjunct Assistant Professor, Department
of Radiology, University of Central Florida
School of Medicine, Florida Hospital,
Orlando, Florida

GUILLAUME WAVREILLE, MD, MSc
Service de Chirurgie de la Main et du
Membre Supérieur, Centre de Consultations
et d'Imagerie de l'Appareil Locomoteur,
Lille, France

JOSEPH D. ZUCKERMAN, MD
Walter A.L. Thompson Professor of Orthopedic
Surgery, Department of Orthopaedic Surgery,
New York University Hospital for Joint
Diseases, New York, New York

---

† Deceased.

Contents

pathophysiological or mechanical cause of the impingement. These include poster-osuperior impingement, anterosuperior impingement, anterior impingement, and entrapment of the long head of the biceps tendon. The objective of this article is to review magnetic resonance imaging findings of each of the 4 types of internal impingement syndromes and discuss the pathophysiology behind the impingement.

Magnetic resonance (MR) imaging is the primary diagnostic imaging modality for the evaluation of patients with suspected internal derangement of the shoulder joint. Awareness and understanding of the complex anatomy of the shoulder articulation and the ability to recognize normal anatomic variants and potential imaging pitfalls are critical to accurate interpretation of conventional and arthrographic MR imaging studies. This review discusses the normal anatomy and anatomic variants of the glenoid labrum, articular cartilage, and glenohumeral ligaments. An improved understanding of normal anatomy, biomechanics, and variants will help to avoid potential pitfalls in the interpretation of noncontrast and arthrographic shoulder MR imaging examinations.

The rotator interval is an anatomically defined triangular area located between the coracoid process, the superior aspect of the subscapularis, and the anterior aspect of the supraspinatus. It is widely accepted that the rotator interval structures fulfill a role in biomechanics and pathology of the glenohumeral joint and long head biceps tendon. However, there is ongoing debate regarding the biomechanical details and the indications for treatment. A better understanding of rotator interval anatomy and function will lead to improved treatment of rotator interval abnormalities, and guide the indications for imaging and surgical intervention.

The extreme range of motion at the shoulder, high velocities and stresses, and repetitive nature of the throwing motion place the throwing athlete at risk for a wide range of pathologic entities. The treating orthopedist must fully understand the biomechanics of the throwing cycle and how it contributes to the potential injuries in the throwing shoulder during each phase of the throwing motion. The goal of orthopedic care and rehabilitation is to allow the throwing athlete to return symptom free to the preinjury level of competition.

The glenohumeral joint provides the greatest range of motion of any joint in the human body. Over the past several decades, histologic studies, biomechanical studies, and improved arthroscopic techniques have contributed to improved knowledge and treatment of glenohumeral joint abnormalities. Continuing advances in magnetic resonance technology have allowed for improved noninvasive visualization of the stabilizers of the shoulder. This article reviews the concept of glenohumeral joint microinstability and its relationship with superior labrum anterior and posterior (SLAP) lesions, reviews the role of the labrum as a stabilizer of the shoulder, and focuses on the diagnosis and classification of SLAP lesions.

prompt treatment, which is critical for joint preservation in the case of infection, for maximal therapeutic efficacy of disease-modifying drugs in the case of rheumatoid arthritis, and for expediting symptomatic relief in the cases of CPPD deposition disease and HAD.

---

† Deceased.

Magnetic Resonance Imaging Clinics of North America

THE CLINICS ARE NOW AVAILABLE ONLINE!

Access your subscription at:
www.theclinics.com

Preface

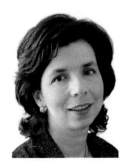

Jenny T. Bencardino, MD
Guest Editor

The unique anatomy and range of motion of the shoulder joint can present a diagnostic challenge. Careful physical examination and radiographic findings often provide important clues in the differential diagnosis and, in many instances, may be sufficient for the assessment of patients with shoulder pain and/or instability. However, characterization of soft tissue injuries and radiographically occult osseous pathology at the shoulder often benefits from the use of MR imaging, a technique that over the past two decades has secured its place as a very important tool in the diagnostic workup of internal derangements affecting the shoulder joint.

The clinical applicability of MR imaging of the shoulder has benefited greatly from the routine use of high field strength magnets and dedicated multi-channel coils as well as from the recent technical developments on 3D imaging acquisition techniques, biochemical imaging of cartilage and metal reduction artifact sequences. Drs Renata La Rocca Vieira, Leon Rybak, and Michael Recht's "Technical Update on MRI of the Shoulder" provides the reader with a cutting-edge, state-of-the-art review on this topic.

Drs Brady Huang and Donald Resnick in their article "Novel Concepts in MR Imaging of the Rotator Cuff Tendons and Their Footprints" bring to light relatively new anatomical and histological descriptions, which have crucial implications in the etiology and pathogenesis of rotator cuff failure as well as important applications in the clinical manifestations and treatment of rotator cuff disease.

"The Rotator Cable: MR Evaluation and Clinical Correlation" by Drs Soterios Gyftopoulos, Jenny Bencardino, Igor Immerman, and Joseph Zuckerman reviews the anatomy and explores the potential biomechanical function of the rotator cable in both the intact and the torn rotator cuff as well as the potential role that the integrity of the rotator cable can play in the treatment selection of patients with rotator cuff tears.

Dr Michael Tuite, in his article "MR Imaging of Rotator Cuff Disease and External Impingement," thoroughly reviews the role of MR imaging as a diagnostic tool in the identification of rotator cuff disease and pathology of the coracoacromial arch associated with external impingement.

"Internal Impingement Syndromes" are often observed in the throwing athletic population. Drs Luis Beltran and Javier Beltran clearly describe the constellation of findings on MR imaging and MR arthrography characteristic for anterior, anterosuperior, posterosuperior, and long head of biceps tendon entrapment syndromes.

Drs Kevin Dunham, Jenny Bencardino, and Andrew Rokito, in their article "Anatomic Variants and Pitfalls of the Labrum, Glenoid Cartilage, and Glenohumeral Ligaments," stress the importance of in-depth understanding of normal anatomy, biomechanics, and variants of the shoulder joint in order to avoid potential pitfalls in the interpretation of noncontrast and arthrographic shoulder MR examinations.

"The Rotator Interval and Long Head of Biceps Tendon: Anatomy, Function, Pathology, and MR Imaging" by Drs Yoav Morag, Asheesh Bedi, and David Jamadar thoroughly covers current concepts, allowing for a better understanding of the rotator interval anatomy and function aimed to provide improved treatment for rotator interval pathology and guide the indications for imaging and surgical intervention.

The pathology of the throwing shoulder is a relatively common problem in Sports Medicine practice

Magn Reson Imaging Clin N Am 20 (2012) xv–xvi
doi:10.1016/j.mric.2012.01.015

affecting both the professional and the recreational athlete. "The Throwing Shoulder: The Orthopedist Perspective" by Drs Randy Cohn and Laith Jazrawi explores the biomechanics of the throwing cycle as well as the clinical manifestations and treatment of typical shoulder injuries that affect throwing athletes.

Drs Eric Chang, Evelyne Fliszar, and Christine Chung, in their article entitled "SLAP Lesions and Microinstability," review the challenging concept of shoulder microinstability and its association with SLAP injuries using both clinical and structural perspectives. Emphasis is made in the imaging evaluation of the group of abnormalities that affect the superior labrum as well as the supporting structures of the superior half of the shoulder joint.

"MR Imaging of Glenohumeral Instability" by Drs Peter MacMahon and William Palmer covers the ever-challenging topic of diagnostic imaging evaluation of the labral capsular complex in the setting of acute dislocation and chronic instability with special insights into the biomechanics of the shoulder joint and treatment implications.

MR imaging of the shoulder joint following surgical treatment of external impingement, rotator cuff disease, and labral capsular injuries is covered thoroughly by Drs Laura Bancroft, Christopher Wasyliw, Christopher Pettis, and Timothy Farley in their article "Postoperative Shoulder MR Imaging." The authors review the features of successful shoulder surgery as well as MR findings that should alert to the possibility of postoperative complications.

"Imaging of the Pediatric Shoulder" by Drs Nancy Chauvin, Camilo Jaimes, Tal Laor, and Diego Jaramillo offers a comprehensive update on the principal tenets of MR imaging of the growing shoulder. The article provides insight into the normal appearance of the glenohumeral osseous and soft tissue structures as well as a thorough review of the pathologic conditions that may affect the pediatric shoulder joint.

Drs A. Ross Sussmann, Jodi Cohen, George Nomikos, and Mark Schweitzer provide up-to-date concepts in the imaging evaluation of inflammatory and infectious shoulder arthropathies including a thorough review of the pathophysiology, clinical manifestations, and treatment of crystal deposition diseases, rheumatoid arthritis, and infectious arthritis of the shoulder joint.

Drs Jean-François Budzik, Guillaume Wavreille, Vittorio Pansini, Antoine Moraux, Xavier Demondion, and Anne Cotten provide a clinical-based review of "Entrapment Neuropathies of the Shoulder" including the anatomy and pathophysiology of the involved nerves as well as the MR imaging features of winging scapular deformity and neurogenic pain syndromes affecting the shoulder girdle.

The journey as guest editor for this issue of the *Magnetic Resonance Imaging Clinics of North America* "Update on the Shoulder" issue has been both inspiring and rewarding thanks to the excellent contributions of so many experts in the fields of sports medicine, orthopedics, and musculoskeletal radiology. My utmost gratitude goes out to all the authors and also to Sarah Barth and her team at Elsevier for their support. I have no doubt that the readers will find this collection of articles a useful up-to-date reference tool on MR imaging of the shoulder during their daily clinical practice.

Jenny T. Bencardino, MD
Department of Radiology
New York University School of Medicine
New York University Hospital for Joint Diseases
Sixth Floor
301 East 17th Street
New York, NY 10003, USA

E-mail address:
Jenny.Bencardino@nyumc.org

Dedication

To my husband Alvand and my children Dario and Avan, the force behind my inspiration.

To my parents Teresa and Libardo, with eternal gratitude. To Dr. Zehava Sadka Rosenberg and Dr. Javier Beltran for their unwavering trust and support.

Magn Reson Imaging Clin N Am 20 (2012) xvii
doi:10.1016/j.mric.2012.01.016

mri.theclinics.com

Erratum

With regard to the article "Congenital cardiovascular malformations: Noninvasive imaging by MRI in neonates," by Rajesh Krishnamurthy and Edward Lee, which appeared in *Magnetic Resonance Imaging Clinics of North America,* Nov 2011 19(4): 813–22 (doi: 10.1016/j.mric.2011.08.002), the publisher would like to clarify that Dr Lee's full name is Edward Y. Lee.

Magn Reson Imaging Clin N Am 20 (2012) xviii
doi:10.1016/j.mric.2012.03.002
1064-9689/12/$ – see front matter © 2012 Elsevier Inc. All rights reserved.

Technical Update on Magnetic Resonance Imaging of the Shoulder

Renata La Rocca Vieira, MD[a],*, Leon D. Rybak, MD[a],
Michael Recht, MD[b]

KEYWORDS

• Shoulder • Magnetic resonance imaging • Technique

Magnetic resonance (MR) imaging with its exquisite soft tissue discrimination and multiplanar capabilities is the imaging modality of choice in the evaluation of the painful shoulder. In many cases, the study is ordered to evaluate for shoulder pain of unknown cause. Conversely, when the source of symptoms is already clear based on physical examination and plain radiography, the examination is ordered to exclude any concomitant condition that would preclude surgery, dictate an alternative surgical approach, or could be addressed at the time of surgery. MR imaging has proved to be invaluable, particularly when addressing issues regarding the rotator cuff, articular cartilage, and labroligamentous structures.

Since the initial use of MR imaging, there has been continued progress with respect to the hardware and software, as well as innovations in the use of contrast agents and patient positioning. This article reviews the present state of MR imaging of the shoulder, highlighting recent advances and discussing controversies with regard to their relative strengths and weaknesses when appropriate. Specifically, we address the use of 3-T MR imaging, arthrography, unique positions adapted for evaluating different portions of the joint capsule, imaging of hardware in the postoperative patient, three-dimensional (3D) imaging techniques, and functional imaging.

IS BIGGER REALLY BETTER?

Imaging at 3-T

Clinical 3-T MR imaging has been one of the fastest growing sectors of the MR imaging market since 2003.[1] This is in large part because of the advantage afforded by the inherent increase in signal-to-noise ratio (SNR) at 3-T and the potential to increase diagnostic accuracy through improved image quality. This improvement may come in the form of higher spatial resolution, speed, or optimization of contrast.

Signal and SNR increase linearly with field strength at frequencies less than 250 MHz.[2,3] Thus, with all other parameters unchanged, going from 1.5- to 3-T results in a 2-fold increase in SNR. This advantage is particularly advantageous when imaging the shoulder joint, a deep portion of anatomy that is difficult to position at the isocenter of the magnet. However, as with many things in MR imaging, there are trade-offs. These include the need to minimize the increased energy deposition or specific absorption rate at greater field strengths and countering the artifacts, which can be more prominent at 3-T compared with 1.5-T.

Artifacts are also accentuated at a higher magnet strength, including chemical shift. The frequency shift between water and fat responsible for chemical shift artifact is increased from 224 Hz at 1.5-T to 448 Hz at 3-T. With respect to the

The authors have nothing to disclose.

[a] Department of Radiology, New York University School of Medicine, 301 East 17th Street, New York, NY 10003, USA
[b] Department of Radiology, New York University School of Medicine, 560 First Avenue, New York, NY 10016, USA
* Corresponding author.
E-mail addresses: Renata.Vieira@nyumc.org, relarocca@gmail.com

Magn Reson Imaging Clin N Am 20 (2012) 149–161
doi:10.1016/j.mric.2012.01.005

images produced, this frequency shift is translated to a pixel shift. To maintain the same pixel shift at 3-T compared with 1.5-T, doubling the receiver bandwidth is indicated. This strategy increases the range of frequencies in each pixel and decreases the size of the pixel shift. Because SNR is inversely proportional to the square root of the receiver bandwidth, this results in a decrease of SNR by 44%.

Another important factor to be considered is that when the field strength increases the T1 of many tissues also increases. Longer T1 values imply that at a given time of repetition (TR), the degree of saturation increases, resulting in a loss of signal. It is thus necessary to increase the TR in most cases when using a 3-T magnet to maintain adequate T1 contrast. Because most sequences used in evaluation of the shoulder rely on intermediate weighting, this phenomenon at 3-T is not so critical.

The development of phased array coils with a greater number of elements and more flexible designs that allow positioning closer to the anatomy of interest has provided a method for gaining increased signal. The increased signal available at 3-T and with the use of phased array coils has opened the way to the use of parallel imaging of the shoulder. Parallel imaging involves the use of the individual elements in a coil to achieve spatial localization, thus reducing the number of phase encoding steps and providing adequate K space filling. However, the trade-off occurs in the form of SNR, because the information from the various coil elements is used independently as opposed to being combined. This situation results in a decrease of SNR proportional to the square root of the temporal resolution. This decreased SNR limits the use of parallel imaging to situations in which there is adequate signal, such as the use of phased array coils and 3-T magnets.

The early results on MR imaging of the shoulder at 3-T have been promising. Magee and Williams[4] retrospectively evaluated 100 MR images of the shoulder at 3-T. Comparing the results with arthroscopy, they found a sensitivity of 90% and specificity of 100% for the detection of SLAP (superior labrum from anterior to posterior) tears. The sensitivity and specificity for tears of the anterior labrum was 89% and 100% and for posterior labral tears was 86% and 100%. These results are comparable and, in many cases, better than those previously reported for the sensitivity and specificity for detecting labral tears at 1.5-T (44%–100% and 66%–100%, respectively).[5–10]

Regarding rotator cuff lesions, Magee and Williams[4] retrospectively reviewed 150 shoulder MR images at 3-T for the assessment of supraspinatus tendon tears. Comparing with arthroscopy, they found a sensitivity and specificity for detection of full-thickness tears of 98% and 96% and for partial-thickness tears of 92% and 100%. Previous studies have shown conventional MR imaging of the shoulder at 1.5-T to have a sensitivity and specificity in the range of 84% to 100% and 86% to 98% for detection of full-thickness supraspinatus tendon tears and sensitivity and specificity in the range of 35% to 92% and 85% to 97% for partial-thickness tears.[7,11–17] This seems to imply comparable performance with respect to full-thickness tears and an improvement with respect to the detection of partial-thickness tears. However, to our knowledge, there is no controlled study showing a significant diagnostic improvement of 3-T over 1.5-T for shoulder lesions.

In our experience, the increased signal afforded by the use of 3-T imaging has allowed for finer matrices and increased in-plane resolution, resulting in better overall image quality and more detailed evaluation of fine intra-articular structures, creating greater diagnostic confidence, particularly with respect to labral (**Fig. 1**) and chondral lesions (**Fig. 2**) as well as partial rotator cuff tears.

Table 1 summarizes the protocol for shoulder MR imaging at 3-T at our institution.

TO INJECT OR NOT TO INJECT
The Arthrography Question

Over time, it has become the standard of practice at many imaging centers to request MR

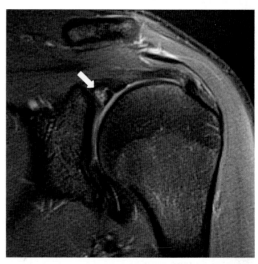

Fig. 1. 3-T MR image of the left shoulder of a 20-year-old man with shoulder pain. Coronal oblique, fluid-sensitive, fat-suppressed image of the shoulder showing a SLAP tear in detail (*white arrow*).

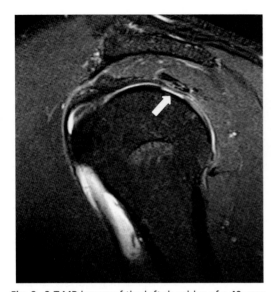

Fig. 2. 3-T MR image of the left shoulder of a 40-year-old man with shoulder pain. Sagittal oblique, fluid-sensitive, fat-suppressed sequence of the shoulder showing a full-thickness cartilage defect along the posterosuperior margin of the humeral head (*white arrow*). Cartilage lesions can be difficult to detect in the glenohumeral joint because of thin cartilage layers over closely apposed curved surfaces.

arthrographic examinations, particularly in the postoperative patient or when evaluating for undersurface tears of the rotator cuff as well as when the presence of intra-articular bodies and lesions of the glenoid cartilage and labroligamentous structures is suspected.[18–35] Arthrography can be performed using direct or indirect techniques.

Direct MR arthrography (D-MRA) of the shoulder is an invasive procedure that is well tolerated by most patients.[36] It involves the injection of a contrast solution into the shoulder joint to distend the capsule and outline the intra-articular structures, thereby improving their delineation and evaluation at subsequent MR imaging (**Fig. 3**).

Most arthrographic examinations involve the injection of dilute gadolinium (Gd) solution in a concentration of 1 to 2 mmol/L.[37,38] Needle placement for intra-articular contrast injection is usually achieved with fluoroscopic or sonographic guidance. Iodinated contrast can be included in the solution to confirm needle placement and confirm an intra-articular injection. Many radiologists choose an anterior approach for evaluation of suspected lesions of the posterior labroligamentous structures and a posterior approach when the symptoms point to involvement of the anterior labrum and capsule. This strategy is used to prevent inadvertent extravasation injection of contrast material, thus obscuring important findings.[24,39] The rotator interval approach has been advocated by others as an alternative anterior mode of access, resulting in a lower probability of injury to key intra-articular structures.[40] Ultrasonography has been used to guide both posterior and rotator interval approaches.[41,42]

Indirect MR arthrography (I-MRA) is based on the principle that intravenous contrast material diffuses into the joint space over time, producing an arthrographic effect. In I-MRA, Gd-based contrast in a concentration of 0.1 mmol/kg is injected intravenously and MR imaging is performed after a delay. Intravenous Gd diffuses from the capillary bed into the interstitial space of the synovium and then leaks into the joint space. The arthrographic effect is dependent on the permeability of the synovial membrane, which is increased in inflammatory conditions, such as rheumatoid arthritis and infection, as well as in the setting of trauma or previous surgery.[43] Factors affecting passage of contrast material between the blood vessels and synovial fluid include a pressure differential between these spaces and the viscosity of the intra-articular fluid.[44] Effusions under tension or those with fluid of increased viscosity (eg, hemorrhagic or purulent material) result in a decreased rate of contrast diffusion into the joint. Other factors that can

Table 1					
Suggested protocol for 3-T MR imaging of the shoulder					
Sequence	TR (ms)	Echo Time (ms)	Slice (mm)	Matrix (%)	Field of View (mm)
Axial proton density	3030	33	2.0	256 × 100	140 × 140
Coronal T2 fat-saturated	3500	72	3.0	256 × 151	140 × 140
Coronal proton density	4500	32	2.0	320 × 75	140 × 140
Sagittal T2 fat-saturated	5000	62	2.5	320 × 75	140 × 140
Sagittal T1	600	11	2.5	320 × 90	140 × 140

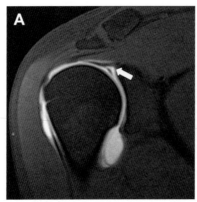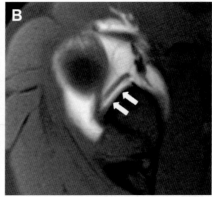

Fig. 3. (*A*, *B*) 1.5-T D-MRA of the right shoulder of a 29-year-old woman with shoulder pain shows the SLAP tear with contrast filling the defect (*white arrow* in *A*). On the axial image (*B*), the classic Oreo cookie sign (*white arrows* in *B*) is noted, with contrast filling the gap between the labrum and glenoid.

lead to suboptimal I-MRA include lack of joint effusion, synovial fibrosis, premature scanning time, or extravasation.[45]

Increasing the dose of contrast material administered intravenously may increase the diffusion gradient, but has been shown to have a limited effect.[28,43,46] Other methods of promoting blood flow to the joint, including exercise, have been used.[47] When a traditional technique is used, a delay of 15 minutes is sufficient. In the presence of a tense or viscous joint effusion, delay times should be increased.

With I-MRA, there can be enhancement of vessels and extra-articular structures, including synovial lined spaces such as tendon sheaths and bursae. Another potential drawback of the method is the lack of adequate capsular distension.

For both D-MRA and I-MRA, the subsequent MR imaging protocol usually consists of T1-weighted fat-suppressed sequences in various planes as well as at least 1 fluid-sensitive fat-suppressed sequence for detection of marrow edema or extra-articular fluid collections. T1-weighted imaging without fat suppression may also be used to capitalize on the signal of the Gd solution and allow for superior contrast in areas delineated by high signal fat.

With respect to clinical performance, D-MRA has been shown to have sensitivity and specificity for detection of labral tears in the range of 80% to 100% and 50% to 100%, respectively, regardless of tear location.[48,49] Chandnani and colleagues[50] found sensitivities for MR imaging and D-MRA of 93% and 96%, respectively, but found the D-MRA better at detecting detached labral fragments (96% vs 46%). Waldt and colleagues[51] found the sensitivity and specificity for detection of all labral tears with D-MRA to be 88% and

91% and Magee and colleagues[52] reported the detection of 9 labral tears in a population of 20 athletes not noted on conventional MR imaging.[51,52] D-MRA has performed particularly well with respect to SLAP tears, with sensitivities of 90% to 100% reported.[53,54]

With regard to the rotator cuff, D-MRA has performed well with respect to full-thickness tears with sensitivities close to 100%.[16,55] D-MRA has also proved more accurate in the detection of partial-thickness undersurface tears of the supraspinatus, with sensitivities and specificities of 80% to 84% and 96% to 97%, respectively.[55,56]

D-MRA is believed to be particularly useful in the postoperative patient. Probyn and colleagues[57] studied a population of 40 patients with recurrent instability after previous capsular repair. Their results indicated sensitivity and specificity in diagnosis of labral tears of 96.2% and 81.8%, and in detecting rotator cuff injury of 94.1% and 81.8%, respectively.

Additional benefits that have been reported for D-MRA include better depiction of the structures of the rotator interval and accurate depiction of lesions involving the proximal biceps tendon.[25,58]

There are not so many reports addressing the clinical efficacy of I-MRA. Wallny and colleagues[59] reported sensitivity and specificity in the diagnosis of labral injuries of 90% and 89%, respectively, compared with 79% and 67% for noncontrast MR imaging. Dinauer and colleagues[60] compared I-MRA with MR imaging with respect to superior labral tears and found it to be more sensitive (84%–91% vs 66%–85%) but less specific (58%–71% vs 75%–83%), with a slightly improved overall accuracy (78%–86% vs 70%–83%). Yagci and colleagues[61] reported sensitivity and specificity for detection of all rotator cuff tears at

I-MRA as 100% and 77.8% to 88.9%, respectively, compared with 73.3% to 80% and 66.7% to 88.9% for MR imaging.

A search of the literature revealed only 1 direct comparison between D-MRA and I-MRA of the shoulder. The investigators found no statistically significant difference between the 2 modalities in the evaluation of tears of the labrum and rotator cuff.[62]

The increased use of 3-T imaging has raised the question of whether arthrography is necessary at higher field strengths. Magee[19] retrospectively evaluated 150 conventional MR imaging and D-MRA examinations at 3-T in the same patients. Using arthroscopy as the gold standard, Magee found that D-MRA showed a statistically significant (P<.05) improvement in sensitivity for detection of partial articular-sided supraspinatus tears, anterior labral tears, and SLAP tears. Major and colleagues[63] compared conventional MR imaging and D-MRA at 3-T with arthroscopy for detection

of labral tears in 22 patients and found a sensitivity of 67% and 83% for the MR imaging and D-MRA, respectively.

PUTTING A NEW TWIST ON THINGS
Novel Imaging Positions

The use of various shoulder positions at MR imaging has been extensively discussed in the literature.[28,30,64–75] These positions have been used for the most part in conjunction with MR arthrography because there seems to be an additive effect with respect to displacing otherwise occult labral tears away from the glenoid rim. The abducted externally rotated (ABER) position (**Fig. 4**) has been shown to place the anterior band of the inferior glenohumeral ligament under tension, facilitating inspection of the anteroinferior capsulolabral complex. Cvitanic and colleagues[66] retrospectively assessed the integrity of the anterior glenohumeral ligament in 256 patients using

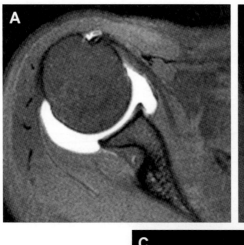
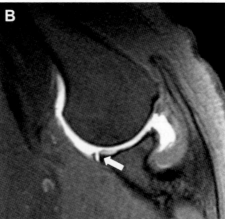
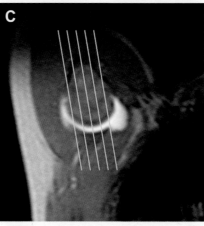

Fig. 4. (A–C) 1.5-T D-MRA of the right shoulder of a 30-year-old woman with shoulder pain. On the axial image (A), there is no evidence of labral tear. However, on the ABER view (B), the partially detached tear of the anteroinferior labrum is well seen as a result of traction on the adjacent capsule (*white arrow*), with contrast filling the defect at the level of the labral base. (C) Scout view with lines showing the plane of acquisition for the ABER view.

both conventional axial and ABER positions at D-MRA at 1.5-T and correlated the results with findings at surgery. These investigators found a sensitivity and specificity of 89% and 95% for the ABER view compared with 48% and 91% for the conventional positions, with an even greater sensitivity and specificity of 96% and 97% when both were used. Borrero and colleagues[76] studied the usefulness of the ABER position at D-MRA for the detection of a posterosuperior labral peel back injury, an injury described in the overhead athlete, and found a sensitivity of 73% and specificity of 100%. Sugimoto and colleagues[77] reported the usefulness of the ABER view at D-MRA in showing detachment of the anteroinferior capsular structures in postoperative patients.

The ABER view has also been shown to improve conspicuity of partial undersurface tears of the supraspinatus at both I-MRA and D-MRA.[18,70] Lee and Lee[69] reported increased sensitivity for the detection of the horizontal component of an undersurface tear of the supraspinatus at D-MRA from 21% to 100% using the ABER position as opposed to relying on the traditional coronal oblique view.

The flexed, adducted, and internal rotated (FADIR) position view is another novel technique that has been shown to have value in certain clinical scenarios. Chiavaras and colleagues[64] performed a retrospective review of 9 patients who were imaged using FADIR positioning at D-MRA. Although arthroscopic correlation was not available in all cases, the investigators found that the FADIR view increased diagnostic confidence in confirming, excluding, or better characterizing a posteroinferior labral abnormality in all 9 patients.

In our institution, the ABER and FADIR positions are added to the protocol for MR arthrographic examinations of the shoulder to evaluate the anteroinferior and posterior capsulolabral structures, respectively. Up to 20% of patients are not able to assume these positions because of pain or apprehension.[68]

GOING HEAVY METAL
Imaging of Hardware

Imaging in the postoperative patient presents unique challenges. Many of the fixation devices used by orthopedic surgeons contain metal, and instruments used at the time of surgery can leave metal shavings behind. In the case of shoulder arthroplasty, the problems of imaging around metal take on even greater importance. Metal can result in large areas of magnetic field inhomogeneity, local gradient-induced eddy currents on metal surfaces, and radiofrequency (RF) shielding effects.[78] Of these factors, metal-induced field inhomogeneities result in the most severe artifacts. Knowledge of these artifacts and techniques used to reduce them has become essential.

Factors to consider in imaging of patients with metallic surgical devices or arthroplasty include the composition of the hardware, the orientation of the hardware in relation to the direction of the main magnetic field (B_0), the type of pulse sequence, the strength of the magnetic field, and imaging parameters (voxel size, field of view, image matrix, and slice thickness).

Ferromagnetic materials, which have high magnetic susceptibility, produce greater artifacts than titanium alloys. Magnetic field inhomogeneities change the phase and frequency of local spins. The result is misregistration and loss of signal, with associated distortion of the shape of the metallic object, predominantly along the frequency axis.[79] It is important to swap phase and frequency direction when required, so as not to obscure the area of clinical interest.

The radiologist cannot control for the type of metal; however, certain changes in the imaging protocol can help reduce the degree of artifact. Whenever possible, the hardware should be positioned parallel to the main magnetic field. Turbo spin echo (TSE) or fast spin echo (FSE) sequences should always be chosen and gradient echo (GRE) sequences avoided. This strategy is because the multiple 180° refocusing pulses help reduce the amount of field inhomogeneity and distortion. The lowest interecho spacing should be achieved so as to minimize the time between the 180° pulses. This spacing can be achieved, at the expense of signal, by increasing (in most cases doubling) the bandwidth (**Fig. 5**), which reduces the frequency sampling time and makes it possible to reduce the echo time. Using longer echo trains, a high-resolution matrix and decreased slice thickness can also be helpful. If fat suppression is required, inversion recovery sequences are preferred to frequency-selective fat-saturation sequences, which rely on field homogeneity.

In imaging of shoulder arthroplasty, the eccentric location of the shoulder relative to the isocenter of the imaging bore and the large spherical humeral component contribute to the more severe susceptibility artifact observed compared with knee or hip arthroplasty.[80]

Although considered the sequence of choice in cases of hardware imaging, FSE or TSE techniques still lead to spatially dependent artifacts (eg, signal voids and pile-ups) as a result of a nonlinear frequency-position mapping caused by metal-induced field inhomogeneities.[78]

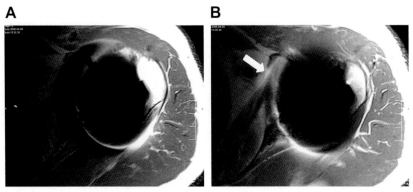

Fig. 5. (*A, B*) Patient's status after shoulder arthroplasty with clinical suspicion for subscapularis tendon tear. (*A*) Significant susceptibility artifact precludes the evaluation of the subscapularis tendon. (*B*) After doubling the bandwidth, the subscapularis tendon is better visualized (*white arrow*).

Recently, new metal reduction artifact techniques in high-field MR imaging magnets have been introduced, including slice encoding for metal artifact correction (SEMAC), view-angle tilting (VAT), and multiacquisition variable-resonance image combination (MAVRIC).[78,81–84] The SEMAC technique, which was introduced by Lu and colleagues,[78] is a modified spin echo sequence that uses VAT and slice-direction phase encoding to correct both in-plane and through-plane artifacts. Hargreaves and colleagues[85] found that SEMAC imaging combined with standard echo-train imaging, parallel imaging, partial-Fourier imaging, and inversion recovery techniques offered flexible image contrast with reduction of metal-induced artifact in scan times less than 11 minutes. With the MAVRIC technique, multiple 3D FSE image datasets are acquired at different frequency bands, offset from the dominant proton frequency, and the images combined, resulting in decreased susceptibility artifact.[81] Chen and colleagues[82] evaluated SEMAC and MAVRIC in 25 postoperative knees and found both effectively reduced artifact extent compared with FSE. A hybrid SEMAC-MAVRIC technique has also been proposed.[86]

Because these imaging techniques are recent developments, there has not been much written about their performance in the clinical setting. Hayter and colleagues[81] performed a retrospective comparison of MAVRIC with FSE images in the evaluation of patients who had undergone hip, shoulder, or knee arthroplasty. They found visualization of the synovium, periprosthetic bone, and supraspinatus tendon to be significantly better on MAVRIC images than on FSE images. More research on the clinical efficacy of these techniques needs to be conducted before they can be used in routine clinical practice.

TAKING IT TO NEW DIMENSIONS
3D Volumetric Imaging

To date, 3D sequences have found their greatest clinical use in evaluation of articular cartilage. Because volumetric imaging has a cost with respect to time, most of these sequences have used fast GRE techniques. These sequences can be broken down into bright-fluid and dark-fluid techniques depending on the signal intensity of the synovial fluid and relative contrast with the articular cartilage.

Many types of 3D GRE sequences including spoiled gradient recalled echo, GRE, double-echo steady state, and fast imaging with steady-state precession (FISP) have been used in imaging of the shoulder joint.[87–91] Lee and colleagues[87] found fat-suppressed GRE to be more sensitive than conventional spin echo T1-weighted sequences with respect to the evaluation of labral tears at D-MRA of the shoulder. Oh and colleagues[88] prospectively compared the diagnostic accuracy of 3D GRE isotropic with conventional FSE sequences at 3-T I-MRA for the diagnosis of labral and rotator cuff lesions. These investigators found no statistically significant difference in sensitivities and specificities using both methods. Magee found that 3D fast GRE isotropic imaging provided the same clinical information as conventional imaging at 3 T with decreased imaging times.[89] Jung and colleagues[90] compared the diagnostic accuracy of 3D fat-suppressed fast GRE using isotropic voxels with traditional two-dimensional (2D) FSE sequences at MR arthrography with respect to the diagnosis of labral lesions. These investigators also found no significant difference in sensitivity and specificity.

More recently, 3D FSE sequences including SPACE (sampling perfection with applications oriented contrast using different flip angle evolutions) (**Fig. 6**) and CUBE have been successfully used, leading to more traditional TSE or FSE contrast. These sequences use long echo trains and parallel imaging to reduce scan time. Variable flip angle modulation is used to constrain T2 decay over an extended echo train, which allows intermediate-weighted images of the joint to be acquired with minimal blurring.[92]

There are few published data regarding the use of 3D FSE sequences in the shoulder. Rybak and colleagues[93] assessed the performance of the SPACE sequence using intermediate-weighted fat-suppressed technique and near isotropic voxels compared with a standard 2D protocol in D-MRA at 1.5-T. Although they found the 3D images to suffer from mildly increased blurring, they allowed for greater confidence in assessing small curved structures such as the proximal biceps tendon and curved portions of the labrum, as well as abnormalities related to partial articular-sided tears of the supraspinatus and posterior labral tears.

In our opinion, these techniques have shown great promise as an adjunct to more traditional MR imaging of the shoulder and can be used selectively to answer specific questions. The possibility of multiplanar reconstruction after image acquisition is an intriguing one both with respect to time savings as well as tailored imaging planes. However, more research is required with regard to the sensitivity and specificity for detection of lesions.

MORE THAN JUST ANATOMY
Biochemical Imaging

Much recent research in MR imaging in the musculoskeletal system has focused on articular cartilage and osteoarthritis (OA).[94] With advances in coil design and field strength, it has become possible to provide exquisite detail with regard to morphologic alterations in cartilage structure. However, the shoulder presents significant challenges in this respect. The cartilage over the glenohumeral joint is between 1- and 1.8-mm thick, which translates to 1 to 2 voxels at the resolution of most clinically used protocols. The curved shape and closely apposed congruent surfaces of the humeral head accentuate the partial volume averaging inherent in most 2D MR protocols.[95] Despite these problems, investigators have reported good sensitivities and specificities for detecting cartilage lesions. Hayes and colleagues,[96] using both MR imaging and D-MRA images, reported an overall sensitivity and specificity of 87.2% and 80.6% in detection of articular cartilage lesions in patients with known instability. Guntern and colleagues[97] studied patients with clinical subacromial impingement with D-MRA. Correlating with arthroscopy, they found a moderate sensitivity and specificity of 53% to 100% and 51% to 87% for humeral lesions and 75% and 63% to 66% for glenoid lesions. Dietrich and colleagues,[98] using a 3D water-excitation true FISP sequence at D-MRA, found improvement in detection of cartilage lesions, which they attributed to thinner slices and increased SNR with the 3D technique.

Investigators have now turned their attention to the search for more sensitive methods for detecting early alterations in the ultrastructure of the cartilage that precede these gross morphologic changes. The MR imaging sequences that have been developed to assess the ultrastructure are targeted at assessing the proteoglycan content as well as collagen orientation and concentration. Most studies dealing with functional imaging have been focused on the knee, where OA is particularly prevalent, the cartilage is thick, and the articular surfaces relatively flat. We are aware of only a few preliminary studies evaluating functional

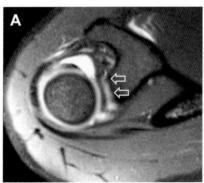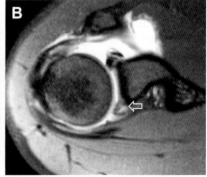

Fig. 6. (A, B) SPACE sequence of the right shoulder. 1-mm-thick axial reconstruction obtained from the 3D data set showing excellent signal and resolution in outlining a SLAP tear (*open arrows* in A and B).

MR imaging of the glenohumeral cartilage.[99–101] Yet, it is important for the imager to be familiar with these techniques because they will almost certainly be applied in all areas of joint imaging once perfected.

The T2 mapping technique assesses the zonal structure of the collagen component of articular cartilage. The orientation of the collagen within the radial, intermediate, and superficial zones helps to dictate the T2 values in these areas. The highly organized orientation in the radial and superficial zones where the fibers are oriented perpendicular and parallel to the subchondral plate, respectively, results in shorter T2 values. In contrast, the random orientation of the collagen fibers in the intermediate zone results in longer T2 values. These findings form the basis for T2 mapping in which changes in T2 values can herald changes in collagen content and structure. T2 mapping can be implemented in a routine clinical environment without hardware modifications or the need for contrast. In a preliminary study, Maizlin and colleagues[100] successfully reported the feasibility of T2 mapping in the glenohumeral joint in routine clinical imaging in 27 shoulders.

The T1ρ technique assesses low-frequency interactions between hydrogen and proteoglycan macromolecules in free water. Referred to as spin lattice relaxation in the rotating frame, it uses clusters of RF pulses to lock magnetization in the transverse plane, followed by additional RF pulses to drive longitudinal recovery. Capturing several values allows the slope of the decay function to be solved and either gray-scale or color-coded maps created. T1ρ has been shown to correlate to proteoglycan content and fixed charge density in clinical OA specimens at 4 T.[102] Similar to T2 mapping, T1ρ mapping can also be performed without the need for an exogenous contrast agent or hardware modifications. In a pilot study, La Rocca Vieira and colleagues[101] successfully assessed the normal T1ρ values of cartilage in the glenohumeral joint of 4 asymptomatic volunteers at 3-T. However, this study was limited by lack of arthroscopic correlation and small sample size.

Delayed Gd-enhanced MR imaging of cartilage (dGEMRIC) has been used to estimate the glycosaminoglycan (GAG) content of cartilage. In early cartilage degeneration, these negatively charged GAG molecules are depleted. When negatively charged Gd salts are injected intravenously, they replace the negative charge vacated by these GAG molecules. By measuring T1 relaxation times after the intravenous administration of the T1 shortening agent, Gd, a map of the areas of GAG depletion can be obtained. The dGEMRIC technique requires a double dose of Gd and an adequate delay to allow for absorption by the cartilage. Most protocols incorporate a brief period of exercise (approximately 10 minutes) followed by a 30-minute to 90-minute delay. Using the dGEMRIC technique, Wiener and colleagues[99] investigated the contrast dynamics in hyaline and fibrous cartilage of the glenohumeral joint after intra-articular injection of gadopentate dimeglumine in 5 cadaveric shoulders. These investigators found a significant decrease in T1 15 minutes after intra-articular contrast injection with more rapid accumulation of contrast in the hyaline as opposed to labral cartilage. This information, although preliminary, shows the feasibility of performing dGEMRIC in the shoulder and might aid in determining the optimal timing after contrast injection for data acquisition. More research regarding the efficacy and usefulness of these relatively novel techniques for assessing early cartilage degeneration in the shoulder needs to be conducted until it can be used clinically.

Improvement in both hardware and software has opened up new opportunities in MR imaging of the shoulder. MR imaging at 3-T has become a reality, with the prospect of 7-T imaging on the horizon. The art of MR arthrography continues to improve, aided by the use of novel imaging positions. New techniques for 3D imaging, the reduction of metal artifacts, and biochemical imaging of cartilage hold great promise.

REFERENCES

1. Mosher TJ. Musculoskeletal imaging at 3T: current techniques and future applications. Magn Reson Imaging Clin North Am 2006;14(1):63–76.

2. Collins CM, Smith MB. Signal-to-noise ratio and absorbed power as functions of main magnetic field strength, and definition of "90 degrees" RF pulse for the head in the birdcage coil. Magn Reson Med 2001;45(4):684–91.

3. Edelstein WA, Glover GH, Hardy CJ, et al. The intrinsic signal-to-noise ratio in NMR imaging. Magn Reson Med 1986;3(4):604–18.

4. Magee TH, Williams D. Sensitivity and specificity in detection of labral tears with 3.0-T MRI of the shoulder. AJR Am J Roentgenol 2006;187(6): 1448–52.

5. Legan JM, Burkhard TK, Goff WB 2nd, et al. Tears of the glenoid labrum: MR imaging of 88 arthroscopically confirmed cases. Radiology 1991; 179(1):241–6.

6. Green MR, Christensen KP. Magnetic resonance imaging of the glenoid labrum in anterior shoulder instability. Am J Sports Med 1994;22(4):493–8.

7. Iannotti JP, Zlatkin MB, Esterhai JL, et al. Magnetic resonance imaging of the shoulder. Sensitivity, specificity, and predictive value. J Bone Joint Surg Am 1991;73(1):17–29.

8. Murray PJ, Shaffer BS. Clinical update: MR imaging of the shoulder. Sports Med Arthrosc 2009;17(1):40–8.

9. Gusmer PB, Potter HG, Schatz JA, et al. Labral injuries: accuracy of detection with unenhanced MR imaging of the shoulder. Radiology 1996; 200(2):519–24.

10. Garneau RA, Renfrew DL, Moore TE, et al. Glenoid labrum: evaluation with MR imaging. Radiology 1991;179(2):519–22.

11. Kneeland JB, Middleton WD, Carrera GF, et al. MR imaging of the shoulder: diagnosis of rotator cuff tears. AJR Am J Roentgenol 1987;149(2):333–7.

12. Singson RD, Hoang T, Dan S, et al. MR evaluation of rotator cuff pathology using T2-weighted fast spin-echo technique with and without fat suppression. AJR Am J Roentgenol 1996;166(5):1061–5.

13. Zlatkin MB, Iannotti JP, Roberts MC, et al. Rotator cuff tears: diagnostic performance of MR imaging. Radiology 1989;172(1):223–9.

14. Quinn SF, Sheley RC, Demlow TA, et al. Rotator cuff tendon tears: evaluation with fat-suppressed MR imaging with arthroscopic correlation in 100 patients. Radiology 1995;195(2):497–500.

15. Reinus WR, Shady KL, Mirowitz SA, et al. MR diagnosis of rotator cuff tears of the shoulder: value of using T2-weighted fat-saturated images. AJR Am J Roentgenol 1995;164(6):1451–5.

16. Toyoda H, Ito Y, Tomo H, et al. Evaluation of rotator cuff tears with magnetic resonance arthrography. Clin Orthop Relat Res 2005;439:109–15.

17. Balich SM, Sheley RC, Brown TR, et al. MR imaging of the rotator cuff tendon: interobserver agreement and analysis of interpretive errors. Radiology 1997; 204(1):191–4.

18. Jung JY, Jee WH, Chun HJ, et al. Magnetic resonance arthrography including ABER view in diagnosing partial-thickness tears of the rotator cuff: accuracy, and inter- and intra-observer agreements. Acta Radiol 2010;51(2):194–201.

19. Magee T. 3-T MRI of the shoulder: is MR arthrography necessary? AJR Am J Roentgenol 2009; 192(1):86–92.

20. Chundru U, Riley GM, Steinbach LS. Magnetic resonance arthrography. Radiol Clin North Am 2009;47(3):471–94.

21. Catalano OA, Manfredi R, Vanzulli A, et al. MR arthrography of the glenohumeral joint: modified posterior approach without imaging guidance. Radiology 2007;242(2):550–4.

22. Chung CB, Corrente L, Resnick D. MR arthrography of the shoulder. Magn Reson Imaging Clin North Am 2004;12(1):25–38, v–vi.

23. Steinbach LS, Palmer WE, Schweitzer ME. Special focus session. MR arthrography. Radiographics 2002;22(5):1223–46.

24. Chung CB, Dwek JR, Feng S, et al. MR arthrography of the glenohumeral joint: a tailored approach. AJR Am J Roentgenol 2001;177(1):217–9.

25. Chung CB, Dwek JR, Cho GJ, et al. Rotator cuff interval: evaluation with MR imaging and MR arthrography of the shoulder in 32 cadavers. J Comput Assist Tomogr 2000;24(5):738–43.

26. Roger B, Skaf A, Hooper AW, et al. Imaging findings in the dominant shoulder of throwing athletes: comparison of radiography, arthrography, CT arthrography, and MR arthrography with arthroscopic correlation. AJR Am J Roentgenol 1999;172(5): 1371–80.

27. Oh CH, Schweitzer ME, Spettell CM. Internal derangements of the shoulder: decision tree and cost-effectiveness analysis of conventional arthrography, conventional MRI, and MR arthrography. Skeletal Radiol 1999;28(12):670–8.

28. Wintzell G, Larsson H, Larsson S. Indirect MR arthrography of anterior shoulder instability in the ABER and the apprehension test positions: a prospective comparative study of two different shoulder positions during MRI using intravenous gadodiamide contrast for enhancement of the joint fluid. Skeletal Radiol 1998;27(9):488–94.

29. Stoller DW. MR arthrography of the glenohumeral joint. Radiol Clin North Am 1997;35(1):97–116.

30. Tirman PF, Bost FW, Steinbach LS, et al. MR arthrographic depiction of tears of the rotator cuff: benefit of abduction and external rotation of the arm. Radiology 1994;192(3):851–6.

31. Schweitzer ME. MR arthrography of the labral-ligamentous complex of the shoulder. Radiology 1994;190(3):641–4.

32. Fritz RC, Stoller DW. Fat-suppression MR arthrography of the shoulder. Radiology 1992;185(2):614–5.

33. Flannigan B, Kursunoglu-Brahme S, Snyder S, et al. MR arthrography of the shoulder: comparison with conventional MR imaging. AJR Am J Roentgenol 1990;155(4):829–32.

34. Gundry CR, Schils JP, Resnick D, et al. Arthrography of the post-traumatic knee, shoulder, and wrist. Current status and future trends. Radiol Clin North Am 1989;27(5):957–71.

35. Resnick D. Shoulder arthrography. Radiol Clin North Am 1981;19(2):243–53.

36. Giaconi JC, Link TM, Vail TP, et al. Morbidity of direct MR arthrography. AJR Am J Roentgenol 2011;196(4):868–74.

37. Kopka L, Funke M, Fischer U, et al. MR arthrography of the shoulder with gadopentetate dimeglumine: influence of concentration, iodinated contrast material, and time on signal intensity. AJR Am J Roentgenol 1994;163(3):621–3.

38. Engel A. Magnetic resonance knee arthrography. Enhanced contrast by gadolinium complex in the rabbit and in humans. Acta Orthop Scand Suppl 1990;240:1–57.

39. Farmer KD, Hughes PM. MR arthrography of the shoulder: fluoroscopically guided technique using a posterior approach. AJR Am J Roentgenol 2002;178(2):433–4.

40. Depelteau H, Bureau NJ, Cardinal E, et al. Arthrography of the shoulder: a simple fluoroscopically guided approach for targeting the rotator cuff interval. AJR Am J Roentgenol 2004;182(2):329–32.

41. Gokalp G, Dusak A, Yazici Z. Efficacy of ultrasonography-guided shoulder MR arthrography using a posterior approach. Skeletal Radiol 2010;39(6):575–9.

42. Souza PM, Aguiar RO, Marchiori E, et al. Arthrography of the shoulder: a modified ultrasound guided technique of joint injection at the rotator interval. Eur J Radiol 2010;74(3):e29–32.

43. Vahlensieck M, Sommer T, Textor J, et al. Indirect MR arthrography: techniques and applications. Eur Radiol 1998;8(2):232–5.

44. Bergin D, Schweitzer ME. Indirect magnetic resonance arthrography. Skeletal Radiol 2003;32(10):551–8.

45. Morrison WB. Indirect MR arthrography: concepts and controversies. Semin Musculoskelet Radiol 2005;9(2):125–34.

46. Peh WC, Cassar-Pullicino VN. Magnetic resonance arthrography: current status. Clin Radiol 1999;54(9):575–87.

47. Vahlensieck M, Peterfy CG, Wischer T, et al. Indirect MR arthrography: optimization and clinical applications. Radiology 1996;200(1):249–54.

48. Schulte-Altedorneburg G, Gebhard M, Wohlgemuth WA, et al. MR arthrography: pharmacology, efficacy and safety in clinical trials. Skeletal Radiol 2003;32(1):1–12.

49. Bencardino JT, Beltran J, Rosenberg ZS, et al. Superior labrum anterior-posterior lesions: diagnosis with MR arthrography of the shoulder. Radiology 2000;214(1):267–71.

50. Chandnani VP, Yeager TD, DeBerardino T, et al. Glenoid labral tears: prospective evaluation with MRI imaging, MR arthrography, and CT arthrography. AJR Am J Roentgenol 1993;161(6):1229–35.

51. Waldt S, Burkart A, Imhoff AB, et al. Anterior shoulder instability: accuracy of MR arthrography in the classification of anteroinferior labroligamentous injuries. Radiology 2005;237(2):578–83.

52. Magee T, Williams D, Mani N. Shoulder MR arthrography: which patient group benefits most? AJR Am J Roentgenol 2004;183(4):969–74.

53. Amin MF, Youssef AO. The diagnostic value of magnetic resonance arthrography of the shoulder in detection and grading of SLAP lesions: comparison with arthroscopic findings. Eur J Radiol 2011. [Epub ahead of print].

54. Applegate GR, Hewitt M, Snyder SJ, et al. Chronic labral tears: value of magnetic resonance arthrography in evaluating the glenoid labrum and labralbicipital complex. Arthroscopy 2004;20(9):959–63.

55. Waldt S, Bruegel M, Mueller D, et al. Rotator cuff tears: assessment with MR arthrography in 275 patients with arthroscopic correlation. Eur Radiol 2007;17(2):491–8.

56. Meister K, Thesing J, Montgomery WJ, et al. MR arthrography of partial thickness tears of the undersurface of the rotator cuff: an arthroscopic correlation. Skeletal Radiol 2004;33(3):136–41.

57. Probyn LJ, White LM, Salonen DC, et al. Recurrent symptoms after shoulder instability repair: direct MR arthrographic assessment–correlation with second-look surgical evaluation. Radiology 2007;245(3):814–23.

58. Zanetti M, Weishaupt D, Gerber C, et al. Tendinopathy and rupture of the tendon of the long head of the biceps brachii muscle: evaluation with MR arthrography. AJR Am J Roentgenol 1998;170(6):1557–61.

59. Wallny T, Sommer T, Steuer K, et al. Clinical and nuclear magnetic resonance tomography diagnosis of glenoid labrum injuries. Unfallchirurg 1998;101(8):613–8 [in German].

60. Dinauer PA, Flemming DJ, Murphy KP, et al. Diagnosis of superior labral lesions: comparison of noncontrast MRI with indirect MR arthrography in unexercised shoulders. Skeletal Radiol 2007;36(3):195–202.

61. Yagci B, Manisali M, Yilmaz E, et al. Indirect MR arthrography of the shoulder in detection of rotator cuff ruptures. Eur Radiol 2001;11(2):258–62.

62. Jung JY, Yoon YC, Yi SK, et al. Comparison study of indirect MR arthrography and direct MR arthrography of the shoulder. Skeletal Radiol 2009;38(7):659–67.

63. Major NM, Browne J, Domzalski T, et al. Evaluation of the glenoid labrum with 3-T MRI: is intraarticular contrast necessary? AJR Am J Roentgenol 2011;196(5):1139–44.

64. Chiavaras MM, Harish S, Burr J. MR arthrographic assessment of suspected posteroinferior labral lesions using flexion, adduction, and internal rotation positioning of the arm: preliminary experience. Skeletal Radiol 2010;39(5):481–8.

65. Brossmann J, Preidler KW, Pedowitz RA, et al. Shoulder impingement syndrome: influence of shoulder position on rotator cuff impingement–an anatomic study. AJR Am J Roentgenol 1996;167(6):1511–5.

66. Cvitanic O, Tirman PF, Feller JF, et al. Using abduction and external rotation of the shoulder to

increase the sensitivity of MR arthrography in revealing tears of the anterior glenoid labrum. AJR Am J Roentgenol 1997;169(3):837–44.

67. Kwak SM, Brown RR, Trudell D, et al. Glenohumeral joint: comparison of shoulder positions at MR arthrography. Radiology 1998;208(2):375–80.

68. Choi JA, Suh SI, Kim BH, et al. Comparison between conventional MR arthrography and abduction and external rotation MR arthrography in revealing tears of the antero-inferior glenoid labrum. Korean J Radiol 2001;2(4):216–21.

69. Lee SY, Lee JK. Horizontal component of partial-thickness tears of rotator cuff: imaging characteristics and comparison of ABER view with oblique coronal view at MR arthrography initial results. Radiology 2002;224(2):470–6.

70. Herold T, Bachthaler M, Hamer OW, et al. Indirect MR arthrography of the shoulder: use of abduction and external rotation to detect full- and partial-thickness tears of the supraspinatus tendon. Radiology 2006;240(1):152–60.

71. Michael JW, Springorum HP, Berzdorf A, et al. Upright MRI of the shoulder demonstrates labrum dynamics. Int J Sports Med 2008;29(12):999–1002.

72. Schreinemachers SA, van der Hulst VP, Jaap Willems W, et al. Is a single direct MR arthrography series in ABER position as accurate in detecting anteroinferior labroligamentous lesions as conventional MR arthrography? Skeletal Radiol 2009;38(7):675–83.

73. Schreinemachers SA, van der Hulst VP, Willems WJ, et al. Detection of partial-thickness supraspinatus tendon tears: is a single direct MR arthrography series in ABER position as accurate as conventional MR arthrography? Skeletal Radiol 2009;38(10):967–75.

74. Iyengar JJ, Burnett KR, Nottage WM, et al. The abduction external rotation (ABER) view for MRI of the shoulder. Orthopedics 2010;33(8):562–5.

75. Yan J, Wang Y, Liu X, et al. Vertical weight-bearing MRI provides an innovative method for standardizing Spurling test. Med Hypotheses 2010;75(6):538–40.

76. Borrero CG, Casagranda BU, Towers JD, et al. Magnetic resonance appearance of posterosuperior labral peel back during humeral abduction and external rotation. Skeletal Radiol 2010;39(1):19–26.

77. Sugimoto H, Suzuki K, Mihara K, et al. MR arthrography of shoulders after suture-anchor Bankart repair. Radiology 2002;224(1):105–11.

78. Lu W, Pauly KB, Gold GE, et al. SEMAC: Slice Encoding for Metal Artifact Correction in MRI. Magn Reson Med 2009;62(1):66–76.

79. Lee MJ, Kim S, Lee SA, et al. Overcoming artifacts from metallic orthopedic implants at high-field-strength MR imaging and multi-detector CT. Radiographics 2007;27(3):791–803.

80. Sperling JW, Potter HG, Craig EV, et al. Magnetic resonance imaging of painful shoulder arthroplasty. J Shoulder Elbow Surg 2002;11(4):315–21.

81. Hayter CL, Koff MF, Shah P, et al. MRI after arthroplasty: comparison of MAVRIC and conventional fast spin-echo techniques. AJR Am J Roentgenol 2011;197(3):W405–11.

82. Chen CA, Chen W, Goodman SB, et al. New MR imaging methods for metallic implants in the knee: artifact correction and clinical impact. J Magn Reson Imaging 2011;33(5):1121–7.

83. Toms AP, Smith-Bateman C, Malcolm PN, et al. Optimization of metal artefact reduction (MAR) sequences for MRI of total hip prostheses. Clin Radiol 2010;65(6):447–52.

84. Kolind SH, MacKay AL, Munk PL, et al. Quantitative evaluation of metal artifact reduction techniques. J Magn Reson Imaging 2004;20(3):487–95.

85. Hargreaves BA, Chen W, Lu W, et al. Accelerated slice encoding for metal artifact correction. J Magn Reson Imaging 2010;31(4):987–96.

86. Koch KM, Brau AC, Chen W, et al. Imaging near metal with a MAVRIC-SEMAC hybrid. Magn Reson Med 2011;65(1):71–82.

87. Lee MJ, Motamedi K, Chow K, et al. Gradient-recalled echo sequences in direct shoulder MR arthrography for evaluating the labrum. Skeletal Radiol 2008;37(1):19–25.

88. Oh DK, Yoon YC, Kwon JW, et al. Comparison of indirect isotropic MR arthrography and conventional MR arthrography of labral lesions and rotator cuff tears: a prospective study. AJR Am J Roentgenol 2009;192(2):473–9.

89. Magee T. Can isotropic fast gradient echo imaging be substituted for conventional T1 weighted sequences in shoulder MR arthrography at 3 Tesla? J Magn Reson Imaging 2007;26(1):118–22.

90. Jung JY, Yoon YC, Choi SH, et al. Three-dimensional isotropic shoulder MR arthrography: comparison with two-dimensional MR arthrography for the diagnosis of labral lesions at 3.0 T. Radiology 2009;250(2):498–505.

91. Xia Y, Zheng S. Reversed laminar appearance of articular cartilage by T1-weighting in 3D fat-suppressed spoiled gradient recalled echo (SPGR) imaging. J Magn Reson Imaging 2010;32(3):733–7.

92. Kijowski R, Gold GE. Routine 3D magnetic resonance imaging of joints. J Magn Reson Imaging 2011;33(4):758–71.

93. Rybak L, La Rocca Vieira R, Shephard T, et al. Comparison of 3D isotropic intermediate-weighted with standard 2D FSE sequences techniques for shoulder arthrography RSNA. Chicago,

2010. Available at: http://rsna2010.rsna.org/search/ search.cfm?action=add&filter=Subspecialty&value= 301102122. Accessed November 20, 2011.

94. Bijlsma JW, Berenbaum F, Lafeber FP. Osteoarthritis: an update with relevance for clinical practice. Lancet 2011;377(9783):2115–26.

95. Polster JM, Schickendantz MS. Shoulder MRI: what do we miss? AJR Am J Roentgenol 2010;195(3): 577–84.

96. Hayes ML, Collins MS, Morgan JA, et al. Efficacy of diagnostic magnetic resonance imaging for articular cartilage lesions of the glenohumeral joint in patients with instability. Skeletal Radiol 2010; 39(12):1199–204.

97. Guntern DV, Pfirrmann CW, Schmid MR, et al. Articular cartilage lesions of the glenohumeral joint: diagnostic effectiveness of MR arthrography and prevalence in patients with subacromial impingement syndrome. Radiology 2003;226(1): 165–70.

98. Dietrich TJ, Zanetti M, Saupe N, et al. Articular cartilage and labral lesions of the glenohumeral joint: diagnostic performance of 3D water-excitation true FISP MR arthrography. Skeletal Radiol 2010;39(5):473–80.

99. Wiener E, Hodler J, Pfirrmann CW. Delayed gadolinium-enhanced MRI of cartilage (dGEMRIC) of cadaveric shoulders: comparison of contrast dynamics in hyaline and fibrous cartilage after intraarticular gadolinium injection. Acta Radiol 2009;50(1):86–92.

100. Maizlin ZV, Clement JJ, Patola WB, et al. T2 mapping of articular cartilage of glenohumeral joint with routine MRI correlation–initial experience. HSS J 2009;5(1):61–6.

101. La Rocca Vieira R, Pakin SK, de Albuquerque Cavalcanti CF, et al. Three-dimensional spin-lock magnetic resonance imaging of the shoulder joint at 3 T: initial experience. Skeletal Radiol 2007; 36(12):1171–5.

102. Regatte RR, Akella SV, Lonner JH, et al. T1rho relaxation mapping in human osteoarthritis (OA) cartilage: comparison of T1rho with T2. J Magn Reson Imaging 2006;23(4):547–53.

Novel Anatomic Concepts in Magnetic Resonance Imaging of the Rotator Cuff Tendons and the Footprint

Brady K. Huang, MD[a,b],*, Donald Resnick, MD[a,b]

KEYWORDS

- Rotator cuff • Footprint • Anatomy • MR imaging

The anatomic and histologic descriptions of the rotator cuff tendons and footprints are continuously evolving, and new discoveries have led to novel concepts in our understanding of rotator cuff tendon pathology. These concepts may be translated into the analysis of these footprints with imaging methods, particularly magnetic resonance (MR) imaging.

FOOTPRINT OF THE SUPRASPINATUS, INFRASPINATUS, AND TERES MINOR TENDONS

Understanding the osseous anatomy of the humeral head is an important requisite for describing the rotator cuff tendon insertions. The classic anatomy of the greater tuberosity of the proximal humerus describes 3 impressions or facets, which have often been designated as superior, middle, and inferior facets or, alternatively, as horizontal, oblique, and vertical facets (**Fig. 1**). As in previous anatomic studies and traditional descriptions, these facets receive the insertional fibers of the supraspinatus, infraspinatus, and teres minor tendons, respectively.[1–4] Some of the most extensive gross anatomic and histologic work was performed by

Clark and Harryman.[5] They found that the rotator cuff tendons fused as one inseparable structure at or near their insertions on the tuberosities of the humerus. The superficial fibers of the tendons generally maintained a parallel relationship with their respective muscle bellies. The supraspinatus and infraspinatus tendons were found to fuse into one inseparable tendon approximately 15 mm from their greater tuberosity insertions. These investigators depicted an interweaving of the supraspinatus and infraspinatus tendons as they coursed toward the greater tuberosity, with some of the anterior fibers of the infraspinatus tendon attaching far anteriorly (**Fig. 2**). However, the actual anterior extent of these fibers was never elucidated.

In addition to their gross descriptions of the rotator cuff tendons, Clark and Harryman[5] described 5 distinct histologic layers of the supraspinatus and infraspinatus tendons: (1) most superiorly, a thin (1 mm in thickness) superficial layer comprising fibers of the coracohumeral ligament; (2) a thicker layer (3–5 mm) of parallel tendon fibers; (3) a deeper layer (3 mm) comprising tendon fibers without uniform orientation, crossing over one another at 45° angles; (4) a layer of loose connective tissue with thick collagen bands, which merge with the coracohumeral

The authors have nothing to disclose.

[a] Division of Musculoskeletal Imaging, San Diego School of Medicine, University of California, San Diego, CA, USA

[b] UCSD Teleradiology and Education Center, 8899 University Center Lane, Suite 370, San Diego, CA 92122, USA

* Corresponding author. UCSD Teleradiology and Education Center, 8899 University Center Lane, Suite 370, San Diego, CA 92122.

E-mail address: bradyhuang@gmail.com

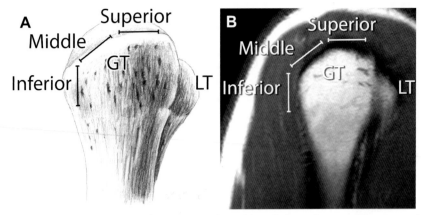

Fig. 1. (*A*) Osseous anatomy of the proximal humerus as viewed from its lateral aspect: 2 bony prominences designated as the greater tuberosity (GT), receiving the insertions of the supraspinatus, infraspinatus, and teres minor tendons, and the lesser tuberosity (LT), receiving the insertion of the subscapularis tendon. The 3 facets of the GT include the superior, middle, and inferior facets, also referred to as the horizontal, oblique, and vertical facets. (*B*) Corresponding oblique sagittal T1-weighted MR image (repetition time [TR]/echo time [TE] = 551/9 ms) obtained at 1.5 T shows the osseous anatomy of the GT and LT.

ligament along the anterior edge of the supraspinatus tendon; and (5) a thin (1.5–2 mm) layer formed by the capsule of the joint, attaching to the greater tuberosity by the Sharpey fibers (**Fig. 3**). In the third layer, the interdigitation of the supraspinatus and infraspinatus tendons resulted in their apparent fusion.

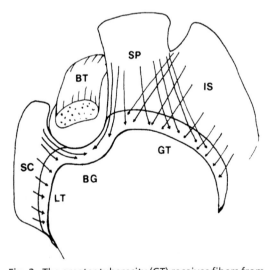

Fig. 2. The greater tuberosity (GT) receives fibers from the supraspinatus (SP) and infraspinatus (IS) tendons, showing an apparent interweaving of the fibers as they insert on the GT. The lesser tuberosity (LT) receives fibers from the subscapularis (SC) tendon. Also, fibers from the SP and SC tendons contribute to the floor of the bicipital groove (BG), which houses the long head of the biceps tendon (BT). (*From* Clark JM, Harryman DT. Tendons, ligaments, and capsule of the rotator cuff. Gross and microscopic anatomy. J Bone Joint Surg Am 1992;74:718; with permission.)

In a cadaveric study by Minagawa and colleagues,[3] a similar pattern of overlap of the supraspinatus and infraspinatus tendons was described. However, these investigators described the supraspinatus tendon as the only tendon inserting on the superior facet of the greater tuberosity, with some fibers inserting on the superior half of the middle facet. The infraspinatus tendon covered the posterior half of the supraspinatus tendon and attached to the entire length of the middle facet.[3] This type of interdigitation of the 2 tendons, which was described by Clark and Harryman[5] and subsequently by Minagawa and colleagues,[3] can be demonstrated on oblique sagittal images through the superior aspect of the cuff (**Fig. 4**).

Clark and Harryman[5] also described the existence of fibrous bands derived from the coracohumeral ligament that reinforced the superficial and deep portions of the supraspinatus and infraspinatus tendons near their greater tuberosity insertions. Regarding the relationship between the undersurface of the supraspinatus and infraspinatus tendons and the joint capsule, these structures adhered tightly near their humeral insertions. A 1-cm-wide thickening of the capsule derived from these fibrous bands of the coracohumeral ligament along the undersurface of the supraspinatus and infraspinatus tendons, located approximately 1.4 cm from the greater tuberosity footprint, was later termed the *rotator cable*, with the intervening portion of the cuff tendons designated as the *crescent*.[6] The muscles, rather than the tendons, of the infraspinatus and teres minor were inseparable just proximal to their myotendinous junctions. The teres minor demonstrated a muscular insertion approximately 2 cm below

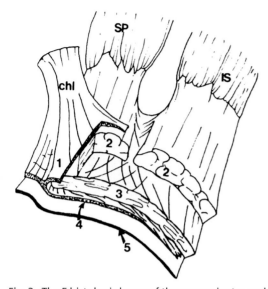

Fig. 3. The 5 histologic layers of the supraspinatus and infraspinatus tendons. Note that the coracohumeral ligament (CHL) forms an envelope around the tendons beginning at the anterior edge of the supraspinatus tendon (SP), forming layers 1 and 4. Layers 2 and 3 form the bulk of the tendon fibers, with the interweaving of the SP and infraspinatus (IS) tendons in layer 3. Layer 5, the deepest layer, is formed by the joint capsule. (*From* Clark JM, Harryman DT. Tendons, ligaments, and capsule of the rotator cuff. Gross and microscopic anatomy. J Bone Joint Surg Am 1992;74:723; with permission.)

its tendinous insertion on the greater tuberosity, a finding that can be demonstrated on MR images (**Fig. 5**).

More recently, the concept of separate tuberosity attachments of the rotator cuff tendons has been reexamined, specifically regarding the shared footprint of the supraspinatus and infraspinatus tendons. In a cadaveric study, Mochizuki and colleagues[7] revised the conventional understanding of this anatomy by demonstrating a relatively small, triangular, anteromedial footprint of the supraspinatus tendon at the superior facet and a comparatively large, trapezoidal footprint of the infraspinatus tendon occupying the anterolateral portion of the superior facet and the entire middle facet (**Fig. 6**). Again, this configuration can be depicted on oblique sagittal MR images (see **Fig. 4**). This arrangement led the investigators to conclude that the development of infraspinatus muscle atrophy in the setting of apparently isolated supraspinatus tendon tear may be related to the far anterior insertion of the infraspinatus tendon and that the infraspinatus muscle may be more biomechanically important during shoulder abduction than previously thought (**Fig. 7**).[7]

A possible related entity that has been recently described by Lunn and colleagues[8] is that of a novel lesion of the infraspinatus characterized by musculotendinous disruption, edema, and late fatty infiltration (**Fig. 8**). In their series of 19 patients, the investigators found full-thickness disruptions of the infraspinatus at the musculotendinous junction in 8 patients, within the tendon in 9 patients, and at an inconclusive site in 2 patients. These patients presented with acute pain, especially at night, with weakness of external rotation of the shoulder. This pathologic lesion was seen in middle-aged patients, with a mean age of 47.7 years, and more often in women than men. These investigators found a high incidence of accompanying rotator cuff pathology, including calcific tendinitis, tendinosis, and partial-thickness tears. Approximately 50% of their patients also reported a history of minor trauma, typically a fall on an outstretched arm. Only 1 of the 6 patients who underwent computed tomography (CT) arthrography demonstrated communication of contrast agent between the glenohumeral joint and the myotendinous junction of the infraspinatus.

Nimura and colleagues[9] further studied the contribution of the joint capsule and found that the capsule attached to the greater tuberosity beneath the supraspinatus, infraspinatus, and superior portion of the teres minor tendons. They described a biconcave area of attachment of the capsule medial to the rotator cuff tendons (**Fig. 9**). The thinnest portion of this capsular attachment was approximately 11 mm posterior to the anteriormost margin of the greater tuberosity, near the tapered posterior margin of the supraspinatus tendon, where it measured approximately 3.5 mm in width, which is in contrast to areas in which the capsular attachment was more robust, measuring as thick as 9 mm, located between the border of the infraspinatus and teres minor tendons. These investigators cited a study by Kim and colleagues,[10] which demonstrated that the most common site for degenerative rotator cuff tears was in an area 13 to 17 mm posterior to the biceps tendon. Thus, the thinnest capsular attachment on the greater tuberosity may be at risk for the development of these degenerative tears. Most partial-thickness tears of the rotator cuff tendons involve the articular side.[11–17] Earlier studies reported that most degenerative rotator cuff tendon tears affected the anterior portion of the supraspinatus tendon, with subsequent posterior propagation.[10] However, more recent studies have shown tears either isolated to or propagating from the infraspinatus tendon.[18,19] In a study by Goutallier and colleagues,[20] fatty degeneration of the infraspinatus muscle was demonstrated on preoperative CT

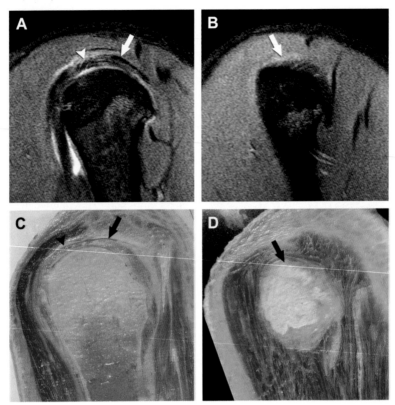

Fig. 4. Oblique sagittal proton density-weighted fat-suppressed images (repetition time [TR]/echo time [TE] = 3067/32 ms) obtained at 3 T at the level of the bicipital groove (*A*) and more laterally at the level of the greater tuberosity facets (*B*). Corresponding oblique sagittal cadaveric sections (*C, D*). The supraspinatus (*arrowhead*) and infraspinatus (*arrow*) tendons are identified separately on the more central images (*A, C*), whereas more peripherally, the fibers appear to interdigitate. In particular, the anterior fibers of the infraspinatus tendon appear to overlap those of the supraspinatus tendon and occupy the posterior half of the horizontal facet of the greater tuberosity (*B, D*).

scans, occurring in the context of large anterosuperior cuff tears that did not appear to involve the infraspinatus tendon (see **Fig. 7**).

The anatomy of the capsular attachments to the greater tuberosity and their relationship with degenerative cuff tears require that this discussion make reference to the bare area, initially described by DePalma[21] as a region along the posterior aspect of the humeral head between the insertion of the posterolateral capsule and overlying

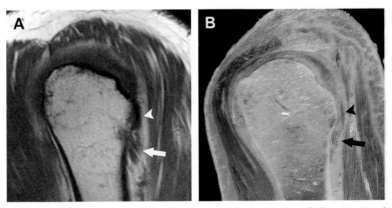

Fig. 5. (*A*) Oblique sagittal T1-weighted image (repetition time [TR]/echo time [TE] = 551/9 ms) obtained at 3 T and (*B*) oblique sagittal cadaveric section, showing the upper tendinous insertion of the teres minor (*arrowhead*) at the vertical facet of the greater tuberosity, with a muscular insertion (*arrow*) inferiorly at the surgical neck.

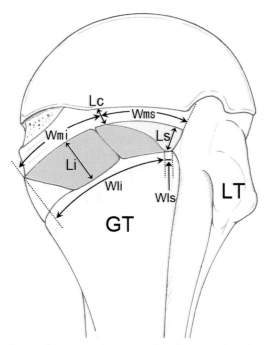

Fig. 6. The supraspinatus tendon footprint (*pink*) is depicted by a triangular area on the greater tuberosity (GT), whereas the footprint of the infraspinatus tendon (*purple*) is depicted by a larger trapezoidal area occupying the lateral portion of the horizontal facet. (*From* Mochizuki T, Sugaya H, Uomizu M, et al. Humeral insertion of the supraspinatus and infraspinatus. New anatomic findings regarding the footprint of the rotator cuff. J Bone Joint Surg Am 2008;90:966; with permission.)

synovial membrane and the articular surface of the humeral head. He reported that this sulcus increased in size from the third decade and theorized that retraction of the capsule and synovium was a phenomenon that occurred with age. The relationship between the bare area and the anatomy of the capsular attachment to the greater tuberosity described by Nimura remains to be elucidated. Perhaps there is gradual attrition of the capsular attachment with advancing age, resulting in an increasing bare area (**Fig. 10**).

Although not explicitly stated, the findings of Nimura and colleagues[9] may explain why degenerative rotator cuff tendon tears, even massive ones, appear to involve the teres minor tendon less often or not at all.[22–25] They found that the capsular attachment to the greater tuberosity was thickest at the posterior margin of the infraspinatus tendon, at the border with the teres minor tendon.[9] Also, the posterior extent of the capsular attachment was to the upper half of the teres minor tendon, whereas the lower half of the teres minor tendon had a muscular attachment on the surgical neck of the humerus without covering the articular capsule. These 2 anatomic findings may help contribute to a more structurally stable posteroinferior cuff.

The clinical significance of the footprint of the superior cuff has gained attention regarding the types of fixation that are used in the surgical repair of tendon tears. A conventional single-row suture anchor technique may not adequately reproduce

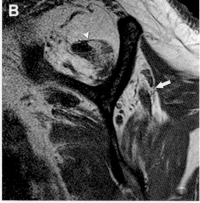

Fig. 7. Supraspinatus tendon footprint tear, with infraspinatus atrophy in a 78-year-old man with shoulder pain. (*A*) Oblique sagittal intermediate-weighted image (repetition time [TR]/echo time [TE] = 2800/56 ms) obtained at 3 T through the greater tuberosity facets demonstrates a full-thickness tear of the supraspinatus tendon (*arrowhead*), with a tendinotic but otherwise intact infraspinatus tendon (*arrow*). (*B*) Oblique sagittal T1-weighted image (TR/TE = 694/10 ms) at the level of the rotator cuff muscle bellies reveals both supraspinatus (*arrowhead*) and infraspinatus (*arrow*) muscle atrophy. (*Courtesy of* K. Chen, MD, San Diego, CA.)

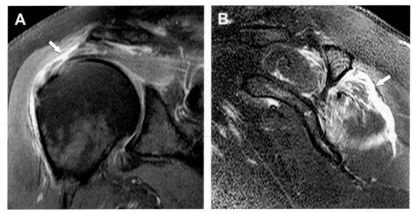

Fig. 8. Imaging appearance of the novel lesion of the infraspinatus muscle and tendon in a 61-year-old woman with worsening shoulder pain. (*A*) Oblique coronal proton density-weighted image (repetition time [TR]/echo time [TE] = 2300/29 ms) obtained at 1.5 T through the oblique facet of the greater tuberosity shows full-thickness tearing of the infraspinatus tendon near the footprint with minimal retraction of the torn tendon (*arrow*). (*B*) Oblique sagittal T2-weighted image (TR/TE = 3500/97 ms) at the level of the glenohumeral joint demonstrating significant intramuscular and extramuscular edema centered about the myotendinous junction of the infraspinatus (*arrow*). Edema is seen to a lesser degree about the supraspinatus muscle.

the anatomy of the native footprint and, in some cases, has been shown to be biomechanically inferior to a double-row suture anchor technique.[26,27] In recent literature reviews, the structural benefit of the double-row technique has been acknowledged; however, there seems to be little difference in the actual functional outcomes when comparing the benefits of single- and double-row procedures, except for a possible benefit of double-row techniques in the treatment of patients with massive cuff tears.[28,29] Further, prospective, randomized controlled trials with longer term follow-up are necessary before any useful conclusions regarding the functional outcomes of reconstructing the rotator cuff footprint are made.

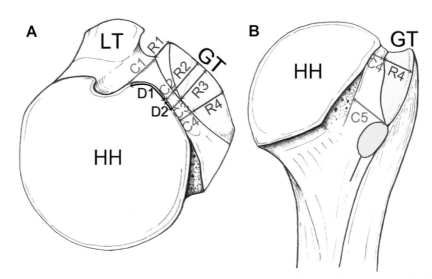

Fig. 9. Schematic illustration of the footprints in the greater tuberosity (GT) as seen from the superior (*A*) and posterior (*B*) aspects of the humerus. C1 to C5 represent the anterior to posterior extent of the capsular insertion deep to the rotator cuff tendons, with C2 representing the minimum width of the capsule. The footprint of the supraspinatus tendon spans R1 through R3, with C3 representing the width of the capsule at the posterior margin of the supraspinatus tendon. R4 represents the maximum width of the infraspinatus tendon footprint, whereas C5 represents the width of the capsular attachment at the posterior margin of the infraspinatus tendon footprint. LT, lesser tuberosity; HH, humeral head. (*From* Nimura A, Kato A, Yamaguchi K, et al. The superior capsule of the shoulder joint complements the insertion of the rotator cuff. J Shoulder Elbow Surg 2011 Aug 3. [Epub ahead of print]; with permission.)

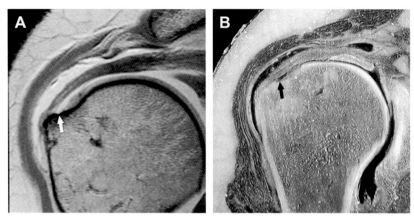

Fig. 10. The bare area of the humeral head in a cadaveric specimen. (*A*) Oblique coronal T1-weighted MR arthrogram (repetition time [TR]/echo time [TE] = 550/10 ms) obtained at 1.5 T shows the bare area representing the area of the footprint lateral to the edge of the articular cartilage that is not covered by tendon fibers (*arrow*). Note the absence of any torn, retracted articular-sided fibers along the undersurface of the tendon. (*B*) Corresponding oblique coronal cadaveric specimen showing the bare area (*arrow*).

FOOTPRINT OF THE SUBSCAPULARIS TENDON

Although a great deal of literature on the investigation of the superior cuff has been published, the anatomy of the subscapularis tendon footprint has garnered only recent attention. The subscapularis tendon may be injured because of falls on an outstretched arm, anterior glenohumeral joint dislocations, or subcoracoid impingement.[30] Tears of the subscapularis tendon were once thought to be uncommon, comprising 3.5% to 8% of rotator cuff tendon tears; however, with the advancement of arthroscopy, subscapularis tendon tears have been found to be much more common with a prevalence of up to 50% reported during arthroscopic rotator cuff repairs.[31] Clark and Harryman[5] demonstrated that the subscapularis had a muscular insertion approximately 2 cm below the lesser tuberosity at the surgical neck of the proximal humerus, similar to the insertion of the teres minor tendon.[5] This arrangement can also be depicted on MR images (**Fig. 11**). These investigators also reported a tendinous slip derived from the upper portion of the subscapularis tendon that passed under the biceps tendon to join with the fibers from the supraspinatus tendon, forming the floor of the biceps tendon sheath (**Fig. 12**). Similar to the supraspinatus tendon, the coracohumeral ligament sends fibers

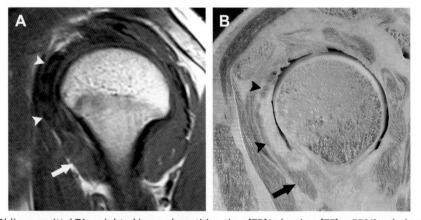

Fig. 11. (*A*) Oblique sagittal T1-weighted image (repetition time [TR]/echo time [TE] = 550/9 ms) obtained at 1.5 T showing that the attachment of the subscapularis muscle to the humerus comprises an upper tendinous insertion (*arrowheads*) in the lesser tuberosity and a muscular insertion inferiorly in the surgical neck (*arrow*). (*B*) Corresponding oblique sagittal cadaveric section demonstrating the same anatomy with an upper tendinous insertion (*arrowheads*) and a lower muscular insertion (*arrow*).

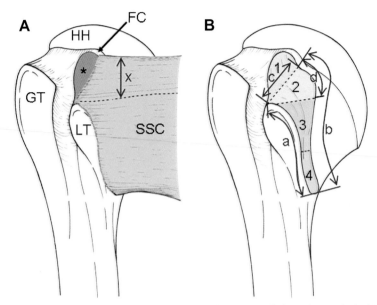

Fig. 12. Anatomic depiction showing the broader superior footprint of the subscapularis (SSC) tendon, with a relatively tapered inferior footprint and a thin muscular insertion below the lesser tuberosity (LT) in the surgical neck of the humerus. (*A*) The tendinous slip (*asterisk*) derived from the most cranial fibers of the intramuscular tendons (X) inserts on the fovea capitis (FC) above the LT. (*B*) Schematic representation of the footprint showing the tendinous slip (1), the insertion of the cranial-most fibers of the intramuscular tendons (2), the lower tendinous insertion (3), and the muscular insertion below the LT (4). GT, greater tuberosity; HH, humeral head. (*From* Arai R, Sugaya H, Mochizuki T, et al. Subscapularis tendon tear: an anatomic and clinical investigation. Arthroscopy 2008;24(9):997–1004; with permission.)

that reinforce the subscapularis tendon in the interval between the subscapularis and supraspinatus tendons. Thus, the subscapularis tendon plays a critical role in stabilizing the biceps tendon. The superior and middle glenohumeral ligaments also run deep to the subscapularis tendon from the medial to lateral edges of the tendon. The subscapularis tendon itself typically comprises 4 to 6 thick collagen bundles extending from the muscle belly medial to the lesser tuberosity.[5]

Since the investigations by Clark and Harryman,[5] more recent studies have attempted to characterize the subscapularis tendon footprint.[30,32–35] The shape of the footprint has been described as being akin to a human ear, a comma, and even the state of Nevada, with the common theme being that the subscapularis tendon has a broader superior insertion and tapered inferior insertion. Prior studies also document the presence of an inferior muscular insertion that occupies the lower third of the footprint, with the upper two-thirds being tendinous. One of these cadaveric studies[34] formally assessed the dimensions of the bare area, between the end of the articular cartilage and the most medial aspect of the subscapularis insertion, similar to that of the superior cuff. This bare area was of variable size,

from as little as 2.9 mm to as much as 17.5 mm in width in a superior-inferior dimension. An anatomic and clinical study by Arai and colleagues[32] confirmed the presence of the upper tendinous slip described by Clark and Harryman,[5] located above the lesser tuberosity and attaching to the area designated as the fovea capitis of the humerus. Arai and colleagues[32] also recognized the important role of the most cranial part of the subscapularis tendon and its tendinous slip in the stability of the biceps tendon. They saw no unstable biceps tendons in the presence of an intact subscapularis tendon in their clinical cases. Conversely, in cases of an unstable biceps tendon, they found no intact subscapularis tendons.

SUMMARY

Knowledge of the precise anatomic characteristics of the footprints of the rotator cuff tendons continues to evolve. These anatomic characteristics are fundamental to the understanding of the pathogenesis of cuff failure, clinical manifestations of such failure, and development of the optimal treatment protocols. Regarding the greater tuberosity, recent literature suggests that the infraspinatus tendon may occupy a more substantial portion of the anterior facet than previously thought and may explain the occurrence of infraspinatus muscle atrophy in the context of an apparently isolated supraspinatus tendon tear. The capsular contribution to the footprint may also be more substantial than previously described and may help maintain the integrity of the supraspinatus, infraspinatus, and teres minor tendons. A relatively narrow zone of the capsule in the region of the posterior fibers of the supraspinatus tendon may explain the subsequent development of degenerative tears in this location. Finally, the subscapularis tendon footprint plays an important role in the biceps tendon stability, by means of an upper tendinous slip derived from the cranial-most fibers of the intramuscular tendon. Subscapularis tendon tears are also more prevalent than previously described, their increasing discovery being likely related to the growing popularity of shoulder arthroscopy.

REFERENCES

1. Curtis AS, Burbank KM, Tierney JJ, et al. The insertional footprint of the rotator cuff: an anatomic study. Arthroscopy 2006;22:603–9.
2. Dugas JR, Campbell DA, Warren RF, et al. Anatomy and dimensions of rotator cuff insertions. J Shoulder Elbow Surg 2002;11:498–503.
3. Minagawa H, Itoi E, Konno N, et al. Humeral attachment of the supraspinatus and infraspinatus tendons: an anatomic study. Arthroscopy 1998;14: 302–6.
4. Ruotolo C, Fow JE, Nottage WM. The supraspinatus footprint: an anatomic study of the supraspinatus insertion. Arthroscopy 2004;20:246–9.
5. Clark JM, Harryman DT. Tendons, ligaments, and capsule of the rotator cuff. Gross and microscopic anatomy. J Bone Joint Surg Am 1992;74:713–25.
6. Burkhart SS, Esch JC, Jolson RS. The rotator crescent and rotator cable: an anatomic description of the shoulder's "suspension bridge". Arthroscopy 1993;9:611–6.
7. Mochizuki T, Sugaya H, Uomizu M, et al. Humeral insertion of the supraspinatus and infraspinatus. New anatomical findings regarding the footprint of the rotator cuff. J Bone Joint Surg Am 2008;90: 962–9.
8. Lunn JV, Castellanos-Rosas J, Tavernier T, et al. A novel lesion of the infraspinatus characterized by musculotendinous disruption, edema, and late fatty infiltration. J Shoulder Elbow Surg 2008;17(4): 546–53.
9. Nimura A, Kato A, Yamaguchi K, et al. The superior capsule of the shoulder joint complements the insertion of the rotator cuff. J Shoulder Elbow Surg 2011. [Epub ahead of print].
10. Kim HM, Dahiya N, Teefey SA, et al. Location and initiation of degenerative rotator cuff tears: an analysis of three hundred and sixty shoulders. J Bone Joint Surg Am 2010;92:1088–96.
11. Ellman H. Diagnosis and treatment of incomplete rotator cuff tears. Clin Orthop 1990;254:64–74.
12. Gartsman GM. Arthroscopic acromioplasty for lesions of the rotator cuff. J Bone Joint Surg Am 1990;72:169–80.
13. Gartsman GM. Arthroscopic treatment of rotator cuff disease. J Shoulder Elbow Surg 1995;4:228–41.
14. Itoi E, Tabata S. Incomplete rotator cuff tears. Results of operative treatment. Clin Orthop 1992;284: 128–35.
15. Olsewski JM, Depew AD. Arthroscopic subacromial decompression and rotator cuff debridement for stage II and stage III impingement. Arthroscopy 1994;10:61–8.
16. Ryu RK. Arthroscopic subacromial decompression: a clinical review. Arthroscopy 1992;8:141–7.
17. Weber SC. Arthroscopic debridement and acromioplasty versus mini-open repair in the management of significant partial-thickness tears of the rotator cuff. Orthop Clin North Am 1997;28:79–82.
18. Shimizu T, Itoi E, Minagawa H, et al. Atrophy of the rotator cuff muscles and site of cuff tears. Acta Orthop Scand 2002;73:40–3.
19. Wening JD, Hollis RF, Hughes RE, et al. Quantitative morphology of full thickness rotator cuff tears. Clin Anat 2002;15:18–22.
20. Goutallier D, Postel JM, Bernageau J, et al. Fatty muscle degeneration in cuff ruptures. Pre- and postoperative evaluation by CT scan. Clin Orthop Relat Res 1994;304:78–83.
21. DePalma AF. Surgery of the shoulder. 3rd edition. Philadelphia: JB Lippincott; 1973.
22. Burkhart SS, Danaceau SM, Pearce CE Jr. Arthroscopic rotator cuff repair: analysis of results by tear size and by repair technique-margin convergence versus direct tendon-to-bone repair. Arthroscopy 2001;17:905–12.
23. Gartsman GM, Khan M, Hammerman SM. Arthroscopic repair of full-thickness tears of the rotator cuff. J Bone Joint Surg Am 1998;80:832–40.
24. Hanusch BC, Goodchild L, Finn P, et al. Large and massive tears of the rotator cuff: functional outcome and integrity of the repair after a mini-open procedure. J Bone Joint Surg Br 2009;91:201–5.
25. Murray TF Jr, Lajtai G, Mileski RM, et al. Arthroscopic repair of medium to large full-thickness rotator cuff tears: outcome at 2- to 6-year follow-up. J Shoulder Elbow Surg 2002;11:19–24.
26. Lo IK, Burkhart SS. Double-row arthroscopic rotator cuff repair: re-establishing the footprint of the rotator cuff. Arthroscopy 2003;19:1035–42.
27. Baums MH, Buchhorn GH, Spahn G, et al. Biomechanical characteristics of single-row repair in

comparison to double-row repair with consideration of the suture configuration and suture material. Knee Surg Sports Traumatol Arthrosc 2008;16:1052–60.

28. Saridakis P, Jones G. Outcomes of single-row and double-row arthroscopic rotator cuff repair: a systematic review. J Bone Joint Surg Am 2010;92: 732–42.

29. Wall LB, Keener JD, Brophy RH. Clinical outcomes of double-row versus single-row rotator cuff repairs. Arthroscopy 2009;25:1312–8.

30. D'Addesi LL, Anbari A, Reish MW, et al. The subscapularis footprint: an anatomic study of the subscapularis tendon insertion. Arthroscopy 2006;22:937–40.

31. Denard PJ, Burkhart SS. A new method for knotless fixation of an upper subscapularis tear. Arthroscopy 2011;27:861–6.

32. Arai R, Sugaya H, Mochizuki T, et al. Subscapularis tendon tear: an anatomic and clinical investigation. Arthroscopy 2008;24:997–1004.

33. Arai R, Mochizuki T, Yamaguchi K, et al. Functional anatomy of the superior glenohumeral and coracohumeral ligaments and the subscapularis tendon in view of stabilization of the long head of the biceps tendon. J Shoulder Elbow Surg 2010;19: 58–64.

34. Ide J, Tokiyoshi A, Hirose J, et al. An anatomic study of the subscapularis insertion to the humerus: the subscapularis footprint. Arthroscopy 2008;24: 749–53.

35. Richards DP, Burkhart SS, Tehrany AM, et al. The subscapularis footprint: an anatomic description of its insertion site. Arthroscopy 2007;23:251–4.

The Rotator Cable: Magnetic Resonance Evaluation and Clinical Correlation

Soterios Gyftopoulos, MD[a],*, Jenny T. Bencardino, MD[a], Igor Immerman, MD[b], Joseph D. Zuckerman, MD[b]

KEYWORDS

- Rotator cable • Rotator cuff • MR imaging • Shoulder injury

The rotator cable was first described in a study by Clark and Harryman[1] as a fibrous band coursing along the undersurface of the supraspinatus and infraspinatus tendons perpendicular to their fibers and continuous with the coracohumeral ligament anteriorly. Burkhart and colleagues[2,3] confirmed the presence of this structure and named it the cable, a descriptive term related to its biomechanical role in these investigators' model of rotator cuff function and failure. The rotator cuff tendon fibers extending distal to the lateral margin of the cable to the greater tuberosity attachment were named the crescent (**Fig. 1**).[2–5]

Based on Burkhart's biomechanical studies,[3,4] 2 different types of functioning rotator cuff tendons have been described: cable-dominant and crescent-dominant. The cable-dominant rotator cuff was theorized to occur in older persons whose cable absorbs the stress produced by the supraspinatus and infraspinatus tendons while shielding the crescent fibers. The crescent would undergo atrophy and thinning related to the shielding, while assuming a markedly reduced role in the biomechanical function of the rotator cuff. Alternatively, the cable would undergo hypertrophy as it assumed the major role in biomechanical functioning. A crescent-dominant rotator cuff was theorized to occur in younger patients. In this scenario, there was no stress shielding of the crescent by the cable and no associated cable hypertrophy.[3,4] Thus, the

cable would not play a major role in the biomechanical function of the rotator cuff.

The rotator cable also plays an important part in Burkhart's model of a rotator cuff tear, in which it functions as the loaded cable of a suspension bridge (**Fig. 2**). In this model, the cable absorbs the compressive and tensile stress produced by the supraspinatus and infraspinatus tendons. The compressive stress is transmitted to its anterior and posterior osseous insertions that serve as the supporting towers where the stress is dissipated. The tensile stress is absorbed and dissipated by the cable itself. According to this model, stress is transferred from the cuff muscles to the rotator cable as a distributed load, thereby stress-shielding the thinner, avascular crescent tissue, particularly in older persons.[2,5] The cable and its osseous insertions also serve as medial to lateral and anterior to posterior barriers in this model, limiting the propagation of tears involving the crescent while preserving the rotator cuff function.[2–5]

ANATOMY
Gross/Histology

There have been several studies describing the gross and magnetic resonance (MR) anatomy of the rotator cable.[6–10] Gross studies have shown a close anatomic relationship between the rotator cable and the coracohumeral ligament.[1,6,7] The

[a] Department of Radiology, New York University Hospital for Joint Diseases, 301 East 17th Street, New York, NY 10003, USA
[b] Department of Orthopaedic Surgery, New York University Hospital for Joint Diseases, 301 East 17th Street, New York, NY 10003, USA
* Corresponding author. 222 East 34th Street, Apartment 1615, New York, NY 10016.
E-mail address: Soterios20@gmail.com

Magn Reson Imaging Clin N Am 20 (2012) 173–185
doi:10.1016/j.mric.2012.01.007

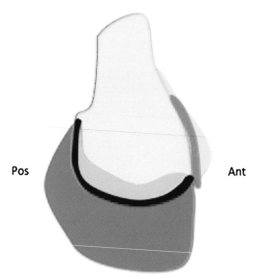

Pos   **Ant**

Fig. 1. Rotator cable. The rotator cable is shown as a blue curvilinear band coursing along the supraspinatus and infraspinatus tendons (*green*). The anterior insertion is at the anterior margin of the supraspinatus tendon adjacent to the biceps tendon (*orange*) and the posterior insertion is found along the posterior margin of the infraspinatus tendon. The crescent fibers (*light green*) extend from the margin of the cable to their insertion onto the greater tuberosity.

coracohumeral ligament arises from the rotator interval and envelops the rotator cuff with superficial and deep limbs (**Fig. 3**). The superficial limb is diminutive and lies along the bursal surface of the tendons. The deep limb is thought to represent the cable and tends to be a larger, thicker structure. The anterior insertion site of the cable is found at the greater tuberosity along the anterior margin of the supraspinatus tendon, just posterior to the biceps tendon. The cable then extends posteriorly perpendicular to the long axis of the supraspinatus and infraspinatus tendon fibers, interposed between the rotator cuff undersurface and the joint capsule. The posterior margin of the cable inserts along the inferior border of the infraspinatus tendon. The cable forms the medial margin of a crescent-shaped area that includes the distal fibers of the supraspinatus and infraspinatus, known as the crescent, located approximately 1.1 to 1.5 cm from the greater tuberosity.[3,6] Studies have shown variable degrees of thickness and width of the cable ranging between 1.2 to 4.7 mm and 4.5 to 12.1 mm, respectively.[3,6] The crescent includes the critical zone, a hypovascular region of the rotator cuff that tends to undergo attritional change and degenerative tearing over time.[11–13] Histologic examination has demonstrated the cable as a fibrillar

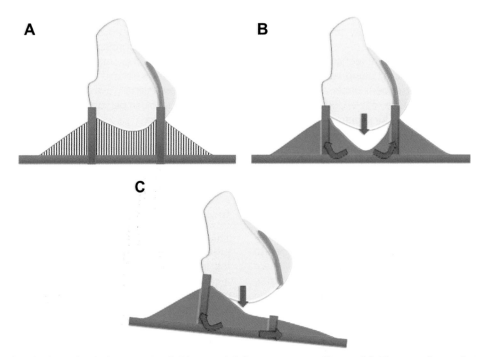

Fig. 2. (*A–C*) Biomechanical suspension-bridge model for a rotator cuff tear. (*A*) The anterior and posterior attachments of a tear correspond to the anterior and posterior supports at either end of the cable, and the free edge of the tear corresponds to the cable. (*B*) As long as the cable's insertions are intact, cuff fibers can continue to act as a compressor of the humeral head because the load is distributed along the cable to its insertions (*red arrows*). (*C*) If the tear extends to and involves one of the insertions, the cuff loses its compressive ability and becomes biomechanically unstable.

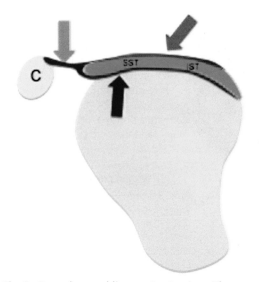

Fig. 3. Coracohumeral ligament extensions. The coracohumeral ligament (*orange arrow*) has 2 extensions that course along the bursal and articular surfaces of the supraspinatus (SST) and infraspinatus (IST) tendons; and a smaller superficial limb (*red arrow*) and a larger, deeper limb that correspond to the rotator cable (*blue arrow*). C, coracoid process.

collagenous structure separate from the supraspinatus and infraspinatus tendon fibers.[6,7]

Imaging

Several studies have examined the imaging appearance of the rotator cuff cable.[6,8,9] The rotator cuff cable is consistently seen on an ultrasonogram as a fibrillar structure coursing perpendicular to the supraspinatus and infraspinatus tendons.[6] The rotator cuff cable can be seen in all the main imaging planes used in MR imaging. In both the coronal oblique and the abducted, externally rotated (ABER) planes, the rotator cable appears as a region of hypointense signal intensity along the undersurface of the supraspinatus and infraspinatus tendons that is continuous with the coracohumeral ligament (**Fig. 4**). The oblique coronal plane provides a cross-sectional view of the rotator cable, and therefore is most useful in the assessment of its craniocaudal thickness and width. In this plane, the cable is typically seen as a rounded focus of hypointense signal on all pulse sequences varying in craniocaudal size from 1 to 5 mm (**Figs. 5** and **6A**). In some instances, however, the cable appears as a broad, dotted line (see **Fig. 6B**). In the authors' experience, a prominent cable is more often visualized among individuals in the fifth to seventh decades of life, who undergo MR imaging of the shoulder in a search for rotator cuff disease. In these cases, the presence of an undersurface fraying and a shallow tearing of the

rotator cuff may help highlight the margins of the cable, increasing its conspicuity. Differentiating the rotator cable from the retracted lateral edge of an articular surface partial tear of the supraspinatus tendon can be challenging, and the authors find triangulating the suspected cable in the axial plane most useful. A true cable will be seen extending from its anterior attachment in the greater tuberosity to its posterior oblique facet insertion in the axial images as opposed to the more focal changes seen in a retracted tear of the supraspinatus articular surface. In young adults, the cable may not be as easily discriminated from the adjacent rotator cuff tendon fibers. Inconsistent visualization of the cable in the setting of partial and full-thickness tears of the rotator cuff has been reported.[9]

Kask and colleagues[8] demonstrated consistent MR imaging visualization of all or parts of the cable in cadaver specimens, with the axial plane providing the most information. In particular, the middle portion of the cable, defined as the segment along the undersurface of the supraspinatus tendon, was seen best in the axial plane. In the axial plane, the body of the cable is seen as a linear or slightly curvilinear region of hypointense signal located approximately 1 to 1.5 cm medial to the outer cortical margin of the greater tuberosity (**Fig. 7A**). Care should be taken to assess for the presence of the cable at the level of the supraspinatus anterior and posterior intramuscular tendons, because the coracoacromial ligament can sometimes be seen coursing over the rotator cuff with the same orientation in consecutive higher axial sections. In the authors' experience, confirmation of the presence of the rotator cable in the oblique coronal plane by triangulation with the axial images is of great clinical utility.

In the sagittal plane, the cable appears as a continuous longitudinal band of hypointense signal oriented in the anteroposterior direction of variable thickness along the articular margin of the supraspinatus and infraspinatus tendons (see **Fig. 7B**). In this plane, the cable is continuous with the coracohumeral ligament anteriorly.

In the ABER plane, the coracohumeral ligament component of the biceps pulley must be identified at the level of the rotator interval and proximal margin of the bicipital groove (**Fig. 8A**). The cable can then be tracked from this point along the undersurface of the rotator cuff tendons, supraspinatus anteriorly and infraspinatus posteriorly, respectively (see **Fig. 8B–F**). Sheah and colleagues[9] visualized the cable as a minimal thickening of the undersurface of the supraspinatus tendon located approximately 1.1 to 1.5 cm medial from the greater tuberosity. These investigators

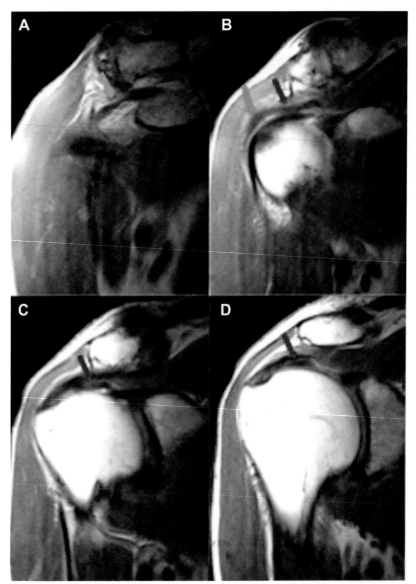

Fig. 4. (*A–D*) Rotator cable in the oblique coronal plane (proton-density weighted image). (*A*) The coracohumeral (CH) ligament originates from the coracoid process (*orange arrow*). (*B*) As it courses posteriorly, the CH ligament gives off the rotator cable (*blue arrow*), which blends and inserts anteriorly with the anterior margin of the supraspinatus tendon adjacent to the long head of biceps tendon (*green arrow*). (*C, D*) The rotator cable continues its course posteriorly along the undersurface of the supraspinatus and infraspinatus tendons (*blue arrows*).

most consistently visualized the cable in the ABER position in both the intact and torn rotator cuff (see **Fig. 8; Fig. 9**). In Sheah's series, the cable was not identified on the non-ABER MR arthrographic images of persons with intact rotator cuffs. In the authors' experience, however, the edges and insertions of the cable can be estimated in 1 or more of the imaging planes in a large proportion of individuals with and without rotator cuff tears who undergo MR imaging evaluation of the shoulder.

PATHOLOGY

MR imaging has been proven to be a reliable and accurate imaging method in the diagnosis and characterization of rotator cuff tears.[14–17] Its role in the evaluation of the rotator cuff cable is not as well defined. Most literature describes the use of the rotator cable and its modifications as a secondary sign of rotator cuff tearing more than as a primary site of pathologic condition.

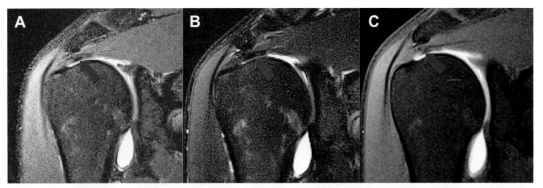

Fig. 5. Rotator cable on different pulse sequences. The rotator cable is demonstrated as a focal region of hypo-intense signal along the undersurface of the supraspinatus tendon (*blue arrow*) on the proton-density (*A*; repetition time [TR] 1000, echo time [TE] 50), fat-suppressed T2 (*B*; TR 3800, TE 79), and fat-suppressed T1 arthrogram (*C*; TR 446, TE 8.6) coronal oblique images in the same patient.

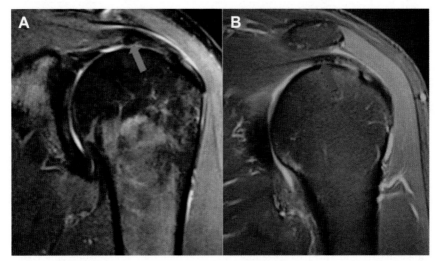

Fig. 6. Variations in width and thickness of rotator cable. Coronal oblique fat-suppressed proton-density (*A*) and T2-weighted (*B*) images in 2 different patients demonstrate a narrow thick cable (*red arrow* in *A*) and thin, broad rotator cable (*blue arrow* in *B*).

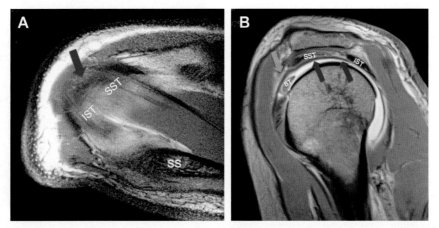

Fig. 7. (*A, B*) Rotator cuff cable in a cadaveric specimen. (*A*) The rotator cable is seen as a curvilinear band of hypointense signal intensity along the undersurface of the supraspinatus (SST) and infraspinatus (IST) tendons (*blue arrow*). (*B*) The rotator cable (*blue arrows*) extends from the coracohumeral ligament (*orange arrow*) and courses along the undersurface of the supraspinatus (SST) and infraspinatus (IST) tendons in this sagittal T1-weighted image. BT, biceps tendon; SS, scapular spine.

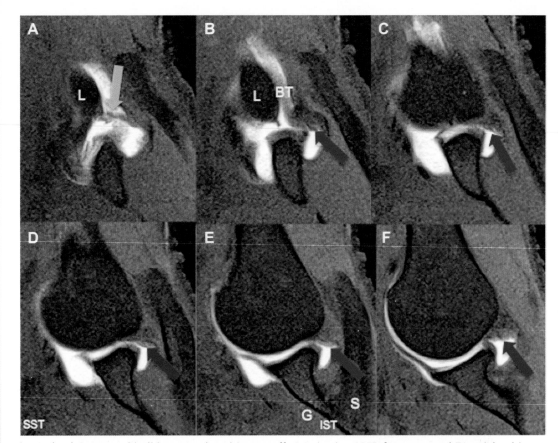

Fig. 8. (*A–F*) Rotator cable (*blue arrows*) and intact cuff. Consecutive ABER fat-suppressed T1-weighted images demonstrate the superior sling of the biceps pulley comprising the coracohumeral ligament fibers (*orange arrow*) providing the roof of the biceps tendon and in continuity with the cable along the undersurface of the supraspinatus (SST) and infraspinatus (IST) tendons. BT, biceps tendon; G, greater tuberosity; L, lesser tuberosity; P, coracoid process.

Sheah and colleagues[9] best identified the cable on non-ABER images in the setting of articular surface rotator cuff tears. Hence, they suggested that visualization of the cable on non-ABER images should prompt the radiologist to look for a partial-thickness tear of the rotator cuff. Towers and colleagues[18] measured the medial displacement of the cable in the setting of rotator cuff tearing and found an association between the position of the rotator cable relative to the greater tuberosity and the cross-sectional involvement of the tear at surgery. Oblique coronal fat-suppressed T2-weighted images were used to locate the image on which the articular surface of the cable was the farthest from the lateral margin of the greater tuberosity. Cable distance of less than 1.7 cm was associated with the absence of tears greater than 30% in cross section, and a cable distance of 3 cm was associated with the absence of tears less than 50%. The correlation coefficient between cable distance and cross section of the tear was 91%. Therefore, a cutoff

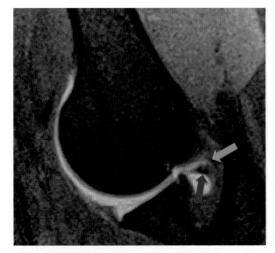

Fig. 9. Rotary cuff cable and articular surface supraspinatus tendon tear. ABER fat-suppressed T1-weighted image demonstrates the rotator cable (*blue arrow*) along the undersurface of torn, retracted supraspinatus tendon articular surface fibers (*green arrow*).

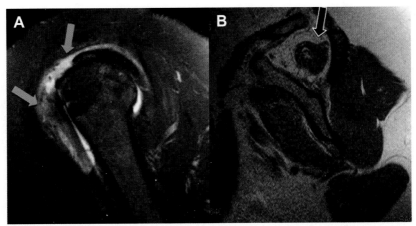

Fig. 10. Anterosuperior rotator cuff tear. (*A*) Oblique sagittal fat-suppressed T2-weighted image demonstrates a full-thickness tear of the anterior supraspinatus tendon fibers (*green arrow*) extending across the rotator interval into the superior subscapularis tendon fibers (*orange arrow*). (*B*) There is advanced fatty degeneration and retraction of the supraspinatus muscle (*black arrow*) on this sagittal oblique T1-weighted image.

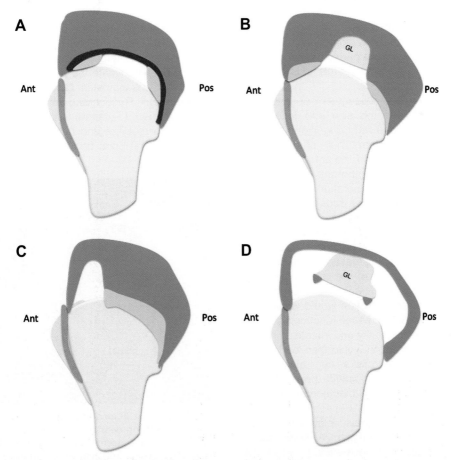

Fig. 11. (*A–D*) Rotator cuff tear shapes. (*A*) Crescent-shaped tear. (*B*) U-shaped tear. (*C*) L-shaped tear. (*D*) Massive tear. Rotator cuff, green; rotator cable, blue; rotator crescent, light green; biceps tendon, orange. GL, glenoid.

value of 1.7 cm in medial displacement of the cable was found to be most useful when differentiating between the small partial tears and the more extensive partial tears.

The association between tearing of the anterior cable attachment and altered biomechanics of the glenohumeral joint was reported by Su and colleagues.[19] Significant anterior and anterosuperior glenohumeral translation was seen in the setting of insertional tears involving the supraspinatus and superior half of the subscapularis tendons with loads of 40 and 50 N. No significant translation was found with isolated supraspinatus tendon tears. Based on the established anatomy of the cable, a tear that propagates from the supraspinatus tendon through the superior aspect of the subscapularis tendon has to involve the anterior attachment of the cable (**Fig. 10**). Even when not directly visualized in the images, the MR diagnosis of anterosuperior rotator cuff tears can thus suggest rotator cable compromise and associated altered glenohumeral joint mechanics (**Fig. 11**). An association between the visualization of the cable in the presence of a partial-thickness supraspinatus tendon tear and a negative Jobe test was noted by Macarini and colleagues.[10] This association suggested a possible biomechanical role for the cable in the setting of a partial-thickness supraspinatus tendon tear, although this finding was not statistically significant.

A study by Kim and colleagues[20] described the relationship between the size and location of a rotator cuff tear and fatty degeneration of the rotator cuff musculature. Their study demonstrated that the integrity of the anterior supraspinatus tendon was an important factor in the development of fatty degeneration of supraspinatus muscle. Specifically, the odds of fatty degeneration of supraspinatus muscle were increased when there was tearing of the anterior margin of the tendon. One of the investigators' hypotheses to explain this finding was based on the presence of the anterior insertion of the rotator cable into these anterior fibers. It was hypothesized that injury to the anterior insertion would weaken the cable, leading to its decreased functioning, resulting in rotator cuff instability and increased muscle retraction. This retraction would then lead to fatty degeneration of the rotator cuff musculature. Although indirect, these findings provide further support for the important biomechanical role of the cable (see **Fig. 11**).

The rotator cable may also play a role in the configuration of rotator cuff tears. As stated earlier, a rotator cuff tear can be modeled after a suspension bridge, with the free margin of the tear corresponding to the cable and the anterior and posterior attachments of the tear corresponding to the supports at each end of the cable's span. The rotator cable can limit the extension of a tear in both the anterior-posterior and medial-lateral planes.[2–5] The barrier-like effect of the cable can shape the extent of tearing, most commonly resulting in a crescent-type tear (see **Fig. 11**). Tears in a cable-deficient rotator cuff would not be limited in extent and could propagate in both the anterior-posterior and medial-lateral planes, which could result in variously shaped cuff tears, most commonly U-shaped, L-shaped, and massive contracted tears (see **Fig. 11**).

Crescent-shaped tears have an excellent medial to lateral mobility, regardless of the size, and can be repaired directly to bone with minimal tension (**Figs. 12–14**).[21] U-shaped tears extend much farther medially, with the apex of the tear adjacent to or medial to the superior glenoid rim (**Fig. 15**). In a study by Sallay and colleagues,[22] the U-shaped rotator cuff tear appeared to be the most common end result of the other types of rotator cuff tears. L-shaped tears are similar to U-shaped tears; however, in the L-shaped tear, one of the leaves is more mobile than the other leaf and can be more easily brought to the bone bed and to the other leaf (**Fig. 16**). L-shaped tears can extend anteriorly into or near the rotator interval (anterior L-shaped tear), or posteriorly into the posterior supraspinatus/anterior infraspinatus tendons (posterior L-shaped tear).[21] Recognizing a longitudinal type of tear (U-shaped, L-shaped) is critical because attempting to mobilize and repair the apex of the tear to a lateral bone bed will result in extreme

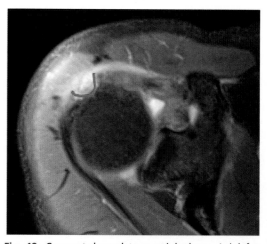

Fig. 12. Crescent-shaped tear, axial plane. Axial fat-suppressed proton-density image of the left shoulder demonstrates a crescent-shaped tear (*red line*) with narrow transverse and narrow longitudinal components located at the junction of the supraspinatus and the infraspinatus tendons.

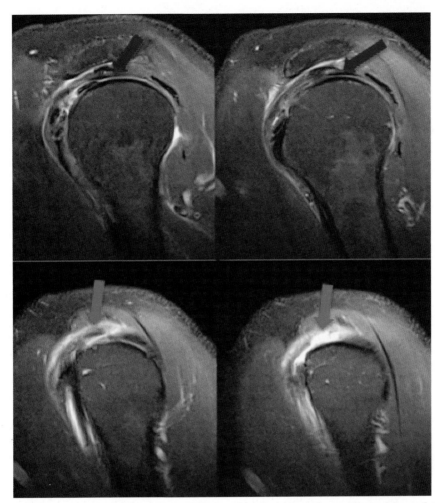

Fig. 13. Crescent-shaped tear, sagittal oblique plane. Multiple consecutive sagittal oblique fat-suppressed T2-weighted images of the right shoulder in the same patient as in **Fig. 12** demonstrates a crescent-shaped full-thickness tear at the junction of the supraspinatus and infraspinatus tendons (*red arrows*). The coracohumeral ligament arises from the coracoid process and extends along the undersurface of the supraspinatus and infraspinatus tendons as the rotator cable (*blue arrows*).

tensile forces in the repaired cuff margin, leading to tensile overload and subsequent tendon failure. Therefore, tears with a deep longitudinal component respond best to repair techniques using margin convergence. Massive, contracted, rotator cuff tears demonstrate no mobility from medial to lateral or from anterior to posterior, and therefore cannot be repaired directly to bone or side to side with margin convergence (**Fig. 17**).[21]

CLINICAL SIGNIFICANCE

Arthroscopically, the cable appears as a thickening at the distal margin of the undersurface of the rotator cuff (**Fig. 18**). It can be routinely seen in the arthroscopy of the intact rotator cuff.[3] In cases of massive rotator cuff tears, the rindlike rotator cable can be easily identified after debridement of the thin crescent tissue (**Fig. 19**). The presence of an intact rotator cable may change the clinical approach to a massive tear of the rotator cuff, particularly in elderly patients. In this context, the ability to identify the rotator cable with MR imaging can provide a great benefit to the surgeon not only in evaluating the patient as a candidate for operative management but also in planning the procedure to be performed.

The concept of a functional rotator cuff tear describes rotator cuffs that are anatomically deficient, yet biomechanically sound because of the action of the rotator cable in transmitting the forces between the anterior and posterior margins of the tear, thereby allowing for force coupling between internal and external rotators of the

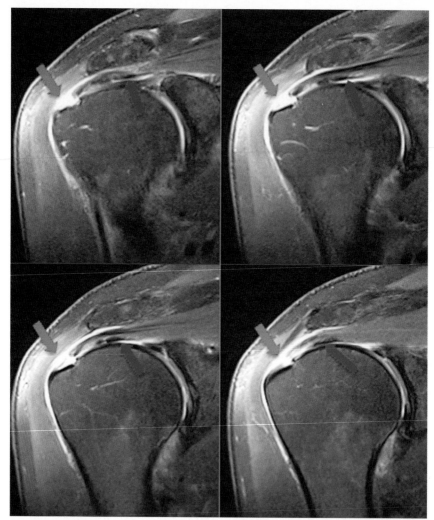

Fig. 14. Crescent-shaped tear, coronal oblique plane. Multiple consecutive coronal oblique fat-suppressed T2-weighted images of the right shoulder from the same patient as in **Figs. 12** and **13** demonstrate a crescent-shaped full-thickness tear at the junction of the supraspinatus and infraspinatus tendons (*red arrows*). The rotator cable courses along the undersurface of the supraspinatus and infraspinatus tendons (*blue arrows*).

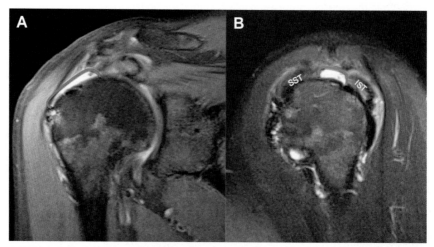

Fig. 15. (*A, B*) U-shaped tear. A fluid-filled cuff defect is seen at the junction of the supraspinatus and infraspinatus tendons on coronal (*A*) and sagittal (*B*) oblique fat-suppressed T2-weighted images of the right shoulder. The U-shape is defined by a long longitudinal component (*red line*) compared with a narrow transverse component (*blue line*), and is typically found at the junctional zone of the supraspinatus and infraspinatus tendons.

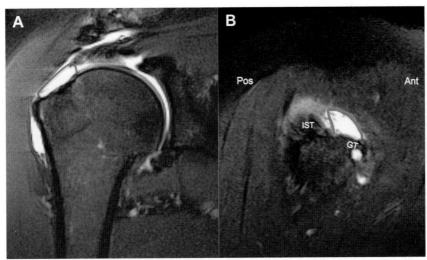

Fig. 16. (*A, B*) Anterior L-shaped tear. An anterior L-shaped tear is seen within the supraspinatus tendon on coronal (*A*) and sagittal (*B*) oblique fat-suppressed T2-weighted images of the right shoulder. The anterior L-shape is defined by a long longitudinal component (*red line*) compared with a narrow transverse component (*blue line*) as well as the location within the anterior half of the rotator cuff insertion onto the greater tuberosity (GT). IST, infraspinatus tendon.

shoulder.[23,24] Although complete surgical repair of rotator cuff tears should be the goal, certain massive tears cannot be adequately repaired. In these cases, Burkhart and colleagues[24] have shown that partial repair can lead to acceptable results, provided the force-couple and the rotator cable are restored. In a study of 14 patients with an average follow-up of 21 months, the authors achieved an average postoperative University of California, Los Angeles (UCLA) score of 27.6, with 8 good or excellent results (compared with an average preoperative UCLA score of 9.8). In another study, Burkhart[25] showed that simple arthroscopic debridement and decompression could lead to good results in patients with painful, but functional rotator cuff tears.

The clinical evidence for a partial repair is further supported by a biomechanical study by Halder and colleagues.[26] In their study, tears involving one-third to two-thirds of the supraspinatus tendon resulted in minimal decreases in force transmission. A significant decrease in force transmission through the rotator cuff occurred only after detachment of the entire supraspinatus tendon,

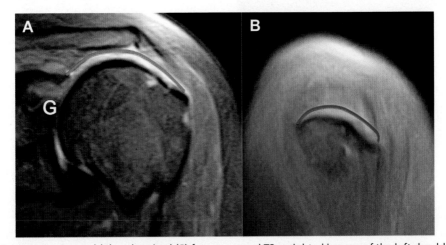

Fig. 17. Massive tear. Coronal (*A*) and sagittal (*B*) fat-suppressed T2-weighted images of the left shoulder demonstrate a massive, retracted cuff tear with long longitudinal (*red line*) and wide transverse components (*blue line*). The tendon fibers are retracted to the level of the glenoid (G), and the greater tuberosity facets are bare.

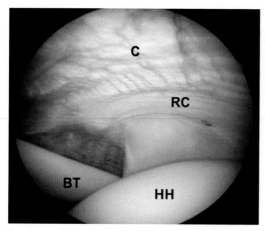

Fig. 18. Rotator cable on arthroscopy. Arthroscopic view of the rotator cable (RC) coursing along the undersurface of the rotator cuff (C). BT, biceps tendon; HH, humeral head. (*Courtesy of* Brian J. Cole, MD, MBA.)

thereby affecting the rotator cable. Furthermore, an attempt to restore the rotator cable with a side-to-side repair after the complete excision of the supraspinatus tendon restored force transmission to 90% of the original value.

The identification of the rotator cable on MR imaging can provide valuable information to the surgeon. In the case of an elderly patient with a functional painful rotator cuff tear, the presence of an intact rotator cable suggests that the patient may benefit from an arthroscopic debridement and decompression. Conversely, in patients with massive rotator cuff tears and a disrupted rotator cable, consideration should be given to the restoration of the rotator cable via a partial repair.

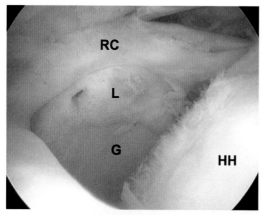

Fig. 19. Rotator cable in the setting of a massive cuff tear on arthroscopy. The rotator cable (RC) is retracted to the level of the superior glenoid rim in this 57-year-old woman with a massive rotator cuff tear who underwent arthroscopic debridement. G, glenoid; L, labrum; HH, humeral head.

SUMMARY

The rotator cable is an extension of the coracohumeral ligament coursing along the undersurface of the supraspinatus and infraspinatus tendons. The rotator cable is thought to play a role in the biomechanical function of the intact and torn rotator cuff, and possibly in the configuration of rotator cuff tears. It can be seen on all the imaging planes used for conventional MR imaging of the shoulder. Clinically, the integrity of the rotator cable can play a role in treatment selection for patients with a rotator cuff tear.

ACKNOWLEGMENTS

The authors would like to thank Donald Resnick and Michael Recht for their help in editing the manuscript.

REFERENCES

1. Clark JM, Harryman DT II. Tendons, ligaments, and capsule of the rotator cuff. J Bone Joint Surg Am 1992;74:713–25.
2. Burkhart SS. Fluoroscopic comparison of kinematic patterns in massive rotator cuff tears: a suspension bridge model. Clin Orthop 1992;284:144–52.
3. Burkhart SS, Esch JC, Jolson RS. The rotator crescent and rotator cable: an anatomic description of the shoulder's "suspension bridge". Arthroscopy 1993;9:611–6.
4. Burkhart SS. Reconciling the paradox of rotator cuff repair versus debridement: a unified biomechanical rationale for the treatment of rotator cuff tears. Arthroscopy 1994;10:4–19.
5. Jensen KL, Williams GR, Russell IJ, et al. Current concepts—rotator cuff tear arthropathy. J Bone Joint Surg 1999;81:1312–24.
6. Morag Y, Jacobson JA, Lucas D, et al. US appearance of the rotator cable with histologic correlation: preliminary results. Radiology 2006;241:485–91.
7. Fallon J, Blevins FT, Vogel K, et al. Functional morphology of the supraspinatus tendon. J Orthop Res 2002;20:920–6.
8. Kask K, Kolts I, Lubienski A, et al. Magnetic resonance imaging and correlative gross anatomy of the ligamentum semicirculare humeri (rotator cable). Clin Anat 2008;21:420–6.
9. Sheah K, Bredella MA, Warner JJ, et al. Transverse thickening along the articular surface of the rotator cuff consistent with the rotator cable: identification with MR arthrography and relevance in rotator cuff evaluation. Am J Roentgenol 2009; 193:679–86.
10. Macarini L, Muscarella S, Lelario M, et al. Rotator cable at MR imaging: considerations on morphological

aspects and biomechanical role. Radiol Med 2011; 116:102–13.

11. Codman EA, Akerson IB. The pathology associated with rupture of the supraspinatus tendon. Ann Surg 1931;94:348–59.

12. Codman EA. The shoulder: rupture of the supraspinatus tendon and other lesions in or about the sub-acromial bursa. Boston: Thomas Todd; 1934.

13. Opsha O, Malik A, Baltazar, et al. MRI of the rotator cuff and internal derangement. Eur J Radiol 2008; 68:36–56.

14. Zlatkin MB, Iannotti JP, Roberts MC, et al. Rotator cuff tears: diagnostic performance of MR imaging. Radiology 1989;172:223–9.

15. Rafii M, Firooznia H, Sherman O, et al. Rotator cuff lesions: signal patterns at MR imaging. Radiology 1990;177:817–23.

16. Palmer WE, Brown JH, Rosenthal DI. Rotator cuff: evaluation with fat-suppressed MR arthrography. Radiology 1993;188:683–7.

17. Robertson PL, Schweitzer ME, Mitchell DG, et al. Rotator cuff disorders: interobserver and intraob-server variation in diagnosis with MR imaging. Radiology 1995;194:831–5.

18. Towers JD, Borrero CG, Bradley JP, et al. Society of Skeletal Radiology 2011 Annual Meeting [abstracts]. Skeletal Radiol 2011;40:485–515.

19. Su WR, Budoff JE, Luo ZP. The effect of anterosuperior rotator cuff tears on glenohumeral translation. Arthroscopy 2009;25:282–9.

20. Kim HM, Dahiya N, Teefey A, et al. Relationship of tear size and location to fatty degeneration of the rotator cuff. J Bone Joint Surg Am 2010;92:829–39.

21. Davidson J, Burkhart SS. The geometric classification of rotator cuff tears: a system linking tear pattern to treatment and prognosis. Arthroscopy 2010;26: 417–24.

22. Sallay PI, Hunker PJ, Lim JK. Frequency of various tear patterns in full-thickness tears of the rotator cuff. Arthroscopy 2007;23:1052–9.

23. Burkhart SS. Shoulder arthroscopy. New concepts. Clin Sports Med 1996;15:635–53.

24. Burkhart SS, Nottage WM, Ogilvie-Harris DJ, et al. A partial repair of irreparable rotator cuff tears. Arthroscopy 1994;10:363–70.

25. Burkhart SS. Arthroscopic debridement and decompression for selected rotator cuff tears. Clinical results, pathomechanics, and patient selection based on biomechanical parameters. Orthop Clin North Am 1993;24:111–23.

26. Halder AM, O'Driscoll SW, Heers G, et al. Biomechanical comparison of effects of supraspinatus tendon detachments, tendon defects, and muscle retractions. J Bone Joint Surg Am 2002;84:780–5.

Magnetic Resonance Imaging of Rotator Cuff Disease and External Impingement

Michael J. Tuite, MD

KEYWORDS

- Rotator cuff disease • Impingement • Tendinopathy
- Shoulder pain

Shoulder pain is the third most common complaint made by patients to their physicians, and is particularly prevalent in older patients.[1] The leading causes of shoulder pain diagnosed after clinical examination in half to two-thirds of these patients are impingement and rotator cuff disease.[2] Many of these patients go on to advanced imaging, and evaluation of the rotator cuff is the most common indication for magnetic resonance (MR) imaging of the shoulder.[3]

This article reviews the etiology of external impingement and rotator cuff tears, and describes the MR imaging appearance of the normal and pathologic rotator cuffs. It focuses on the supraspinatus tendon because this is the tendon involved in 95% of rotator cuff tears, either alone or combined with adjacent infraspinatus or subscapularis tendon tears.[4–7] The internal impingement of the shoulder, which tends to occur in younger overhead-throwing athletes and has a different set of characteristic findings on MR imaging, is not discussed.

ETIOLOGY OF ROTATOR CUFF DISEASE AND EXTERNAL IMPINGEMENT

External impingement, also known as subacromial impingement syndrome or classic shoulder impingement, refers to shoulder pain during the forward elevation of the humerus.[6] The pain is generally caused by compression of the rotator cuff, the long head of the biceps tendon, and the subacromial-subdeltoid (SASD) bursa between the humeral head and the coracoacromial arch.[6,8] Although it was thought in the past that it was the compression of the rotator cuff itself that caused the pain, it was later found that there are few sensory nerve fibers within rotator cuff tendons.[8] The synovial capsule of the glenohumeral joint and SASD bursa are highly innervated, and repeated compression with inflammation and synovitis of these structures is now thought to be the major cause of impingement pain. Impingement pain can be severe in patients with rotator cuff tears that involve the joint or bursal capsule, but can also be seen in patients with completely normal rotator cuffs. Even intrasubstance rotator cuff tears or tendinopathy with focal swelling of the rotator cuff tendon can stretch the adjacent capsule and worsen compression of the joint and/or bursal synovium between the humeral head and the overlying coracoacromial arch, contributing to inflammation and pain.

External impingement of the shoulder is usually classified into 2 types: primary and secondary.[6] The primary type is attributable to abnormalities of the coracoacromial arch that cause mechanical compression on the rotator cuff. These extrinsic abnormalities include a hooked anterior acromion process, inferiorly directed acromioclavicular joint osteophytes, a thick coracoacromial ligament, or an os acromiale. The secondary type is caused by instability or rotator cuff dysfunction, whereby repeated unrestrained cranial displacement of the humeral head compresses the cuff and adjacent structures against the undersurface of the coracoacromial arch. Although isolated secondary

Division of Musculoskeletal Imaging and Intervention, University of Wisconsin School of Medicine and Public Health, Madison, WI, USA
E-mail address: mtuite@uwhealth.org

Magn Reson Imaging Clin N Am 20 (2012) 187–200
doi:10.1016/j.mric.2012.01.011

mri.theclinics.com

external impingement can occur in young people with multidirectional instability or microinstability, it is most common in older patients in whom secondary impingement is combined with primary external impingement. In these older patients the humeral head depressors, such as the pectoralis major and the teres major muscles, gradually become weaker and can no longer counterbalance the deltoid muscle to keep the humeral head centered in the glenoid fossa during arm elevation or abduction. When the deltoid muscle contracts to elevate the arm, the humeral head is pulled cephalad, leading to repeated compression of the rotator cuff, capsule, and bursa against the extrinsic abnormalities of the coracoacromial arch. Primary and secondary external impingement can lead to mechanical wear and shearing forces that tear the tendon fibers, and these worsen when both types of external impingement are present.[9]

Although damage to the tendon would seem to be more likely to the bursal side of the cuff because of pointy coracoacromial abnormalities, several studies have shown that most partial-thickness rotator cuff tears occur on the articular surface of the tendon.[4,5,10,11] Investigators have proposed 3 main reasons for this observation:

- If the structures indenting into the bursal surface of the cuff are blunted, they can cause bulging of the opposite articular surface with tensile stretching of the articular-sided fibers, leading to undersurface fiber failure.[12]
- The articular surface fibers are stiffer and do not stretch well if subjected to a tensile load, and this also causes them to fail earlier.[13,14]
- Several investigators have found that because blood supply is poorer on the articular side of the cuff than on the bursal side, the bursal surface heals, whereas the articular surface does not heal in repetitive microtrauma.[15,16]

Rotator cuff tendons undergo myxoid degeneration with age and therefore become weaker and more susceptible to tearing.[17] Tendons are also known to lose the lubricating material within the tendon that ensures the smooth gliding motion of the tendon fascicles.[18] These changes are referred to as intrinsic degeneration of the rotator cuff. Most investigators believe that repetitive external impingement and intrinsic degeneration combine to cause most rotator cuff tears.[6,19]

MR IMAGING OF THE ROTATOR CUFF

MR imaging of the shoulder is usually performed with the patient supine and the humerus comfortably externally rotated. Slight external rotation aligns the supraspinatus tendon with the blade of the scapula so that it can be optimally evaluated with standard oblique coronal and oblique sagittal planes. If the humerus is allowed to be in internal rotation, the lateral tendon curves out of the oblique coronal plane and causes partial averaging of the tendon with muscle, reducing the accuracy for diagnosing cuff tears.[20]

Although there is no single preferred protocol for imaging the rotator cuff, there are several basic principles. The supraspinatus tendon is the main structure involved in patients with rotator cuff disease and external impingement, so the coronal and sagittal imaging planes should be oriented relative to the long axis of the supraspinatus muscle. High accuracy for diagnosing rotator cuff tears has been reported with fat-suppressed, fast spin-echo, T2-weighted sequences in the oblique, coronal, and oblique sagittal planes.[21–23] A non–fat-suppressed, short echo time (TE) sequence should also be obtained to evaluate for muscle fatty atrophy. There is more variability in the preferred axial pulse sequence, and the selection of the type of sequence usually depends on reader preference and machine capability.

Normal Rotator Cuff Anatomy and MR Appearance

The rotator cuff is a fairly complex structure composed of 4 tendons: the supraspinatus, the infraspinatus, the teres minor, and the subscapularis tendons. Most infraspinatus tears and many subscapularis tendon tears occur adjacent to supraspinatus tendon tears as part of massive rotator cuff tears. Teres minor tendon tears are rare, although denervation atrophy of the teres minor is not uncommon.

The supraspinatus muscle originates from the posterior upper scapula and extends laterally above the scapular spine to insert onto the superior facet of the greater tuberosity of the humerus. The lateral supraspinatus tendon merges with the more posterior infraspinatus tendon in the lateral 1.5 cm prior to insertion, and this forms a tendinous cuff. The supraspinatus has 2 different tendons laterally. The main tendon forms medially within the mid-substance of the muscle but then lies progressively more anteriorly within the muscle as it moves laterally until it forms the anterior half of the supraspinatus portion of the rotator cuff. The more posterior part of the muscle forms a much shorter aponeurosis that is only about 2 cm in length. It merges laterally with the main anterior supraspinatus tendon anteriorly, and with the infraspinatus tendon posteriorly (**Fig. 1**).

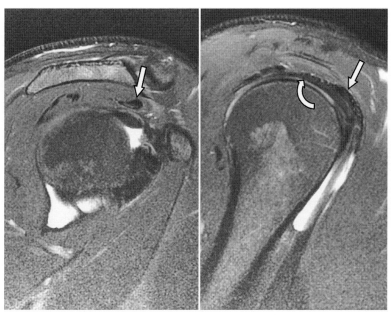

Fig. 1. Normal rotator cuff. Two adjacent oblique sagittal fat-suppressed T2-weighted images demonstrate the anterior main tendon (*arrows*) and the posterior aponeurotic tendon (*curved arrow*) of the supraspinatus.

The rotator cuff tendon is also histologically complex. Clark and Harryman[15] described the 5 layers of the rotator cuff. The 2 layers that form the bursal third of the tendon and the layer forming the articular surface of the cuff contain closely packed, well-organized tendon fibers. The 2 layers in the center of the cuff contain less-organized fibers mixed with connective tissue. This anatomic feature is important when looking at MR images of the rotator cuff because it explains why the 2 surfaces of the cuff are low signal, whereas the central portion is intermediate signal on T2-weighted images (**Fig. 2**).

The various histologic layers of the rotator cuff also result partly from other ligaments combining with the lateral portion of the supraspinatus tendon to form the cuff. For example, the collagen fibers from the joint capsule merge with the undersurface of the supraspinatus tendon to contribute to layer 5. Another important contributor to the rotator cuff is the coracohumeral ligament, which extends posteriorly and divides to send fibers above and below the supraspinatus tendon, thereafter merging with the tendon to form the superficial layer 1 and the deep layer 4 of the rotator cuff.[15] The fibers in layer 4 can form a 1-cm-wide, focally thickened band extending from front to back across the supraspinatus and infraspinatus portions of the cuff, called the ligamentum semicirculare humeri or the rotator cable.[24] The rotator cable can sometimes be seen on MR images as a low-signal band within the cuff, close to the articular surface, running perpendicular to the long axis of the supraspinatus and infraspinatus tendons (**Fig. 3**).

MR IMAGING OF EXTERNAL IMPINGEMENT

External impingement is generally considered to be a clinical diagnosis. The condition is defined as a chronic ache in the lateral aspect of the shoulder aggravated by elevation of the arm.

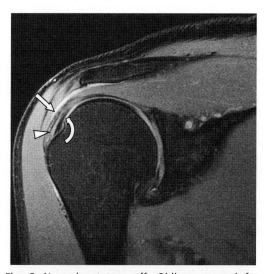

Fig. 2. Normal rotator cuff. Oblique coronal fat-suppressed T2-weighted image shows the low-signal bursal surface (*arrow*) and articular surface (*curved arrow*) layers, and the intermediate-signal central layer (*arrowhead*) of the supraspinatus tendon.

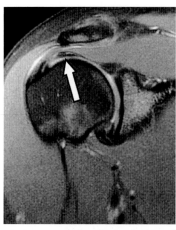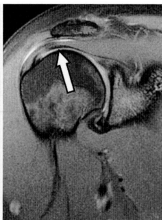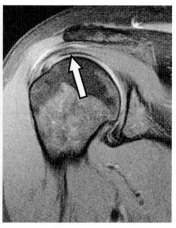

Fig. 3. Rotator cable. Three adjacent oblique coronal fat-suppressed T2-weighted images demonstrate the low-signal rotator cable (*arrows*).

During forward flexion and abduction, patients usually complain of an arc between 60° and 120° in which the pain is most severe. The pain may also be severe at night and can awaken the patient from sleep.[6]

There are 2 physical examination tests used to confirm external impingement. The Neer impingement test involves forward flexion of the arm with the elbow extended to 180°, with pain elicited at maximal elevation. The Hawkins-Jobe test begins with the shoulder flexed forward at 90° and the elbow bent, with pain elicited with internal rotation, abduction, and increased forward flexion. External impingement is further confirmed if there is decreased pain after a lidocaine injection into the SASD bursa, the so-called impingement test.

The MR imaging findings of a patient with external impingement are variable, and can range from normal to tendinopathy to a rotator cuff tear. There are several MR image findings that are useful to note even in patients with no indications of rotator cuff disease. One of these is abnormal fluid in the SASD bursa, which can indicate SASD bursitis and is often present in patients with symptomatic impingement syndrome. Although a small amount of fluid within the bursa is common, an effusion defined by a width greater than 3 mm suggests bursitis.[25] Other findings associated with SASD bursitis include fluid medial to the acromioclavicular (AC) joint or in the anterior portion of the bursa. Another finding that has been associated with impingement pain is a decreased (≤7 mm) acromiohumeral distance in the absence of a rotator cuff tear.[26]

The most controversial MR imaging findings of impingement involve coracoacromial arch structures. Most investigators agree that resecting large AC joint inferior osteophytes and a type 3, downsloping, anterior acromion process, can slow the progression of rotator cuff disease or improve the healing of a surgically repaired tear.[6,27] It is less clear whether abnormalities of the coracoacromial arch by themselves cause external impingement syndrome, or if impingement can be diagnosed on an MR image simply by identifying these abnormalities.[28] The following paragraphs describe the MR imaging appearance and summarize the literature on the main coracoacromial arch abnormalities: AC joint osteophytes, anterior hooked acromion process, lateral downsloping of the acromion, os acromiale, and a thickened coracoacromial ligament.

Several investigators have reported that inferiorly directed AC joint osteophytes (especially those ≥3 mm) are associated with impingement and rotator cuff tears (**Fig. 4**).[29–31] Other investigators, however, found that AC joint osteoarthritis is

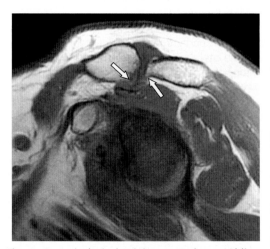

Fig. 4. Acromioclavicular joint osteophytes. Oblique sagittal T1-weighted image shows inferiorly pointed osteophytes (*arrows*) indenting the supraspinatus tendon in a patient with impingement syndrome.

very common in patients who are either asymptomatic or have only AC joint tenderness, and have noted that resection of the AC joint leads to instability of the joint and poor outcomes.[6,32–35] With newer capsule-sparing and coplaning techniques, symptomatic instability of the distal clavicle after AC joint decompression surgery has been reduced.[30,36] Most investigators believe it is useful to note the inferiorly directed osteophytes of the AC joint that are larger than 3 mm and indent the rotator cuff on the MR image, because most surgeons resect them at surgery in patients with external impingement syndrome.[30,37]

Many articles have been written on the hooked or type 3 anterior acromion process (**Fig. 5**). Charles Neer[27,38] popularized the theory that the anterior acromion process was the major extrinsic cause of external impingement and rotator cuff disease. Bigliani and colleagues[39,40] later proposed a classification system for the anterior acromion process as seen on the coracoacromial arch radiographic view, whereby a downward-hooked acromion process was classified as type 3 and was thought to be most associated with rotator cuff tears. Several other investigators have also found an association between a hooked anterior acromion process and rotator cuff tears.[41–47] Some also believe that there is a similar association between a downward-tilted anterior acromion process and rotator cuff tears.[48]

There are many articles, however, that dispute the concept that a hooked anterior acromion process causes subacromial impingement syndrome or rotator cuff tears.[28,49–52] Several articles have argued that many cases of hooked

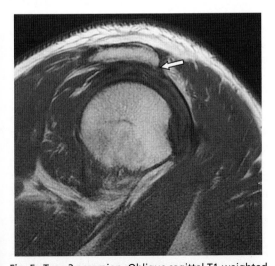

Fig. 5. Type 3 acromion. Oblique sagittal T1-weighted image demonstrates a downsloping anterior acromion process (*arrow*) in a patient with impingement pain.

acromion are actually enthesophytes at the origin of the coracoacromial ligament.[11,53,54] These enthesophytes create an extended, more rigid, anterior lip of the acromion process but do not by themselves indent the supraspinatus tendon. The prevalence of the type 3 acromion process has also been shown to increase with age.[55,56] The association with rotator cuff tears could have occurred because cuff tears are also more common with increasing age or because these enthesophytes are more likely to develop in patients with rotator cuff tears. Several investigators have observed high interobserver variability in classifying the anterior acromion and have noted that slight differences in radiographic technique can alter the appearance and classification assigned to an acromion process.[42,47,57–60]

Matsen and colleagues[6] consider that a downturned, anterior acromion may play a role in impingement pain but only secondarily, with the primary contribution coming from a tight posterior capsule or weak humeral depressors. These investigators propose that a tight posterior capsule or weak humeral head depressors result in a slight anterosuperior shift of the humeral head with arm elevation. Because the humeral head does not remain concentric with the undersurface of the acromion process during arm elevation, the rotator cuff tendon now rubs against and is compressed and abraded by the anterior acromion process, leading to impingement pain and rotator cuff tears.

Whatever the explanation, when treating patients with a rotator cuff tear or external impingement, most surgeons remove the enthesophyte and perform debridement of the downward-curved anterior acromial undersurface to flatten it. This anterior subacromial decompression procedure has been shown to improve impingement pain, even in patients with congenital subacromial stenosis.[6,27,38,39,61,62]

Lateral downsloping of the lateral acromion process has also been described by several investigators as a potential cause of impingement pain.[34,52] Other reports have found that a large lateral extension of the acromion process, or a lateral heel-type spur, can be associated with rotator cuff tears.[28,63] Prior to Neer's 1972 article, many impingement patients had lateral acromion resection but did not achieve much pain relief.[27] Neer showed that impingement pain arises mainly from forward flexion of the arm and not from abduction; he therefore disputed the notion that the lateral aspect of the acromion plays a major role in impingement pain for most patients. Other investigators have confirmed that a lateral downsloping acromion does not correlate with impingement pain or rotator cuff tears.[50,51,64] Most surgeons are reluctant to resect the lateral portion of the acromion process, except in cases where there is severe lateral downsloping, clearly compressing and potentially abrading the rotator cuff.

An unfused anterior acromion process or os acromiale has also been associated with impingement syndrome and rotator cuff tears.[65–77] The theory is that the deltoid muscle attached to a mobile os acromiale contracts and pulls down the os, causing it to bang against the SASD bursa and the rotator cuff to create impingement pain and tears.[78] Some investigators, however, have found no association between os acromiale and rotator cuff tears.[73,79] Even if there is no association, it is important to identify an os acromiale on the MR image especially if there is a pseudarthrosis with fluid signal at the nonunion, because surgeons need to decide whether to resect, fuse, or leave alone the os at the time of arthroscopy (**Fig. 6**).[68,75,76]

MR IMAGING OF ROTATOR CUFF TENDINOPATHY AND INTRATENDINOUS TEARS

Rotator cuff tendinopathy is usually seen in patients older than 40 years, with a reported average age of about 50 years.[80] There are 2 hallmarks of rotator cuff tendinopathy on MR images: (1) abnormal increased signal within the substance of the cuff without extension to either the articular or bursal surface, and (2) swelling or increased thickness of the tendon (**Fig. 7**).[81] The increased signal within the cuff has been shown to be caused by mucoid

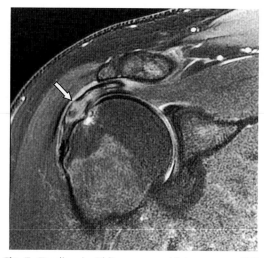

Fig. 7. Tendinosis. Oblique coronal fat-suppressed T2-weighted image shows abnormal high signal and focal swelling (*arrow*) of the supraspinatus tendon, consistent with tendinosis.

and eosinophilic degeneration, splits in the tendon fibers, increased type III collagen, and degradation of mucopolysaccharide with increased glycosaminoglycan and proteoglycan.[17,82] Tendinopathy findings on MR images do not necessarily correlate with pain, but the changes are often seen in patients with impingement syndrome.[80]

There are several pitfalls in accurately diagnosing rotator cuff tendinopathy on MR images,[81] one of which is angular anisotropy, or the magic-angle effect, which causes increased signal within the tendon on low TE images. Overcalling of the magic angle can be reduced by recognizing that it occurs in the downsloping lateral portion of the supraspinatus tendon in which the collagen fibers are oriented about 55° to the static magnetic field, and that the increased signal fades on longer TE T2-weighted images. Another pitfall is the overcalling of the normal intermediate signal in the center of the tendon, resulting from the varied histology of the cuff. Unlike a normal tendon's intermediate signal, tendinopathy usually causes higher signals on T2-weighted images.

Intratendinous partial rotator cuff tears are also called intrasubstance or interstitial tears. It is controversial whether these are a severe form of tendinopathy or should be included in the category of partial-thickness cuff tears. These tears are included in this section because many surgeons prefer to call them intratendinous clefts or fissures and do not believe that these lesions themselves are a significant cause of pain.[83,84] Other investigators, however, have reported improvement in symptoms with incision and tenorrhaphy.[85]

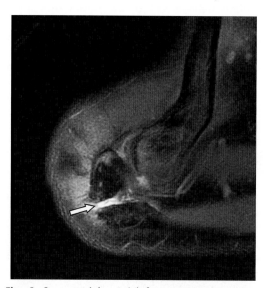

Fig. 6. Os acromiale. Axial fat-suppressed intermediate-weighted image shows a high signal (*arrow*) at the junction of the os acromiale with the scapular spine, which may indicate a mobile os.

Intratendinous tears appear on MR images as fluid signal intensity within the central zone of the tendon without extension to the articular or bursal surface of the cuff (**Fig. 8**). The intratendinous cleft does not communicate with the joint and so will not show high signal intensity on a direct MR arthrogram T1-weighted image. These lesions are often difficult for the surgeon to identify at arthroscopy.[86]

One type of intratendinous tear is a focal cleft at the supraspinatus footprint adjacent to the superior facet of the greater tuberosity, termed a concealed interstitial delamination (CID).[87] In the study by Schaeffeler and colleagues,[87] these focal intratendinous clefts were seen in 23 of 305 MR arthrograms. It is important to distinguish a CID lesion from a rim rent tear, which also appears on MR as a small high-signal focus at the supraspinatus footprint. The distinction is that in a rim rent tear, the abnormal high signal on the MR image extends to the tendon surface.

Intratendinous tears also need to be differentiated from partial-thickness tears with delamination, in which the intratendinous portion of the tear is the most conspicuous finding on the MR images. The articular and bursal surfaces of the cuff should always be carefully inspected to determine if the fluid signal within the tendon extends to the cuff surface. Direct MR arthrogram images can be helpful in distinguishing a noncommunicating intratendinous tear from a partial articular with intratendinous extension tear, or PAINT, lesion (**Fig. 9**).[88]

MR IMAGING OF PARTIAL-THICKNESS ROTATOR CUFF TEARS

One of the most useful roles of MR imaging of the shoulder is in helping clinicians to diagnose rotator cuff tears in patients with impingement pain.

Diagnosing partial-thickness tears in clinical examination is challenging because many of these patients have a normal radiograph and do not have significant weakness of the rotator cuff muscle. Many surgeons operate on patients if the MR image shows a tear and the patient continues to have pain after several months of physical therapy.[6] It should be noted that cuff tears can be present in asymptomatic individuals, so the clinical and imaging findings should be evaluated together.[89,90]

For many surgeons, the important partial-thickness cuff tears are those involving the surface of the cuff, and these are classified as articular surface tears, bursal surface tears, or tears involving the articular and bursal sides of the cuff. Tears involving the articular surface are more common than bursal surface tears by a ratio of about 2:1 to 3:1, whereas tears involving both surfaces are about as common as those only involving the bursal surface.[91,92] Partial-thickness tears appear on fat-suppressed T2-weighted MR images as abnormal increased signals extending to the surface of the rotator cuff (**Fig. 10**). Fortunately, most superficial and deep layers of the cuff are normally low signal on MR images, so the involvement of the cuff surface by a tear is usually apparent.

Although most partial tears can be diagnosed on conventional MR images, investigations have found only moderate accuracy.[23,87,93,94] One reason for this is that partial tears are often small and shallow. Not all tears are fluid-signal intense because they can be filled with fibrovascular tissue, which has only mildly increased signal intensity on T2-weighted images.[95]

There are several factors that can help improve accuracy in diagnosing rotator cuff tears. Articular surface tears are more common than bursal surface tears. Arthroscopic data have also shown that 85% of small rotator cuff tears are in the

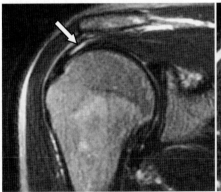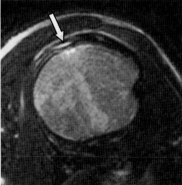

Fig. 8. Intratendinous tear or fissure. Oblique coronal (*left*) and sagittal fat-suppressed T2-weighted (*right*) images demonstrate a linear intrasubstance fissure (*arrows*) within the tendon.

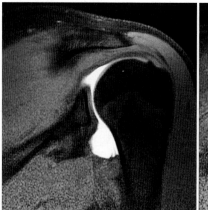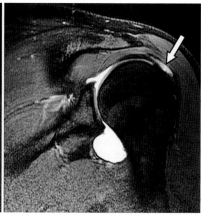

Fig. 9. Intratendinous tear. Oblique coronal fat-suppressed T1-weighted (*left*) and T2-weighted (*right*) images from an MR arthrogram shows a high signal (*arrow*) within the tendon on the T2-weighted image but not on the T1-weighted image. The high signal therefore derives from tendinosis and not from an articular surface partial-thickness tear with delamination.

anterior half of the supraspinatus tendon, and about one-third involve the anterior edge of the tendon.[91] The pretest probability of a mild signal abnormality of the articular surface of the anterior supraspinatus representing a tear is therefore higher than a similar abnormal signal focus involving the bursal portion of the posterior cuff. A secondary sign that can also be helpful is an intramuscular cyst, which is almost always associated with a partial-thickness cuff tear.[96–98]

Small rotator cuff tears can also be difficult to diagnose on MR imaging because the tendon curves downward in the lateral rotator cuff where tears usually occur, and thus is oriented obliquely within the image voxel. One technique that has

been proposed is to obtain an angled oblique sagittal acquisition perpendicular to the lateral rotator cuff, where tears usually occur (**Fig. 11**).[4] The sensitivity of MR imaging for partial tears can also be improved with intra-articular contrast; direct MR arthrography has a 95% accuracy for articular-surface, partial-thickness tears.[99]

Although many partial-thickness cuff tears appear as focal defects on the surface of the supraspinatus tendon in the critical zone, there are several other common appearances. One of these is a rim rent tear, which is a partial–thickness, avulsion-type tear that occurs at the insertion of the cuff onto the greater tuberosity.[91,100] When the rim rent tear involves the articular surface, it is sometimes called a partial articular surface tendon avulsion, or PASTA, lesion. Partial-thickness tears can also extend horizontally within the intratendinous portion of the cuff as delamination tears.[101] When a partial-thickness tear occurs on an articular surface, it can be called a PAINT lesion.[101,102]

MR IMAGING OF FULL-THICKNESS ROTATOR CUFF TEARS

Full-thickness rotator cuff tears are tears that extend from the glenohumeral joint to the subacromial bursa. The classification of rotator cuff tears is somewhat confusing because many of these full-thickness tears are actually partial tendon tears and not complete tears of the entire supraspinatus tendon. Large full-thickness cuff tears may be complete tendon tears if they involve the entire anterior to posterior width of the supraspinatus tendon, and these may lead to muscle atrophy and fatty infiltration.

The accuracy of conventional MR imaging is much higher for full-thickness tears than for

Fig. 10. Articular surface partial-thickness rotator cuff tear. Oblique coronal fat-suppressed T2-weighted image shows a high-signal defect (*arrow*) involving the undersurface of the supraspinatus tendon.

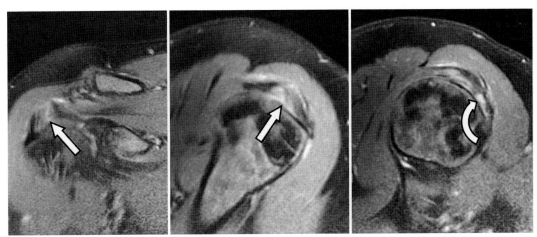

Fig. 11. Articular surface partial-thickness rotator cuff tear. Oblique coronal (*left*), oblique sagittal (*middle*), and angled oblique sagittal (*right*) fat-suppressed T2-weighted images. The oblique coronal image shows a subtle area of increased signal within the cuff while the oblique sagittal image shows a broad area of ill-defined high signal (*arrows*). The angled oblique sagittal image more clearly shows the small articular surface partial tear of the anterior supraspinatus tendon (*curved arrow*) identified at arthroscopy.

partial-thickness tears, with several studies reporting an accuracy of more than 90%.[23,103] The most common MR imaging appearance of a full-thickness tear is a high signal, often fluid signal intensity, extending across the tendon from the glenohumeral joint to the subacromial bursa (**Fig. 12**). Although fluid signal in the tear is common, about 10% of patients have what has been called a low-signal tear in which there is no fluid in the tear.[104] Many of these are chronic rotator cuff tears in patients who have no

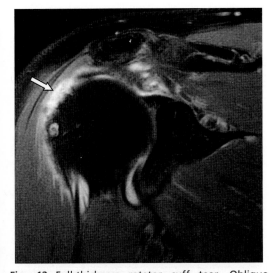

Fig. 12. Full-thickness rotator cuff tear. Oblique coronal fat-suppressed T2-weighted image shows fluid signal intensity extending from the humeral head to the deltoid muscle, indicating a full-thickness supraspinatus tendon tear (*arrow*).

significant effusion; although the humeral head is high-riding so that there is no normal cuff tissue on the MR image between the humeral head and the subacromial bursa (**Fig. 13**).

Most pinpoint, full-thickness, supraspinatus tendon tears occur about 1 cm from the insertion onto the greater tuberosity within the so-called critical zone of the tendon. Although there is some controversy in the literature, several investigators have shown this region to be the site of increased loading, compression, and poorer blood supply, so that the tendon does not heal well after microtrauma.[105–107] These small tears may not enlarge right away because the critical zone is within the rotator crescent lateral to the rotator cable and they are therefore partially protected from tensile forces.[108] Untreated, small, full-thickness tears eventually enlarge.[109] Full-thickness tears can also occur at the footprint of the supraspinatus tendon. These tears may be rim rent tears that have progressed to full-thickness tears, or they may be critical-zone tears that have enlarged with subsequent resorption/mechanical wear of the tendon stump at the insertion.

MR imaging is particularly helpful in identifying muscle atrophy with fatty infiltration in patients with full-thickness, full-width (complete), supraspinatus tendon tears. Several studies have shown that patients with fatty atrophy do less well after rotator cuff repair, and therefore the identification of this problem on the MR image can help determine if a patient is a good candidate for surgery.[110,111] There are two MR imaging measurements of the supraspinatus muscle that allow quantitative grading of atrophy and fatty

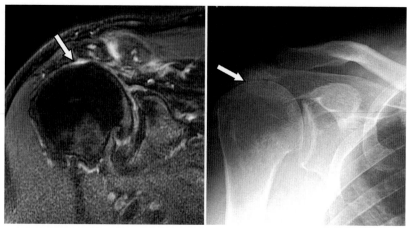

Fig. 13. Low-signal full-thickness rotator cuff tear. Oblique coronal fat-suppressed T2-weighted image (*left*) and Neer anteroposterior radiograph (*right*) show a full-thickness rotator cuff tear (*arrows*) with no tendon between the humeral head and the acromion process.

replacement. One of these is the occupation ratio described by Thomazeau and colleagues,[112] which measures the amount of muscle atrophy. The ratio is determined by measuring on an oblique sagittal image medial to the glenoid (where the scapula appears as a Y shape), the cross-sectional area of the supraspinatus muscle relative to the area of the supraspinatus fossa (defined as the area between the spine and superior blade of the scapula) (**Fig. 14**). An occupation ratio of less than 0.4 indicates severe atrophy. Fatty replacement is also measured on an oblique, sagittal, non–fat-suppressed image. In the grading system of Goutallier and colleagues,[113] a ratio of muscle

to fat of 1:1 is considered moderate fatty infiltration, and more fat than muscle is classified as severe. Patients with severe atrophy and fatty replacement of the cuff have a much higher retear rate after rotator cuff repair.[113]

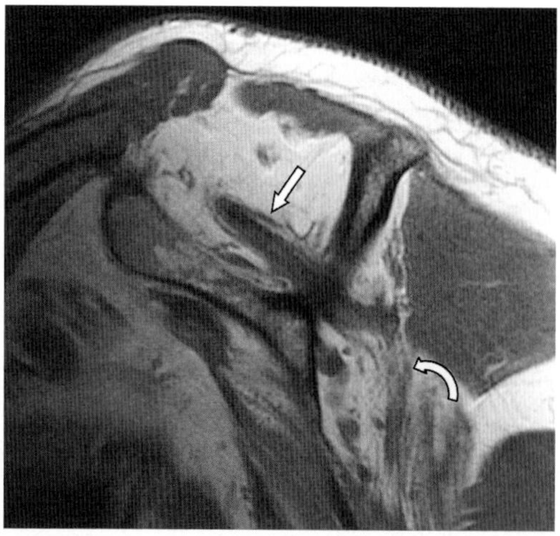

In summary, MR imaging plays a major role in helping to identify rotator cuff disease and in demonstrating the pathology associated with external impingement. Many surgeons rely on MR imaging to assist in decision making and pre-surgical planning for patients with rotator cuff pain.

Fig. 14. Oblique sagittal T1-weighted image medial to the glenoid fossa through the scapular "Y" shows severe atrophy of the supraspinatus muscle (*arrow*) with an occupation ratio of less than 0.4, and severe fat replacement of the infraspinatus muscle (*curved arrow*).

REFERENCES

1. Hambly N, Fitzpatrick P, MacMahon P, et al. Rotator cuff impingement: correlation between findings on MRI and outcome after fluoroscopically guided subacromial bursography and steroid injection. AJR Am J Roentgenol 2007;189(5):1179–84.
2. Michener LA, McClure PW, Karduna AR. Anatomical and biomechanical mechanisms of subacromial impingement syndrome. Clin Biomech (Bristol, Avon) 2003;18(5):369–79.
3. Sher JS, Iannotti JP, Williams GR, et al. The effect of shoulder magnetic resonance imaging on clinical decision making. J Shoulder Elbow Surg 1998;7:205–9.
4. Tuite MJ, Asinger D, Orwin JF. Angled oblique sagittal MR imaging of rotator cuff tears: comparison with standard oblique sagittal images. Skeletal Radiol 2001;30:262–9.
5. Tuite MJ, Yandow DR, DeSmet AA, et al. Diagnosis of partial and complete rotator cuff tears using combined gradient echo and spin-echo imaging. Skeletal Radiol 1994;23(7):541–5.
6. Matsen FA, Arntz CT, Lippitt SB. Rotator cuff. In: Rockwood CA, Matsen FA, editors. The shoulder. Philadelphia: WB Saunders; 1998. p. 755–839.

7. Opsha O, Malik A, Baltazar R, et al. MRI of the rotator cuff and internal derangement. Eur J Radiol 2008;68(1):36–56.

8. Soifer TB, Levy HJ, Soifer FM, et al. Neurohistology of the subacromial space. Arthroscopy 1996;12(2): 182–6.

9. Hallstrom E, Karrholm J. Shoulder kinematics in 25 patients with impingement and 12 controls. Clin Orthop Relat Res 2006;448:22–7.

10. Budoff JE, Nirschl RP, Guidi EJ. Debridement of partial-thickness tears of the rotator cuff without acromioplasty. J Bone Joint Surg Am 1998;80:733–48.

11. Ozaki J, Fujimoto S, Nakagawa Y, et al. Tears of the rotator cuff of the shoulder associated with pathological changes in the acromion: a study in cadavers. J Bone Joint Surg Am 1988;70:1224–30.

12. Lo IK, Burkhart SS. The etiology and assessment of subscapularis tendon tears: a case for subcoracoid impingement, the roller-wringer effect, and TUFF lesions of the subscapularis. Arthroscopy 2003;19(10):1142–50.

13. Nakajima T, Rokuuma N, Hamada K, et al. Histologic and biomechanical characteristics of the supraspinatus tendon: reference to rotator cuff tearing. J Shoulder Elbow Surg 1994;3:79–87.

14. Lee SB, Nakajima T, Luo ZP, et al. The bursal and articular sides of the supraspinatus tendon have a different compressive stiffness. Clin Biomech 2000;15(4):241–7.

15. Clark JM, Harryman DT. Tendons, ligaments, and capsule of the rotator cuff. J Bone Joint Surg Am 1992;74(5):713–25.

16. Loehr JF, Uhthoff HK. The microvascular pattern of the supraspinatus tendon. Clin Orthop 1990;254:35–8.

17. Kjellin I, Ho CP, Cervilla V, et al. Alterations in the supraspinatus tendon at MR imaging: correlation with histopathologic findings in cadavers. Radiology 1991;181(3):837–41.

18. Funakoshi T, Martin SD, Schmid TM, et al. Distribution of lubricin in the ruptured human rotator cuff and biceps tendon: a pilot study. Clin Orthop Relat Res 2010;468(6):1588–99.

19. Fu FH, Harner CD, Klein AH. Shoulder impingement syndrome. Clin Orthop 1991;269:162–73.

20. Carroll KW, Helms CA. Magnetic resonance imaging of the shoulder: a review of potential sources of diagnostic errors. Skeletal Radiol 2002;31(7):373–83.

21. Singson RD, Hoang T, Dan S, et al. MR evaluation of rotator cuff pathology using T2-weighted fast spin-echo technique with and without fat suppression. AJR Am J Roentgenol 1996;166(5):1061–5.

22. Vlychou M, Dailiana Z, Fotiadou A, et al. Symptomatic partial rotator cuff tears: diagnostic performance of ultrasound and magnetic resonance imaging with surgical correlation. Acta Radiol 2009;50(1):101–5.

23. de Jesus JO, Parker L, Frangos AJ, et al. Accuracy of MRI, MR arthrography, and ultrasound in the diagnosis of rotator cuff tears: a meta-analysis. AJR Am J Roentgenol 2009;192(6):1701–7.

24. Sheah K, Bredella MA, Warner JJ, et al. Transverse thickening along the articular surface of the rotator cuff consistent with the rotator cable: identification with MR arthrography and relevance in rotator cuff evaluation. AJR Am J Roentgenol 2009;193(3): 679–86.

25. White EA, Schweitzer ME, Haims AH. Range of normal and abnormal subacromial/subdeltoid bursa fluid. J Comput Assist Tomogr 2006;30(2): 316–20.

26. Mayerhoefer ME, Breitenseher MJ, Wurnig C, et al. Shoulder impingement: relationship of clinical symptoms and imaging criteria. Clin J Sport Med 2009;19(2):83–9.

27. Neer CS. Anterior acromioplasty for the chronic impingement syndrome in the shoulder: a preliminary report. J Bone Joint Surg Am 1972;54:41–50.

28. Jia X, Ji JH, Pannirselvam V, et al. Does a positive Neer impingement sign reflect rotator cuff contact with the acromion? Clin Orthop Relat Res 2011; 469(3):813–8.

29. Petersson CJ, Gentz CF. Ruptures of the supraspinatus tendon: the significance of distally pointing acromioclavicular osteophytes. Clin Orthop 1983; 174:143–8.

30. Cuomo F, Kummer FJ, Zuckerman JD, et al. The influence of acromioclavicular joint morphology on rotator cuff tears. J Shoulder Elbow Surg 1998; 7(6):555–9.

31. de Abreu MR, Chung CB, Wesselly M, et al. Acromioclavicular joint osteoarthritis: comparison of findings derived from MR imaging and conventional radiography. Clin Imaging 2005;29(4):273–7.

32. Campbell RS, Dunn A. External impingement of the shoulder. Semin Musculoskelet Radiol 2008;12(2): 107–26.

33. Hardy DC, Vogler JB 3rd, White RH. The shoulder impingement syndrome: prevalence of radiographic findings and correlation with response to therapy. AJR Am J Roentgenol 1986;147(3):557–61.

34. MacGillivray JD, Fealy S, Potter HG, et al. Multiplanar analysis of acromion morphology. Am J Sports Med 1998;26(6):836–40.

35. Weber SC. Arthroscopic debridement and acromioplasty versus mini-open repair in the treatment of significant partial-thickness rotator cuff tears. Arthroscopy 1999;15(2):126–31.

36. Kharrazi FD, Busfield BT, Khorshad DS. Acromioclavicular joint reoperation after arthroscopic subacromial decompression with and without concomitant acromioclavicular surgery. Arthroscopy 2007;23(8): 804–8.

37. Chen AL, Rokito AS, Zuckerman JD. The role of the acromioclavicular joint in impingement syndrome. Clin Sports Med 2003;22(2):343–57.

38. Neer CS. Impingement lesions. Clin Orthop 1983; 173:70–7.

39. Bigliani LU. Impingement syndrome: etiology and overview. In: Watson MS, editor. Surgical disorders of the shoulder. New York: Churchill Livingstone; 1991. p. 237–46.

40. Bigliani LU, Morrison DS, April EW. The morphology of the acromion and its relationship to rotator cuff tears. Orthop Trans 1986;10:228.

41. Tuite MJ, Toivonen DA, Orwin JF, et al. Acromial angle on radiographs of the shoulder: correlation with the impingement syndrome and rotator cuff tears. AJR Am J Roentgenol 1995;165(3):609–13.

42. Peh WC, Farmer TH, Totty WG. Acromial arch shape: assessment with MR imaging. Radiology 1995;195(2):501–5.

43. Farley TE, Neumann CH, Steinbach LS, et al. The coracoacromial arch: MR evaluation and correlation with rotator cuff pathology. Skeletal Radiol 1994;23(8):641–5.

44. Wang JC, Horner G, Brown ED, et al. The relationship between acromial morphology and conservative treatment of patients with impingement syndrome. Orthopedics 2000;23(6):557–9.

45. Tasu JP, Miquel A, Rocher L, et al. MR evaluation of factors predicting the development of rotator cuff tears. J Comput Assist Tomogr 2001;25(2): 159–63.

46. Panni AS, Milano G, Lucania L, et al. Histological analysis of the coracoacromial arch: correlation between age-related changes and rotator cuff tears. Arthroscopy 1996;12(5):531–40.

47. Epstein RE, Schweitzer ME, Frieman BG, et al. Hooked acromion: prevalence on MR images of painful shoulders. Radiology 1993;187(2):479–81.

48. Zuckerman JD, Kummer FJ, Cuomo F, et al. The influence of coracoacromial arch anatomy on rotator cuff tears. J Shoulder Elbow Surg 1992; 1(1):4–14.

49. Hyvönen P, Päivänsalo M, Lehtiniemi H, et al. Supraspinatus outlet view in the diagnosis of stages II and III impingement syndrome. Acta Radiol 2001;42(5):441–6.

50. Chang EY, Moses DA, Babb JS, et al. Shoulder impingement: objective 3D shape analysis of acromial morphologic features. Radiology 2006;239(2): 497–505.

51. Moses DA, Chang EY, Schweitzer ME. The scapuloacromial angle: a 3D analysis of acromial slope and its relationship with shoulder impingement. J Magn Reson Imaging 2006;24(6):1371–7.

52. Banas MP, Miller RJ, Totterman S. Relationship between the lateral acromion angle and rotator cuff disease. J Shoulder Elbow Surg 1995;4(6): 454–61.

53. Fukuda H, Hamada K, Nakajima T, et al. Pathology and pathogenesis of the intratendinous tearing of the rotator cuff viewed from en bloc histologic sections. Clin Orthop Relat Res 1994;304:60–7.

54. Getz JD, Recht MP, Piraino DW, et al. Acromial morphology: relation to sex, age, symmetry, and subacromial enthesophytes. Radiology 1996; 199(3):737–42.

55. Shah NN, Bayliss NC, Malcolm A. Shape of the acromion: congenital or acquired–a macroscopic, radiographic, and microscopic study of acromion. J Shoulder Elbow Surg 2001;10(4):309–16.

56. Speer KP, Osbahr DC, Montella BJ, et al. Acromial morphotype in the young asymptomatic athletic shoulder. J Shoulder Elbow Surg 2001;10(5): 434–7.

57. Mayerhoefer ME, Breitenseher MJ, Roposch A, et al. Comparison of MRI and conventional radiography for assessment of acromial shape. AJR Am J Roentgenol 2005;184(2):671–5.

58. Haygood TM, Langlotz CP, Kneeland JB, et al. Categorization of acromial shape: interobserver variability with MR imaging and conventional radiography. AJR Am J Roentgenol 1994;162(6): 1377–82.

59. Bright AS, Torpey B, Magid D, et al. Reliability of radiographic evaluation for acromial morphology. Skeletal Radiol 1997;26(12):718–21.

60. Jacobson SR, Langlotz CP, Kneeland JB, et al. Reliability of radiographic assessment of acromial morphology. J Shoulder Elbow Surg 1995;4(6): 449–53.

61. Burkhart SS. Congenital subacromial stenosis. Arthroscopy 1995;11(1):63–8.

62. Björnsson H, Norlin R, Knutsson A, et al. Fewer rotator cuff tears fifteen years after arthroscopic subacromial decompression. J Shoulder Elbow Surg 2010;19(1):111–5.

63. Nyffeler RW, Werner CM, Sukthankar A, et al. Association of a large lateral extension of the acromion with rotator cuff tears. J Bone Joint Surg Am 2006;88(4):800–5.

64. Yao L, Lee HY, Gentili A, et al. Lateral down-sloping of the acromion: a useful MR sign? Clin Radiol 1996;51(12):869–72.

65. Barbiera F, Bellissima G, Iovane A, et al. Os acromiale producing rotator cuff impingement and rupture. A case report. Radiol Med 2002;104(4): 359–62.

66. Wright RW, Heller MA, Quick DC, et al. Arthroscopic decompression for impingement syndrome secondary to an unstable os acromiale. Arthroscopy 2000;16(6):595–9.

67. Swain RA, Wilson FD, Harsha DM. The os acromiale: another cause of impingement. Med Sci Sports Exerc 1996;28(12):1459–62.

68. Edelson JG, Zuckerman J, Hershkovitz I. Os acromiale: anatomy and surgical implications. J Bone Joint Surg Br 1993;75:551–5.

69. Park JG, Lee JK, Phelps CT. Os acromiale associated with rotator cuff impingement: MR imaging of the shoulder. Radiology 1994;193(1):255–7.

70. Hutchinson MR, Veenstra MA. Arthroscopic decompression of shoulder impingement secondary to os acromiale. Arthroscopy 1993;9(1):28–32.

71. Mudge MK, Wood VE, Frykman GK. Rotator cuff tears associated with os acromiale. J Bone Joint Surg Am 1984;66(3):427–9.

72. Warner JJ, Beim GM, Higgins L. The treatment of symptomatic os acromiale. J Bone Joint Surg Am 1998;80(9):1320–6.

73. Boehm T, Rolf O, Martetschlaeger F, et al. Rotator cuff tears associated with os acromiale. Acta Orthop 2005;76(2):241–4.

74. Norris TR, Fischer J, Bigliani LU, et al. The unfused acromial epiphysis and its relationship to impingement syndrome. Orthop Trans 1983; 254:39–48.

75. Kurtz CA, Humble BJ, Rodosky MW, et al. Symptomatic os acromiale. J Am Acad Orthop Surg 2006;14(1):12–9.

76. Sahajpal D, Strauss EJ, Ishak C, et al. Surgical management of os acromiale: a case report and review of the literature. Bull NYU Hosp Jt Dis 2007;65(4):312–6.

77. Smith J, Dahm DL, Newcomer-Aney KL. Role of sonography in the evaluation of unstable os acromiale. J Ultrasound Med 2008;27(10):1521–6.

78. Davlin CD, Fluker D. Bilateral os acromiale in a division I basketball player. J Sports Sci Med 2003;2: 175–9.

79. Ouellette H, Thomas BJ, Kassarjian A, et al. Re-examining the association of os acromiale with supraspinatus and infraspinatus tears. Skeletal Radiol 2007;36(9):835–9.

80. Lewis JS. Rotator cuff tendinopathy. Br J Sports Med 2009;43(4):236–41.

81. Sein ML, Walton J, Linklater J, et al. Reliability of MRI assessment of supraspinatus tendinopathy. Br J Sports Med 2007;41(8):e9.

82. Williams GR Jr, Iannotti JP, Rosenthal A, et al. Anatomic, histologic, and magnetic resonance imaging abnormalities of the shoulder. Clin Orthop Relat Res 1996;330(330):66–74.

83. Tuite MJ. Shoulder and humerus: musculotendinous pathology. In: Sonin A, Manaster BJ, editors. Diagnostic imaging: musculoskeletal trauma. Salt Lake City (UT): Amirsys; 2010. p. 72–7.

84. Gartsman GM. Arthroscopic acromioplasty for lesions of the rotator cuff. J Bone Joint Surg Am 1990;72(2):169–80.

85. Uchiyama Y, Hamada K, Khruekarnchana P, et al. Surgical treatment of confirmed intratendinous rotator cuff tears: retrospective analysis after an average of eight years of follow-up. J Shoulder Elbow Surg 2010;19(6):837–46.

86. Lo IK, Gonzalez DM, Burkhart SS. The bubble sign: an arthroscopic indicator of an intratendinous rotator cuff tear. Arthroscopy 2002;18(9):1029–33.

87. Schaeffeler C, Mueller D, Kirchhoff C, et al. Tears at the rotator cuff footprint: prevalence and imaging characteristics in 305 MR arthrograms of the shoulder. Eur Radiol 2011;21(7):1477–84.

88. Lee SY, Lee JK. Horizontal component of partial-thickness tears of rotator cuff: imaging characteristics and comparison of ABER view with oblique coronal view at MR arthrography-initial results. Radiology 2002;224:470–6.

89. Miniaci A, Dowdy PA, Willits KR, et al. Magnetic resonance imaging evaluation of the rotator cuff tendons in the asymptomatic shoulder. Am J Sports Med 1995;23(2):142–5.

90. Sher JS, Uribe JW, Posada A, et al. Abnormal findings on magnetic resonance images of asymptomatic shoulders. J Bone Joint Surg Am 1995;77(1):10–5.

91. Tuite MJ, Turnbull JR, Orwin JF. Anterior versus posterior, and rim rent rotator cuff tears: prevalence and MR sensitivity. Skeletal Radiol 1998;27: 237–43.

92. Chun KA, Kim MS, Kim YJ. Comparisons of the various partial-thickness rotator cuff tears on MR arthrography and arthroscopic correlation. Korean J Radiol 2010;11(5):528–35.

93. Traughber P, Czech M. Accuracy of fat-suppressed MR imaging of the shoulder for detection of partial-thickness rotator cuff tears [letter]. Radiology 1996; 198(1):293.

94. Traughber PD, Goodwin TE. Shoulder MRI: arthroscopic correlation with emphasis on partial tears. J Comput Assist Tomogr 1992;16(1):129–33.

95. Van Dyck P, Gielen JL, Veryser J, et al. Tears of the supraspinatus tendon: assessment with indirect magnetic resonance arthrography in 67 patients with arthroscopic correlation. Acta Radiol 2009; 50(9):1057–63.

96. Manvar AM, Kamireddi A, Bhalani SM, et al. Clinical significance of intramuscular cysts in the rotator cuff and their relationship to full- and partial-thickness rotator cuff tears. AJR Am J Roentgenol 2009;192(3):719–24.

97. Kassarjian A, Torriani M, Ouellette H, et al. Intramuscular rotator cuff cysts: association with tendon tears on MRI and arthroscopy. AJR Am J Roentgenol 2005;185(1):160–5.

98. Sanders TG, Tirman PF, Feller JF, et al. Association of intramuscular cysts of the rotator cuff with tears of the rotator cuff: magnetic resonance imaging findings and clinical significance. Arthroscopy 2000;16:230–5.

99. Waldt S, Bruegel M, Mueller D, et al. Rotator cuff tears: assessment with MR arthrography in 275 patients with arthroscopic correlation. Eur Radiol 2007;17(2):491–8.

100. Vinson EN, Helms CA, Higgins LD. Rim rent tear of the rotator cuff: a common and easily overlooked partial tear. AJR Am J Roentgenol 2007;189(4): 943–6.

101. Walz DM, Miller TT, Chen S, et al. MR imaging of delamination tears of the rotator cuff tendons. Skeletal Radiol 2007;36(5):411–6.

102. Conway JE. Arthroscopic repair of partial-thickness rotator cuff tears and SLAP lesions in professional baseball players. Orthop Clin North Am 2001; 32(3):443–56.

103. Magee T, Williams D. 3.0-T MRI of the supraspinatus tendon. AJR Am J Roentgenol 2006;187(4): 881–6.

104. Rafii M, Firooznia H, Sherman O, et al. Rotator cuff lesions: signal patterns at MR imaging. Radiology 1990;177:817–23.

105. Rudzki JR, Adler RS, Warren RF, et al. Contrast-enhanced ultrasound characterization of the vascularity of the rotator cuff tendon: age- and activity-related changes in the intact asymptomatic rotator cuff. J Shoulder Elbow Surg 2008;17(Suppl 1):96S–100S.

106. Rothman HR, Parke W. The vascular anatomy of the rotator cuff. Clin Orthop 1965;41:176–86.

107. Uhthoff HK, Hammond DI, Sarkar K, et al. The role of the coracoacromial ligament in the impingement syndrome—a clinical, radiological and histological study. Int Orthop 1988;12:97–104.

108. Burkhart SS, Esch JC, Jolson RS. The rotator crescent and rotator cable: an anatomic description of the shoulder's "suspension bridge". Arthroscopy 1993;9(6):611–6.

109. Mays M, Lin D, Gugala Z, et al. Efficacy of repeat shoulder magnetic resonance imaging. Orthopedics 2008;31(6):543.

110. Khoury V, Cardinal E, Brassard P. Atrophy and fatty infiltration of the supraspinatus muscle: sonography versus MRI. AJR Am J Roentgenol 2008;190(4): 1105–11.

111. Tae SK, Oh JH, Kim SH, et al. Evaluation of fatty degeneration of the supraspinatus muscle using a new measuring tool and its correlation between multidetector computed tomography and magnetic resonance imaging. Am J Sports Med 2011;39(3): 599–606.

112. Thomazeau H, Rolland Y, Lucas C, et al. Atrophy of the supraspinatus belly. Assessment by MRI in 55 patients with rotator cuff pathology. Acta Orthop Scand 1996;67(3):264–8.

113. Goutallier D, Postel JM, Bernageau J, et al. Fatty muscle degeneration in cuff ruptures. Pre- and postoperative evaluation by CT scan. Clin Orthop Relat Res 1994;304(304):78–83.

Internal Impingement Syndromes

Luis S. Beltran, MD[a,*], Violeta Nikac, MD[b],
Javier Beltran, MD[b]

KEYWORDS

- Shoulder magnetic resonance • Impingement • Rotator cuff
- Arthrography

Impingement syndromes of the shoulder can be caused by external or internal causes. External causes are due to primary abnormalities in the coracoacromial arch causing extrinsic compression of the subacromial bursa and the rotator cuff, leading to rotator cuff tear and retraction, as first described by Neer in 1972,[1] and including subacromial and subcoracoid impingement. It occurs most commonly in middle-aged nonathletic individuals. Internal causes of impingement are secondary to rotator cuff and capsular dysfunction and are categorized by the location of the impingement and the underlying pathophysiological or mechanical cause of the impingement. These include posterosuperior impingement, anterosuperior impingement, anterior impingement, and entrapment of the long head of the biceps tendon (LHBT) (**Fig. 1**). Although the diagnosis of internal impingement is primarily clinical, magnetic resonance imaging (MRI) can play an important role in confirming clinical suspicion or suggesting the diagnosis. In this article, the authors discuss the MRI evaluation and pathophysiological mechanisms of internal impingement syndromes of the shoulder.

POSTEROSUPERIOR IMPINGEMENT

Posterosuperior impingement, which was first described by Walch and colleagues,[2] refers to contact of the undersurface of the posterosuperior rotator cuff with the posterosuperior labrum when the arm is abducted and externally rotated (ABER), where the cuff can become pinched between the labrum and the greater tuberosity. It occurs most frequently in professional throwing athletes and is attributed to repetitive overhead motion, most commonly in baseball pitchers, tennis players, javelin throwers, and swimmers. Typical symptoms include posterior superior shoulder pain that commences during the late cocking phase of overhead movement and intensifies during the early acceleration phase.[3]

Jobe[4] presented an expanded spectrum of injury occurring in overhead throwing athletes in the setting of posterosuperior impingement, which includes injuries to the superior labrum, the rotator cuff tendon, the greater tuberosity, the inferior glenohumeral ligament, and the superior glenoid bone. He also suggested that internal impingement in throwing athletes may progressively worsen because of gradual stretching of the anterior capsuloligamentous structures, leading to anterior displacement of the humeral head and impingement of the rotator cuff and the posterosuperior labrum between the greater tuberosity of the humerus and the glenoid margin. This theory led to the initial treatment approach for anterior glenohumeral instability using anterior capsulolabral reconstruction; however, results of this treatment were unpredictable.[5] Halbrecht and colleagues[6] disagreed with Jobe's premise of anterior instability worsening internal impingement and showed that glenohumeral instability, where the humeral head is subluxed anteriorly, resulting in decreased contact with the posterosuperior glenoid compared with the reduced position. Therefore, they proposed that anterior instability does not worsen internal impingement but rather lessens it. The role

[a] Department of Radiology, New York University Langone Medical Center, 660 First Avenue, Room 218, New York, NY 10016, USA
[b] Department of Radiology, Maimonides Medical Center, 4802 Tenth Avenue, Brooklyn, NY 11219, USA
* Corresponding author.
E-mail address: Luis.Beltran@nyumc.org

Magn Reson Imaging Clin N Am 20 (2012) 201–211
doi:10.1016/j.mric.2012.01.008
1064-9689/12/$ – see front matter © 2012 Elsevier Inc. All rights reserved.

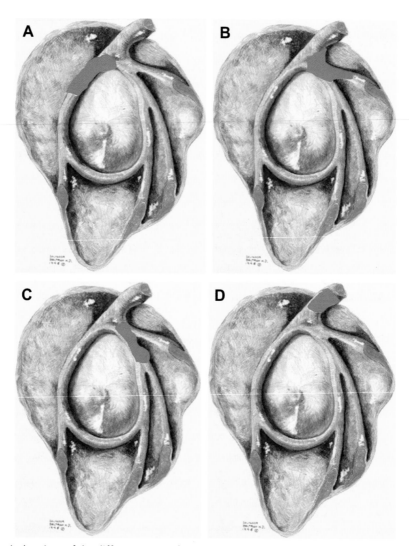

Fig. 1. Schematic drawings of the different types of internal impingement. The red mark indicates the location of the pathology along the bicipital labroligament complex. (*A*) Posterosuperior impingement. (*B*) Anterosuperior impingement (ASI). (*C*) Anterior Impingement. (*D*) Entrapment of the long head of the biceps tendon. (*Courtesy of* Salvador Beltran, MD.)

of anterior capsular laxity as a causative factor in posterosuperior impingement is still controversial.

Burkhart and colleagues[7] proposed that posterosuperior impingement is a normal phenomenon in all shoulders and is not usually pathologic in the disabled throwing shoulder. Rather they proposed that scarring of the posterior joint capsule leads to loss of internal rotation of the humeral head in the throwing athlete, starting a pathologic cascade that results in posterosuperior shift of the glenohumeral rotation point during abduction and external rotation that is maximal in the late cocking phase of throwing. The posterosuperior displacement of the rotation point may be also caused by the thickened posterior capsule moving inferior to the humeral head on abduction and external rotation, according to Burkhart and colleagues.[7] At this point the shift results in maximal shear stress on the posterosuperior labrum and the biceps anchor, resulting in a peel back mechanism that produces a posterior type IIB superior labrum anterior and posterior (SLAP) lesion with posterior extension.[8] This is also referred to as glenohumeral internal rotation deficit (GIRD), because it is believed that the primary initiating event of this cascade of events is scarring of the posterior joint capsule leading to restriction of internal rotation or excessive external rotation. Throwing athletes with

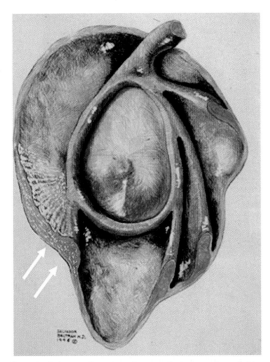

Fig. 2. Schematic glenohumeral internal rotation deficit (GIRD). There is scarring of the posterior joint capsule (*arrows*), which leads to restriction of internal rotation or excessive external rotation. (*Courtesy of Salvador Beltran, MD.*)

GIRD require an increase of the external rotation during the late cocking phase to achieve sufficient throwing power (**Fig. 2**).

The magnetic resonance (MR) and MR arthrographic findings of posterosuperior impingement have been described by several authors,[3,9–15] and they include (**Figs. 3** and **4**): (1) tearing of the posterior undersurface fibers of the supraspinatus tendon and anterior undersurface of the infraspinatus tendon, (2) tearing of the posterosuperior glenoid labrum or type IIB SLAP lesion, (3) humeral head impaction or subcortical humeral head cysts, (4) laxity of the anterior capsule, and (5) thickening of the posterior capsule (**Fig. 5**). It is important to note that when evaluating MR images obtained in the ABER position, nonpathologic entrapment of the articular surface fibers of the supraspinatus tendon occurs in all normal individuals and when isolated this finding does not suggest pathologic impingement. However, if there are additional findings associated with posterosuperior impingement as previously described, then the diagnosis can be suggested on the ABER view.

ANTEROSUPERIOR IMPINGEMENT

Anterosuperior impingement was first described in 2000 by Gerber and Sebesta,[16] who observed internal impingement between the humeral head and the anterior superior glenoid rim on arthroscopy while the patient's arm was horizontally adducted, maximally externally rotated, and anteriorly elevated. This patient had symptoms of anterior superior shoulder pain attributed to repetitive overhead movement thatwas either occupational (masonry) or sports related (pole vaulting). During arthroscopy, partial tears of the deep fibers of the subscapularis tendon along the lesser tuberosity attachment were described, in addition to tearing of the humeral attachments of the coracohumeral and superior glenohumeral ligaments (biceps pulley lesion).

Habermeyer later described anterosuperior impingement as impingement of the long head of

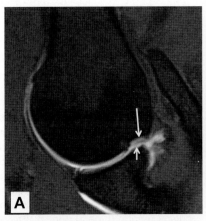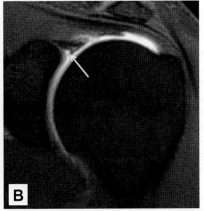

Fig. 3. Posterosuperior impingement: (*A*) T1W fat-suppressed arthrogram in the abduction external rotation (ABER) position. There is entrapment and irregularity of articular surface fibers of the supraspinatus between the humeral head and the glenoid (*long arrow*) and an articular cartilage defect of the adjacent posterior superior aspect of the glenoid (*short arrow*). (*B*) Oblique coronal T1W fat-suppressed arthrogram in the same patient. Posterosuperior labral tear (*arrow*).

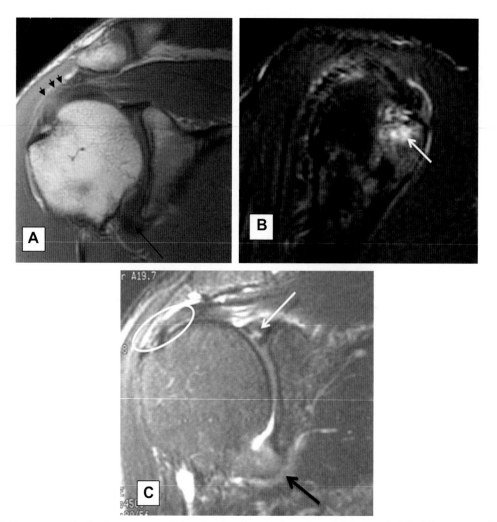

Fig. 4. Posterosuperior impingement and glenohumeral internal rotation deficit (GIRD). (*A*) Oblique coronal T1W image demonstrating capsular fibrosis (*long arrow*), and supraspinatus tear (*short arrows*). (*B*) Water-sensitive sagittal image of the same patient showing microfractures/cysts in the humeral head (*arrow*). (*C*) Coronal oblique fat saturated T2W image of the same patient: GIRD (*black arrow*) with SLAP (*white arrow*) and partial thickness rotator cuff tear (*oval*).

the biceps tendon with the anterosuperior glenoid rim and noted that an important factor for this to develop is the additional partial articular-sided tear of the subscapularis tendon and a lesion of the biceps pulley.[17] Tears of the undersurface of the anterior supraspinatus tendon were also identified. The etiology of the biceps pulley lesion can be traumatic or degenerative. Traumatic causes include a fall on an outstretched arm while the arm is in full internal or external rotation, or while falling backward on the hand or elbow.[18] Degenerative or chronic injury can occur in patients with repetitive overhand activity.[16]

Lesions of the biceps pulley have been classified by Bennett[19] and Habermeyer and colleagues[17] based on lesions involving the subscapularis tendon, superior glenohumeral/medial coracohumeral (SGHL-MCHL) complex, and the lateral coracohumeral ligament (LCHL).

Biceps subluxation and instability was first classified by Bennett in 2001.[19] Bennett has since modified his classification based on subsequent arthroscopic findings.[20] He classifies biceps pulley injuries as involving the intra-articular subscapularis tendon (type 1) (**Fig. 6**), the medial sheath (comprised of the SGHL-MCHL ligament complex) (type 2) (**Fig. 7**), both the medial sheath and subscapularis tendon (type 3) (**Fig. 8**), the supraspinatus and lateral coracohumeral ligament (type 4) (**Fig. 9**), or all structures—intra-articular subscapularis tendon, medial sheath, supraspinatus tendon, and LCHL (type 5) (**Fig. 10**).

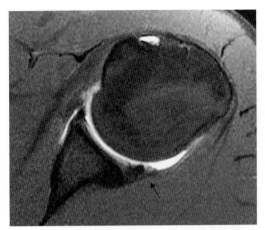

Fig. 5. Glenohumeral internal rotation deficit (GIRD). Axial T1 fat sat magnetic resonance (MR) arthrogram show thickening of the posterior capsule and labral irregularity (*arrow*).

Type 1 lesions are isolated lesions of the subscapularis tendon, and although the medial sheath remains intact, tearing of the subscapularis tendon, which lends structural support to the medial sheath, is sufficient to result in some degree of deformation of the medial sheath allowing the biceps tendon to lie medially within the bicipital groove. Tearing of the medial sheath alone (type 2) results in subluxation of the biceps tendon between the subscapularis tendon and the coracohumeral ligament, which often has the appearance of an intratendinous subluxation. However, if axial and sagittal images are reviewed carefully, an intact subscapularis tendon is seen at its lesser tuberosity insertion. Intra-articular dislocation of the biceps tendon can only occur after both the intra-articular subscapularis tendon and medial sheath are disrupted (type 3).

Articular-sided tears of the anterior supraspinatus tendon that propagate into the rotator interval can result in tearing of the lateral coracohumeral ligament. Although the rotator cuff is not considered to be part of the biceps reflection pulley, the rotator cuff provides important superolateral tension on the medial coracohumeral ligament, as it contributes to the rotator interval capsule by contiguity with the medial coracohumeral ligament. Disruption of the normal tension results in anterior dislocation of the biceps tendon in relation to the subscapularis tendon and coracohumeral ligament (type 4). Tears of the anterior supraspinatus and cranial fibers of the subscapularis tendons (ie, the anterior rotator cuff) are highly associated with biceps tendon pathology, ranging from tendon subluxation or dislocation to partial or complete tendon tears.[21] When there is injury to both the lateral and medial stabilizing structures of the biceps pulley, the biceps tendon is free to dislocate anteriorly or into the joint (type 5).

Habermeyer classified biceps pulley lesions into 4 types (**Fig. 11**). Type 1 lesions are isolated tears of

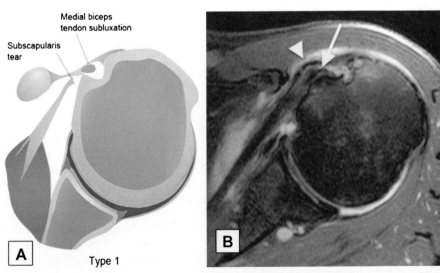

Fig. 6. Bennet type 1 lesion. (*A*) Schematic type 1 Bennet lesion with tear of the intra-articular fibers of the subscapularis tendon and medial subluxation of the biceps tendon. (*B*) Axial T2 image demonstrates medial biceps tendon subluxation (*arrow*). The superficial fibers of the subscapularis tendon are preserved (*arrowhead*). The deep fibers are torn. ([A] *From* Petchprapa CN, Beltran LS, Recht MP, et al. The rotator interval: a review of anatomy, function, and normal and abnormal MRI appearance. Am J Roentgenol 2010;195(3):570; with permission.)

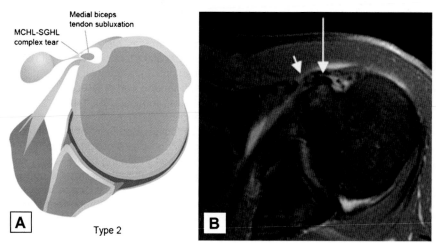

Fig. 7. Bennet type 2 lesion. (*A*) Schematic a Type 2 Bennet lesion with tearing of the medial sheath and medial subluxation of the biceps tendon. (*B*) Axial fat saturated T2W images demonstrating a torn medial sheath (*short arrow*) and medial subluxation of the biceps tendon (*long arrow*). ([A] *From* Petchprapa CN, Beltran LS, Recht MP, et al. The rotator interval: a review of anatomy, function, and normal and abnormal MRI appearance. Am J Roentgenol 2010;195(3):570; with permission.)

the medial sheath or SGHL-MCHL complex along the anterior aspect of the pulley. The supraspinatus and subscapularis tendons are intact, and there is no biceps tendon subluxation. Type 2 lesions involve a pulley lesion in association with a partial-thickness articular surface tear of the anterior fibers of the supraspinatus tendon and mild

medial subluxation of the biceps tendon. Type 3 lesions involve a pulley lesion in association with partial deep tearing of the superior fibers of the subscapularis tendon and subluxation of the biceps tendon, partially extending beyond the containment of the SGHL-MCHL sling. Type 4 lesions involve a pulley lesion in association with partial

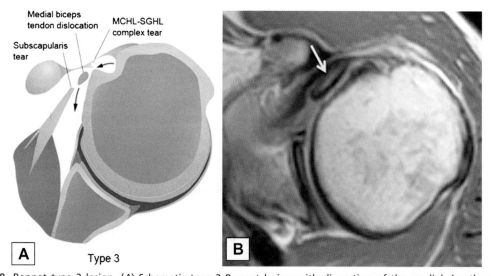

Fig. 8. Bennet type 3 lesion. (*A*) Schematic type 3 Bennet lesion with disruption of the medial sheath, which consists of the medial coracohumeral ligament (MCHL) and superior glenohumeral ligament (SGHL) complex, and a tear of the subscapularis tendon. There is intra-articular dislocation of the biceps tendon. (*B*) Axial proton density image demonstrating resultant intra-articular dislocation of the biceps tendon (*arrow*). ([A] *From* Petchprapa CN, Beltran LS, Recht MP, et al. The rotator interval: a review of anatomy, function, and normal and abnormal MRI appearance. Am J Roentgenol 2010;195(3):570; with permission.)

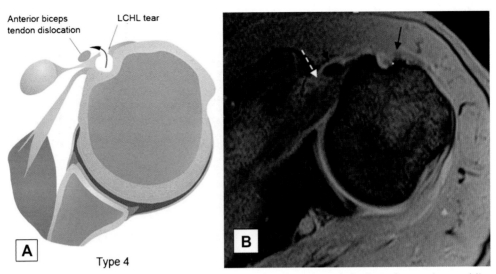

Fig. 9. Bennet type 4. (*A*): Schematic type 4 Bennet lesion with tearing of the lateral coracohumeral ligament (LCHL) and anterior extra-articular dislocation of the biceps tendon. (*B*) Axial gradient echo image with a tear of the LCHL (*arrow*), which normally should be visualized attaching to the greater tuberosity, and extra-articular dislocation of the biceps tendon (*short arrow*), which is located anterior to the subscapularis tendon (*white dotted arrow*). ([A] *From* Petchprapa CN, Beltran LS, Recht MP, et al. The rotator interval: a review of anatomy, function, and normal and abnormal MRI appearance. Am J Roentgenol 2010;195(3):570; with permission.)

articular surface tears of the supraspinatus and subscapularis tendons and medial dislocation of the biceps tendon, which is located anterior to the lesser tuberosity.

ANTERIOR IMPINGEMENT

Anterior impingement occurs when there is contact between the rotator cuff, which has a partial under-surface tear, and the superior labrum just anterior to the biceps anchor. It is important to note that contact between the rotator cuff and the superior labrum is normal when the shoulder is in forward flexion. This has been demonstrated in cadaveric studies that simulated the Neer[22] and Hawkins[23] tests to demonstrate contact between the articular surface of the rotator cuff and the anterosuperior glenoid rim.[24] However, Struhl demonstrated that when there is a tear of the rotator cuff in this area, the contact becomes abnormal, as there is fragmented tissue that is sheared and compressed between the superior humeral head and the glenoid.[25] Anterior impingement occurs in the general nonathletic population, in contrast to posterosuperior impingement, which occurs in elite athletes. The clinical presentation mimics that of subacromial impingement, which includes pain with forward elevation of the arm and overhead use of the arm as well as tenderness over the anterior rotator cuff area. The patients have no signs of instability.

Struhl described arthroscopic findings of partial-thickness tears of the rotator cuff in all 10 patients with anterior internal impingement.[25] This was demonstrated intraoperatively while performing the Hawkins test, which resulted in contact between an abnormal and fragmented rotator cuff with the anterior superior labrum. On preoperative MRI, only 20% of patients showed a partial-thickness rotator cuff tear. Additional findings at arthroscopy included fraying and detachment of the anterosuperior labrum (SLAP IIA) in 60% of patients, and partial subscapularis tears in 20% of patients.

Since anterior impingement can mimic classic subacromial impingement, and since treatment strategies are significantly different, MRI can play an important role in the correct diagnosis and management of these patients by identifying rotator cuff and associated labral pathology in the characteristic location, and ruling out changes associated with classical subacromial impingement.

ENTRAPMENT OF THE LONG HEAD OF THE BICEPS TENDON

Entrapment of the long head of the biceps tendon (LHBT) within the joint and subsequent pain and locking of the shoulder on elevation of the arm were first described by Boileau and colleagues.[26] They evaluated 21 patients who on physical examination had tenderness elicited in the region

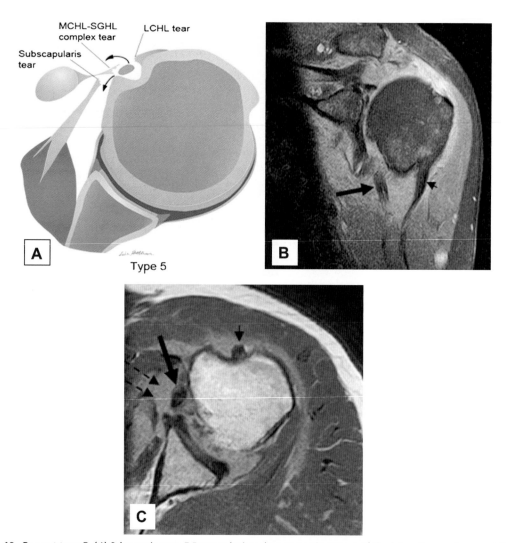

Fig. 10. Bennet type 5. (*A*) Schematic type 5 Bennet lesion demonstrating tears of the lateral coracohumeral liga-ment (LCHL), medial sheath (medial coracohumeral ligament [MCHL] and superior glenohumeral ligament [SGHL] complex) and subscapularis tendon with intra-articular or extra-articular dislocation of the biceps tendon. (*B*) Coronal fat saturated T1W image demonstrating an accessory biceps tendon, which is a rare anatomic variant (*short arrow*) and dislocated biceps tendon (*arrow*). (*C*) Axial T1W image showing the accessory biceps tendon within the bicipital groove (*short arrow*). The dislocated biceps (*arrow*) is seen between fibers of the torn subscapularis (*dotted arrows*). ([A] *From* Petchprapa CN, Beltran LS, Recht MP, et al. The rotator interval: a review of anatomy, function, and normal and abnormal MRI appearance. Am J Roentgenol 2010;195(3):570; with permission.)

overlying the bicipital groove and loss of the final 10° to 20° of passive elevation. On arthrography, they demonstrated the hourglass biceps, which has a characteristic morphology related to hyper-trophy of the intra-articular biceps tendon. During surgery, entrapment of the hypertrophic intra-articular portion of the long head of the biceps tendon was demonstrated in each case with a dynamic intra-operative test (hourglass test) that involved forward elevation of the arm with the elbow extended. They described a characteristic buckling of the tendon,

which was squeezed between the humeral head and the glenoid, resembling an hourglass, as it was squeezed at its middle portion between the humeral head and the glenoid. They attributed the entrap-ment of the tendon to the hypertrophy of the intra-articular portion, which leads to a disproportion between the tendon and the cross-sectional size of the bicipital groove, preventing the tendon from sliding into the groove, leading to its entrapment or mechanical block. In all cases, complete eleva-tion of the arm, which was symmetric to the other

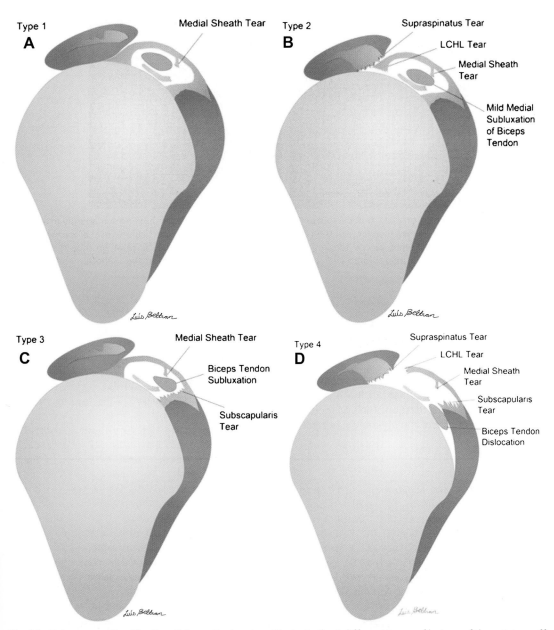

Fig. 11. Habermeyer Classification. Schematic drawings illustrate the 4 different types of lesions of the rotator cuff interval as described by Habermeyer. (*A*) Type 1. Tear of the medial sheath of the coracohumeral ligament without dislocation of the biceps tendon. (*B*) Type 2. Tear of the medial and lateral sheath of the coracohumeral ligament with medial subluxation of the biceps tendon and supraspinatus tendon tear. (*C*) Type 3. Tear of the medial sheath of the coracohumeral ligament with medial subluxation of the biceps tendon and tear of the subscapularis tendon. (*D*) Type 4. Tear of the medial and lateral sheaths of the coracohumeral ligament with tear of the subscapularis and supraspinatus tendons and medial dislocation of the biceps tendon. (*From* Beltran J, Bencardino J, Mellado J, et al. MR arthrography of the shoulder: variations and pitfalls. RadioGraphics 1997;17:1403–12; with permission.)

arm, was restored following resection of the intra-articular portion of the biceps tendon with either biceps tenodesis or tenotomy.

The definitive diagnosis of the hourglass biceps is made primarily by the combination of the appropriate clinical history and surgical findings described. MRI and MR arthrography may suggest the diagnosis with the characteristic hypertrophic morphologic changes of the intra-articular biceps tendon (**Fig. 12**).

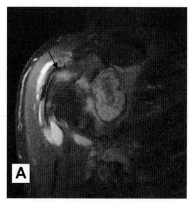 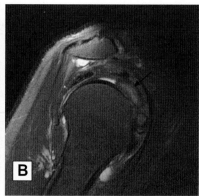

Fig. 12. Hourglass biceps. Coronal (*A*) and sagittal (*B*) fat-saturated T2W images showing a markedly irregularly thickened biceps tendon (*arrow*), which has the resemblance of an hourglass, particularly in the coronal image (*A*). Such a markedly thickened biceps tendon can become entrapped in the bicipital groove, resulting in impingement between the humeral head and glenoid during flexion of the arm at the glenohumeral joint.

SUMMARY

Internal impingement syndromes are relatively frequent in the professional throwing athletic population. Their diagnosis is typically based on combined clinical and arthroscopic evaluation; however MRI and MR arthrography can contribute to the preoperative assessment of these patients by demonstrating a constellation of findings specific for each 1 of the 4 types of impingement syndromes.

REFERENCES

1. Neer CS 2nd. Anterior acromioplasty for the chronic impingement syndrome in the shoulder: a preliminary report. J Bone Joint Surg Am 1972;54(1):41–50.

2. Walch G, Liotard JP, Boileau P, et al. Postero-superior glenoid impingement. Another impingement of the shoulder. J Radiol 1993;74(1):47–50.

3. Giaroli EL, Major NM, Higgins LD. MRI of internal impingement of the shoulder. AJR Am J Roentgenol 2005;185(4):925–9.

4. Jobe CM. Posterior superior glenoid impingement: expanded spectrum. Arthroscopy 1995;11(5):530–6.

5. Jobe FW, Giangarra CE, Kvitne RS, et al. Anterior capsulolabral reconstruction of the shoulder in athletes in overhand sports. Am J Sports Med 1991;19(5):428–34.

6. Halbrecht JL, Tirman P, Atkin D. Internal impingement of the shoulder: comparison of findings between the throwing and nonthrowing shoulders of college baseball players. Arthroscopy 1999;15(3):253–8.

7. Burkhart SS, Morgan CD, Kibler WB. The disabled throwing shoulder: spectrum of pathology part I: path-oanatomy and biomechanics. Arthroscopy 2003; 19(4):404–20.

8. Burkhart SS, Morgan CD. The peel-back mechanism: its role in producing and extending posterior

type II SLAP lesions and its effect on SLAP repair rehabilitation. Arthroscopy 1998;14(6):637–40.

9. Kaplan LD, McMahon PJ, Towers J, et al. Internal impingement: findings on magnetic resonance imaging and arthroscopic evaluation. Arthroscopy 2004;20(7):701–4.

10. Tirman PF, Bost FW, Garvin GJ, et al. Posterosuperior glenoid impingement of the shoulder: findings at MR imaging and MR arthrography with arthroscopic correlation. Radiology 1994;193(2):431–6.

11. Tirman PF, Smith ED, Stoller DW, et al. Shoulder imaging in athletes. Semin Musculoskelet Radiol 2004;8(1):29–40.

12. Tuite MJ. MR imaging of sports injuries to the rotator cuff. Magn Reson Imaging Clin N Am 2003;11(2): 207–19, v.

13. Tuite MJ, Petersen BD, Wise SM, et al. Shoulder MR arthrography of the posterior labrocapsular complex in overhead throwers with pathologic internal impingement and internal rotation deficit. Skeletal Radiol 2007;36(6):495–502.

14. Ouellette H, Labis J, Bredella M, et al. Spectrum of shoulder injuries in the baseball pitcher. Skeletal Radiol 2008;37(6):491–8.

15. Opsha O, Malik A, Baltazar R, et al. MRI of the rotator cuff and internal derangement. Eur J Radiol 2008;68(1):36–56.

16. Gerber C, Sebesta A. Impingement of the deep surface of the subscapularis tendon and the reflection pulley on the anterosuperior glenoid rim: a preliminary report. J Shoulder Elbow Surg 2000;9(6):483–90.

17. Habermeyer P, Magosch P, Pritsch M, et al. Antero-superior impingement of the shoulder as a result of pulley lesions: a prospective arthroscopic study. J Shoulder Elbow Surg 2004;13(1):5–12.

18. Le Huec JC, Schaeverbeke T, Moinard M, et al. Traumatic tear of the rotator interval. J Shoulder Elbow Surg 1996;5(1):41–6.

19. Bennett WF. Subscapularis, medial, and lateral head coracohumeral ligament insertion anatomy. Arthroscopic appearance and incidence of "hidden" rotator interval lesions. Arthroscopy 2001;17(2):173–80.

20. Bennett WF. Correlation of the SLAP lesion with lesions of the medial sheath of the biceps tendon and intra-articular subscapularis tendon. Indian J Orthop 2009;43(4):342–6.

21. Namdari S, Henn RF 3rd, Green A. Traumatic anterosuperior rotator cuff tears: the outcome of open surgical repair. J Bone Joint Surg Am 2008;90(9):1906–13.

22. Neer CS 2nd, Welsh RP. The shoulder in sports. Orthop Clin North Am 1977;8(3):583–91.

23. Hawkins RJ, Hobeika PE. Impingement syndrome in the athletic shoulder. Clin Sports Med 1983;2(2): 391–405.

24. Valadie AL 3rd, Jobe CM, Pink MM, et al. Anatomy of provocative tests for impingement syndrome of the shoulder. J Shoulder Elbow Surg 2000;9(1): 36–46.

25. Struhl S. Anterior internal impingement: an arthroscopic observation. Arthroscopy 2002;18(1):2–7.

26. Boileau P, Ahrens PM, Hatzidakis AM. Entrapment of the long head of the biceps tendon: the hourglass biceps–a cause of pain and locking of the shoulder. J Shoulder Elbow Surg 2004;13(3):249–57.

Anatomic Variants and Pitfalls of the Labrum, Glenoid Cartilage, and Glenohumeral Ligaments

Kevin S. Dunham, MD[a], Jenny T. Bencardino, MD[b],*, Andrew S. Rokito, MD[c]

KEYWORDS

- Shoulder • Variants • Labrum • Glenoid cartilage
- Glenohumeral ligaments

Magnetic resonance (MR) imaging is the primary diagnostic imaging modality for the evaluation of patients with suspected internal derangement of the shoulder joint. Awareness and understanding of the complex anatomy of the shoulder articulation and the ability to recognize normal anatomic variants and potential imaging pitfalls are critical to accurate interpretation of conventional and arthrographic MR imaging studies.[1,2] This review discusses the normal anatomy and anatomic variants of the glenoid labrum, articular cartilage, and glenohumeral ligaments (GHLs). An improved understanding of normal anatomy, biomechanics, and variants helps to avoid potential pitfalls in the interpretation of noncontrast and arthrographic shoulder MR examinations.

LABRUM
Function/Biomechanics

The glenoid labrum acts as a passive stabilizer to the glenohumeral articulation by adding depth to the shallow glenoid fossa.[3] It also serves as a primary attachment site for the GHLs, joint capsule, and long head of the biceps tendon. The labrum demonstrates considerable anatomic variability in its appearance, which may pose a diagnostic challenge to image interpretation.

The labral outline is ovoid in configuration, conforming to the underlying glenoid rim, and is most firmly attached to the glenoid posteriorly and inferiorly.[4] Previous reports have shown the labrum to be predominantly composed of fibrous tissue with some fibrocartilaginous components at the chondrolabral junction.[5,6] At the central interface of the glenoid labrum and the glenoid cartilage, 2 specific types of chondrolabral junctions have been described. There may be an abrupt transition with the labrum demonstrating a free edge margin (type A) or there may be a transition zone where the fibrous labrum blends with the glenoid hyaline cartilage (type B attachment) (**Fig. 1**). Initially the labrum was considered to normally be of low signal intensity on all MR pulse sequences; however, more recent studies have identified areas of increased linear or globular signal intensity in nearly a third of arthroscopically normal labral tissue.[7] In type B attachments, intermediate signal

The authors have nothing to disclose.

[a] Department of Radiology, New York University Langone Medical Center, 560 First Avenue, New York, NY 10016, USA

[b] Department of Radiology, NYU Radiology Associates, New York University Langone Medical Center, 560 First Avenue, New York, NY 10016, USA

[c] Division of Shoulder and Elbow Surgery, Department of Orthopaedic Surgery and Hospital for Joint Diseases, New York University Medical Center, 301 East 17th Street, New York, NY 10003, USA

* Corresponding author.
E-mail address: Jenny.Bencardino@nyumc.org

Magn Reson Imaging Clin N Am 20 (2012) 213–228
doi:10.1016/j.mric.2012.01.014

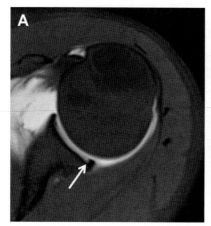
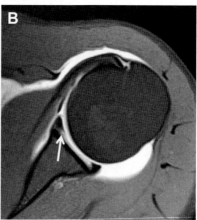

Fig. 1. Type A and B labrum. Axial fat-suppressed T1-weighted (repetition time/echo time, 514/8.6) MR arthrographic images demonstrate type A versus type B labrum. (*A*) Type A labrum characterized by abrupt chondrolabral transition and sharp marginated labral free edge is shown (*arrow*). (*B*) Ill-defined heterogeneous signal at the chondrolabral interface attributed to undercutting of the labral fibrocartilage by glenoid hyaline cartilage typical of a type B labrum is demonstrated (*arrow*).

intensity may be noted at the chondrolabral junction corresponding to the transitional zone of fibrocartilage, which should not be misinterpreted as a labral tear.[8]

Typically considered to be triangular or rounded in cross section, a range of glenoid labral morphologies has been described. Park and colleagues[9] evaluated labral shape on 108 arthrograms of asymptomatic volunteers and found a triangular shape to be most common (anterior, 64%; posterior, 47%) followed by rounded (17%, 33%). Flat, cleaved, notched, or absent labrum was also seen. The labrum typically measures approximately 4 mm in width and 3 mm in thickness; however, broad variation in labral size from 2 to 14 mm between normal individuals exist, thus rendering size criteria of little diagnostic utility.[7]

Superior Labrum

The labrum demonstrates its greatest variation in morphology and attachment above the equator. At the superior labrum, fibers from the proximal origin of the long head of the biceps tendon blend with the labrum forming the biceps labral complex (BLC). Three distinct types of complexes have been described (**Fig. 2**).[4] In a type I BLC, the labrum is firmly attached to the glenoid rim, with no intervening cartilage or central free edge. In a type II BLC, the attachment of the glenoid labrum and biceps tendon to the glenoid occurs more medially and there is continuation of the hyaline cartilage under the labrum accompanied by a small synovial-lined sulcus between the labral free edge and cartilage. In a type III BLC, a prominent triangular meniscoid labrum projects into the joint space and results in a deep recess that may be continuous with a sublabral foramen (**Fig. 3**).

The sublabral sulcus or recess present in type II and III BLCs represents the most frequent normal anatomic variant of the superior labrum. A cadaveric study by Smith and colleagues[10] demonstrated a recess deeper than 2 mm to be present in 39% of specimens. The recess can be identified on routine MR imaging and is enhanced by the presence of a joint effusion or an intra-articular contrast solution.[10] Mischaracterization of this finding as a superior labral anterior-posterior (SLAP) II tear is a potential diagnostic pitfall.[11] Tuite and Orwin[12] described 3 key features of the superior recess to help differentiate it from an SLAP tear: (1) location: a sulcus typically extends only to the most posterior insertion point of the biceps tendon attachment to the labrum and glenoid[13]; (2) contour: a sulcus should demonstrate smooth margins, any irregularity in the contour should be considered suspicious for SLAP tear; and (3) orientation: the direction of increased signal intensity/fluid should extend medially, paralleling the underlying glenoid cartilage; any extension laterally into the substance of the labrum should be considered pathologic. A shallow contrast-filled cleft can sometimes be depicted between the labrum and the biceps, the so-called bicipital labral sulcus (**Fig. 4**).[14]

A second normal anatomic variant of the superior labrum is the sublabral foramen that may be seen in association with a sublabral sulcus or in isolation. Present in 11% of normal patients,[15] the foramen represents a focal developmental

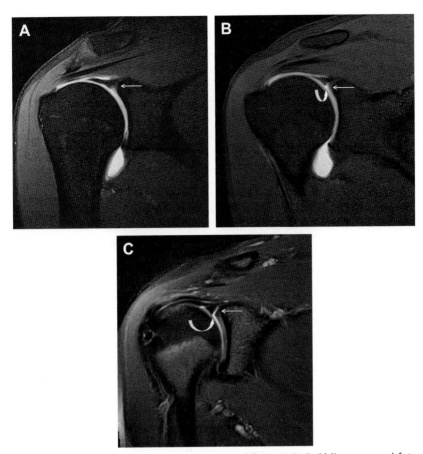

Fig. 2. BLC. Three distinct types of BLC have been described. (*A*) Type I BLC. Oblique coronal fat-suppressed T1-weighted (repetition time/echo time [TR/TE], 446/8.6) MR arthrographic image demonstrates a smooth, firm attachment of the labrum to the superior glenoid (*arrow*) with no intervening sulcus. (*B*) Type II BLC. Oblique coronal fat-suppressed T1-weighted (TR/TE, 446/8.6) MR arthrographic image demonstrates continuation of the hyaline cartilage under the labrum (*arrow*) accompanied by a contrast-filled sulcus between the labral free edge and cartilage (*curved arrow*). (*C*) Type III BLC. Oblique coronal fat-suppressed T2-weighted (TR/TE, 3410/72) image shows a prominent triangular meniscoid labrum outlined by fluid because of a deep sublabral sulcus (*curved arrow*) that parallels the underlying glenoid cartilage (*arrow*) extending through the superior labral base.

detachment of the anterosuperior labrum, which may be confused with an anterior labral tear if care is not taken to note features of this anatomic variant (**Fig. 5**). Again, location is a key factor because the normal foramen is identified along the anterosuperior quadrant between the 1-o'clock to 3-o'clock position. The sublabral foramen can vary in extent from a focal detachment to involvement of the entire anterosuperior quadrant. Initial descriptions of the location of the foramen stated that it should not extend below the level of the midglenoid notch that is present at the physeal line or junction of the superior and middle thirds of the glenoid; however, Tuite and colleagues[16] noted that in some patients a sublabral foramen may extend below the midglenoid notch. Smooth margins of the foramen, no significant displacement (<1–2 mm) of the detached

labrum, and lack of associated traumatic injuries in the adjacent capsuloligamentous structures are additional helpful parameters to distinguish this variant from a labral tear. The sublabral foramen provides a communicating pathway between the glenohumeral joint and the subscapularis recess (**Fig. 6**). Loose bodies may extrude through a sublabral foramen and collect in the subscapularis recess.[17] Constricted joint fluid access to the subscapularis recess through the sublabral foramen should not be misconstrued as a type II SLAP tear with associated paralabral cyst. High origin of the middle and inferior GHLs (MGHL and IGHL) with narrowing of Weitbrecht foramen may promote extension of fluid and/or debris through the sublabral foramen as an alternative path to the subscapularis recess.[18] The presence of high origin of the anterior band of the IGHL

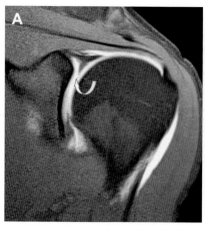
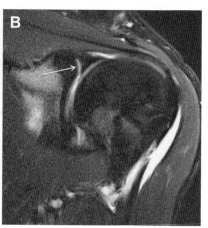

Fig. 3. Sublabral sulcus and meniscoid superior labrum: pseudo-SLAP. (*A*) Meniscoid attachment of the superior labrum is demonstrated on this oblique coronal fat-suppressed T1-weighted (repetition time/echo time [TR/TE], 698/8.6) MR arthrogram. Note a linear focus of contrast extending into the sublabral sulcus (*curved arrow*). (*B*) Corresponding oblique coronal fat-suppressed T2-weighted (TR/TE, 5880/79) image shows hyaline cartilage paralleling the glenoid margin manifested by linear intermediate signal intensity (*arrow*). The diagnosis of a sulcus is supported by the lack of lateral extension of contrast into the substance of the labrum, irregular labral margins, or extension of signal/contrast posterior to the biceps anchor.

was recently reported as a potential imitator of sublabral foramen.[19]

The anterosuperior labrum may also be diminutive or absent. The combination of an absent anterosuperior labrum and a thickened cordlike MGHL is termed the Buford complex; this is a relatively

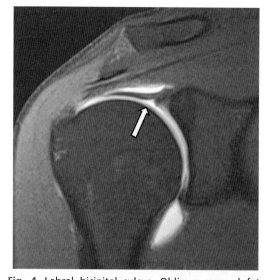

Fig. 4. Labral bicipital sulcus. Oblique coronal fat-suppressed T1-weighted (repetition time/echo time, 446/8.6) MR arthrogram demonstrates a labral bicipital sulcus manifested by a shallow cleft with smooth margins located between the undersurface of the proximal intra-articular biceps tendon and the superior labrum (*arrow*).

uncommon normal variant, occurring in approximately 1.5% of patients (**Fig. 7**).[20,21] This variant is important to recognize because it may also be misinterpreted as a labral tear or a displaced long head of the biceps tendon. Care should be taken to follow the cordlike structure on consecutive axial images cross-referencing them in the sagittal plane.

MR Imaging Technique

The labrum is routinely evaluated in all 3 planes on MR imaging, with the axial plane providing the most diagnostic information and the coronal plane serving an adjunctive role for evaluation of the superior labrum and inferior glenohumeral capsulolabral complex. Several reports have detailed the importance of proper shoulder positioning to optimize evaluation of its complex anatomy and specifically to aid in detection of subtle abnormalities of the glenoid labrum and GHLs. The shoulder is routinely imaged in neutral or slight external rotation. The degree of rotation can be assessed by noting the position of the bicipital grove on axial images. Significant internal rotation should be avoided for conventional MR imaging of the shoulder because it results in medial displacement of the joint capsule and contraction of the subscapularis tendon, both of which may obscure the subjacent anteroinferior labrum. MR imaging of the shoulder with the arm in alternate positions has been advocated to better assess the integrity of specific labroligamentous structures.

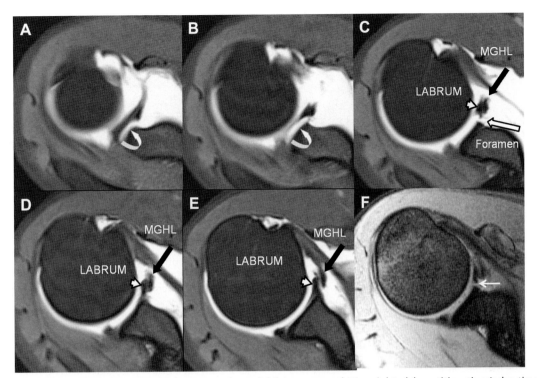

Fig. 5. Sublabral sulcus and foramen. Consecutive axial fat-suppressed T1-weighted (repetition time/echo time [TR/TE], 617/8.6) MR arthrographic images demonstrate the coexistence of a sublabral sulcus and sublabral foramen in a 21-year-old woman. (*A, B*) Note contrast located deep to a smooth superior labrum denoting the sublabral sulcus (*curved arrow*). (*C*) Continuing inferiorly, there is focal detachment of the anterosuperior labrum consistent with sublabral foramen (*open arrow*) with communicating neck of contrast extending from the glenohumeral joint to the subscapularis recess. Note the normal-appearing anterior labrum (*arrowhead*) and MGHL (*black arrow*) (*C–E*). (*F*) Conventional axial gradient echo (TR/TE, 610/15) image of the same patient at a comparable level to image C demonstrates the nonarthrographic appearance to the sublabral foramen (*arrow*) characterized by a smoothly marginated, nondisplaced anterosuperior labrum.

Abduction and External Rotation

Tirman and colleagues[22] originally described the use of abduction and external rotation (ABER) positioning for evaluation of the rotator cuff. Other investigators have since noted improved detection of anteroinferior labral pathology with the ABER technique.[23,24] Imaging is performed using a flexible coil, with the arm above the head, the elbow flexed, and palm facing upward, thus placing tension on the anteroinferior capsulolabral complex and potentially revealing otherwise-occult pathology of the labrum or IGHL (**Fig. 8**). Kwak and colleagues[24] described the ABER position as optimal for evaluation of the IGHL and advocated it as an adjunct to routine imaging examination. In a recent publication, Schreinemachers and colleagues[25] retrospectively compared the sensitivity and specificity of conventional arthrograms with single arthrographic series in ABER position. After reviewing 250 arthrograms with arthroscopic correlation in 92 patients, the investigators found no significant difference in detection of anteroinferior labroligamentous injury. The investigators concluded that limited study with images acquired only in the ABER position could replace the more time-consuming complete examination if there was only a clinical concern for anteroinferior labroligamentous pathology. In another recent investigation, Takubo and colleagues[26] evaluated the nonarthrographic MR imaging technique in ABER position and found comparable sensitivity and specificity to arthroscopy for the identification of a biomechanically intact IGHL. A recognized downside to this and other adjunctive positions is prolonged examination time. In addition, some patients experience discomfort and/or a sensation of instability, particularly with the ABER position, and may not be able to tolerate this portion of the examination.

Flexion, Adduction, and Internal Rotation

Imaging of the shoulder in flexion, adduction, and internal rotation (FADIR) has been advocated to

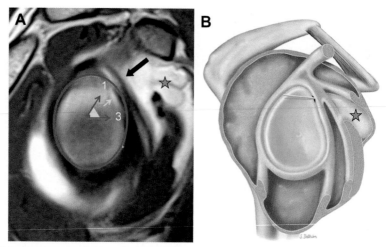

Fig. 6. Sublabral foramen anatomy. (*A*) Oblique sagittal T1-weighted (repetition time/echo time, 512/9.4) MR arthrographic image from same patient in **Fig. 5** demonstrates typical location of the sublabral foramen (*yellow arrow*) between the 1-o'clock and 3-o'clock positions of the anterosuperior labral quadrant, at the site of attachment of the MGHL (*black arrow*), subscapularis recess (*blue star*). (*B*) Anatomic illustration shows the sublabral foramen as a communicating pathway from the glenohumeral joint into the subscapularis recess (*blue star*). (*Courtesy of* Salvador Beltran, MD.)

better evaluate the posterior capsulolabral complex. The FADIR position is achieved by placing the patient's arm across the chest with the hand on the contralateral shoulder. Chiavaras and colleagues[27] evaluated the impact of FADIR position in the detection of posterior labral tears in a recent small preliminary retrospective review and found it to be a useful adjunct to conventional imaging (**Fig. 9**).

Adduction and Internal Rotation

Nonarthrographic MR imaging with the arm in internal rotation may cause redundancy of the anteroinferior capsular structures and obscuration of the underlying labrum, potentially leading to false-negative interpretations.[28] With the administration of intra-articular contrast and distension of the joint, capsular apposition becomes less problematic. Song and colleagues[29] introduced the adduction and internal rotation (ADIR) position at MR arthrography and evaluated its diagnostic performance compared with ABER and neutral position in the assessment of anterior inferior labral lesions. In their retrospective review of patients found to have anteroinferior labroligamentous injury at arthroscopy, the investigators reported that ADIR was superior to ABER and neutral position in the discrimination between subtypes of Bankart injuries.

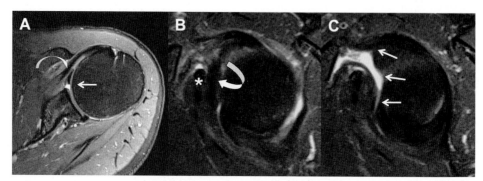

Fig. 7. Buford complex. (*A*) Axial fat-suppressed proton density (repetition time/echo time [TR/TE], 3030/33) image demonstrates cordlike thickening of the MGHL (*curved arrow*) and absence of the anterosuperior labrum (*arrow*) compatible with a Buford complex. (*B, C*) Consecutive oblique sagittal fat-suppressed T2-weighted (TR/TE, 5000/62) images confirm the findings of cordlike thickening of the MGHL (*curved arrow*) coursing deep to the subscapularis tendon (*asterisk*) associated with an absent anterosuperior labrum (*arrows*).

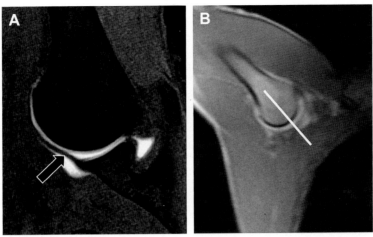

Fig. 8. IGHL in ABER position. (*A*) Oblique axial T1-weighted (repetition time/echo time, 583/8.6) fat-suppressed MR arthrogram with the arm in ABER position demonstrates an intact anterior band of the IGHL under tension (*arrow*). (*B*) Localizer image obtained specifically for the ABER series acquisition with overlying scout line demarcates plane of section in (*A*).

CARTILAGE
Anatomy and Histology

The articular surfaces of the glenoid fossa and the humeral head are lined by hyaline cartilage.

Articular congruity of the glenohumeral joint is improved by normal alterations in the cartilage thickness. There is relative thinning of the articular cartilage of the glenoid centrally and thickening along the periphery. In contradistinction, the

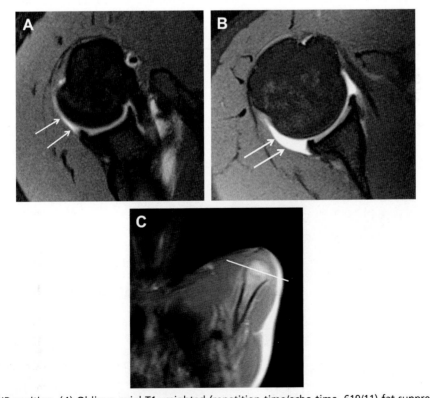

Fig. 9. FADIR position. (*A*) Oblique axial T1-weighted (repetition time/echo time, 619/11) fat-suppressed MR arthrogram with the arm in FADIR position demonstrates increased tension placed on an intact posterior capsulolabral complex (*arrows*) relative to neutral rotation (*B*). (*C*) Localizer image obtained specifically for the FADIR series acquisition with overlying scout line demarcates plane of section in (*A*).

articular cartilage of the humeral head is thicker centrally and thinner near its margins.

A focal well-demarcated articular cartilage defect at the central aspect of the glenoid termed the bare spot has been reported in the surgical and radiologic literature (**Fig. 10**). Burkhart and colleagues[30] reported its consistent location at the central aspect of the inferior glenoid and noted that it provided a useful landmark at arthroscopy to quantify the degree of glenoid bone loss. However, in a subsequent study by Kralinger and colleagues[31] in which 3-dimensional computed tomography of cadaveric specimens was performed, the investigators discovered variation in the location of the bare spot. Evaluation in the pediatric population using MR imaging has also shown some slight but significant variability in the location of the bare spot. Kim and colleagues[32] also noted a considerable lower incidence in the pediatric population supporting the hypothesis that this may be an acquired finding.

Focal thickening of the subchondral bone along the central aspect of the glenoid fossa is an additional normal variant termed the Ossaki tubercle. This is typically accompanied by thinning of the overlying cartilage. These variants should not be mischaracterized as osteochondral injuries. The absence of subchondral bone marrow signal abnormality and lack of intra-articular loose bodies are pertinent negative findings.

A bare area of the humeral head devoid of articular cartilage or sulcus has also been described.

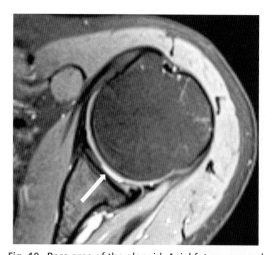

Fig. 10. Bare area of the glenoid. Axial fat-suppressed proton density (repetition time/echo time, 2700/33) image through the midglenoid demonstrates a focal well-demarcated articular cartilage defect (*arrow*) located at the central aspect of the glenoid compatible with bare area. Debate remains whether this represents a normal variant or an acquired lesion.

Located posteriorly between the posterior insertion of the joint capsule and synovial membrane and the adjacent articular cartilage, this bare area may be confused with a Hill-Sachs impaction injury (**Fig. 11**). An additional bare area has been described between the supraspinatus insertion on the greater tuberosity and the adjacent articular cartilage. This bare area is used by surgeons to quantify partial-thickness articular surface tears. Failure to recognize and account for the bare area at imaging may lead to erroneous diagnosis or overestimation of partial thickness supraspinatus tendon tears. In contradistinction, widening of the bare area may be due to loss of the articular cartilage and/or undersurface supraspinatus tear.[33]

Assessment of glenohumeral articular cartilage abnormalities using routing MR imaging and MR arthrography has yielded only moderate diagnostic accuracy, in part because of the curved morphology and relative thinness of the glenohumeral articular cartilage.[34] Improvements in accuracy in identifying cartilage injury and loss have been made by application of advanced cartilage imaging techniques. Dietrich and colleagues[35] retrospectively reviewed performance of 3-dimensional water-excitation true fast imaging with steady-state precession sequence in 75 shoulder MR arthrograms with arthroscopic correlation and found good diagnostic performance. However, this technique was not compared directly with conventional imaging sequences, so it remains unclear if there is a diagnostic advantage. T2 mapping and delayed gadolinium-enhanced MR imaging of cartilage have been recently used to image the glenohumeral joint. These advanced imaging techniques may provide a mechanism to detect degenerative changes of glenohumeral articular cartilage before they are evident on anatomic imaging and theoretically at a stage where they may be reversible.[36,37]

LIGAMENTS

The large size discrepancy between the small glenoid and the large humeral head affords the shoulder joint the largest range of motion in the human body.[3] However, it also renders the joint inherently unstable and susceptible to dislocation and subluxation. Active and passive stabilizers serve to maintain stability of the shoulder.

The GHLs serve as important static stabilizers of the shoulder joint over a wide range of positions. Formed by localized thickenings of the glenohumeral joint capsule, the ligaments extend from the anterior and inferior margins of the capsule to the anatomic neck of the humerus. Three main

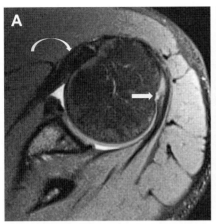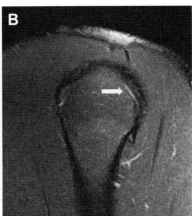

Fig. 11. Bare area of the humerus. (*A*) Axial proton density (repetition time/echo time [TR/TE], 3030/33) fat-suppressed image through the proximal humerus at the level of the subscapularis tendon (*curved arrow*) shows normal bare area of the humerus (*arrow*) close to the posterior capsular insertion and synovial membrane. This finding should not be mistaken for a Hill-Sachs impaction lesion, which would be located more superiorly at and above the level of the coracoid process. (*B*) The bare area (*arrow*) can also be appreciated in the oblique sagittal plane as demonstrated on this T2-weighted (TR/TE, 5000/62) image in the same patient.

ligaments have been described: superior GHL (SGHL), MGHL, and IGHL complex, the IGHL complex formed by anterior and posterior bands and intervening axillary recess.

The capsular mechanism provides the most important contribution to the stability of the glenohumeral joint. The anterior stabilizing structures include the fibrous capsule, GHLs, synovial membrane and recesses, fibrous glenoid labrum, subscapularis muscle and tendon, and scapular periosteum. Three types of anterior capsular insertions have been described according to the proximity of the insertion to the glenoid margin. In a type I configuration, the capsule inserts at the glenoid margin; type II inserts at the glenoid neck; and type III inserts more medially along the scapula. A direct relationship between the degree of medial insertion and glenoid instability has been suggested, with type III capsular insertions being associated more frequently with unstable shoulders.[2] However, care should be taken when evaluating MR arthrograms to not misinterpret overdistention of the joint capsule as a type III capsular insertion.

The posterior stabilizing structures include the posterior capsule, synovial membrane, glenoid labrum and periosteum, and posterior superior tendinous cuff and associated muscles (supraspinatus, infraspinatus, and teres minor). The long head of the biceps tendon and triceps tendon provide additional stability to the glenohumeral articulation as they course about the anterosuperior and inferior aspect of the capsule, respectively.

Several studies have examined the relative contribution of each GHL to stability depending on the position of the arm. Matsen and colleagues[38] and Caspari and Geissler[39] reported the absence of the SGHL and MGHL in a relative high percentage of individuals as an argument against the importance of these structures in maintaining joint stability. By selectively releasing these structures in cadaveric specimens, Turkel and colleagues[40] studied the individual contribution of each GHL at various degrees of abduction and rotation. The investigators concluded that the IGHL is critical in preventing anterior dislocation over a range of positions, especially with the arm abducted at 90°.[40] The validity of these results has been called into question, however, by other researchers who argue that the capsular structures work as a unit, and disrupting even a single component to assess its role in isolation disrupts the synergistic effect of the structures and the unit as a whole.[41]

Others have sought a different approach to study the GHLs. O'Connell and colleagues[41] measured tension of the GHLs in cadavers after application of controlled external torque and concluded that at 90° abduction, the IGHL and MGHL developed the most strain. At 45° abduction, the most strain was also developed by the IGHL and MGHL, but the SGHL was also somewhat tensed. At 0° of arm abduction, the SGHL was found to play a role limiting inferior translation of the humeral head with respect to the glenoid.

There also remains debate in the surgical literature regarding arthroscopic evaluation of the

GHLs. The question posed is whether the capsular structures identified at arthroscopy represent the classically described ligaments versus mere infolding of the joint capsule. In a combined cadaveric live subject study, Pouliart and Gagey[42] systematically examined a total of 300 shoulders for which arthroscopy, open dissection, or both were performed. The investigators reported that in neutral position or low degrees of abduction, the classically described capsular infoldings were identifiable in nearly all cases; however, with higher degrees of ABER, the capsule appeared smooth without distinct ligamentous structures. The investigators concluded that given the positional dependence, the infoldings seen at arthroscopy may not represent the true glenohumeral capsular ligaments.

Moore and colleagues[43] investigated the strain distribution of the IGHL at varying degrees of ABER using strain grid markers in cadaveric specimens. Although these investigators found that the strain on the anterior IGHL increased with external rotation, their results suggest that the capsule acts more as a complex fibrous sheet in a synergistic manner rather than as discrete components.[44]

SGHL

The SGHL extends from the superior glenoid margin and base of the coracoid, just anterior to the biceps tendon and courses inferolaterally to the anterior humerus just superior to the lesser tuberosity at the anatomic neck. The SGHL is nearly invariably present, identified at arthroscopy in 97% of patients[3] and in an arthrographic series by Palmer and colleagues[45] in 98% of patients. On MR imaging, the SGHL can be well visualized on axial planes as a low–signal intensity structure arising from the superior glenoid tubercle and paralleling the coracoid process. Oblique sagittal projection is also useful for demonstrating the normal course of the SGHL just inferior to the coracohumeral ligament and coracoid process.[46]

Variants

Variant origins of the SGHL reported in the radiologic literature include a common origin with the MGHL and/or direct origin from the biceps tendon.[14] Pradhan and colleagues[47] issued a case report of a rare variant in which the SGHL arises from the posterior labrum and overrides the biceps tendon origin without attaching to the anterior labrum or MGHL. The SGHL is normally thin but can become thickened in patients with an underdeveloped or absent MGHL.

MGHL

Of all the GHLs, the MGHL demonstrates the most variability.[3] The ligament may be absent in up to 30% of patients.[48] Initial arthroscopic studies of MGHL anatomy described an origin from the anterior margin of the scapula, just medial to the articular surface. The ligament then courses in an oblique inferolateral direction along the posterior margin of the subscapularis tendon and inserts on the neck of the humerus. In some patients, the ligament may blend with the joint capsule before inserting on the humerus just below the insertion of the SGHL. On MR arthrography, a distinct origin of the MGHL from the anterosuperior labrum has been described.[14] This origin is well demonstrated on axial MR arthrographic images in which the MGHL appears as a hypointense structure separated from the labrum by a small cleft. As the MGHL courses along the labrum, it may be mistaken for an anterior labral tear if care is not taken to follow the structure on continuous axial slices.[14] On more inferior axial images, the MGHL may appear as a rounded or flat hypointense structure that blends with the capsule or may be separate from the capsule. The inferolateral oblique course of the ligament across the anterior capsular space as well as its labral origin and distal capsular merging points are well demonstrated on oblique sagittal MR arthrographic images. Oblique coronal images are less helpful, and the MGHL is not routinely visualized in this plane unless thickened and redundant.[2]

The position and appearance of MGHL on MR imaging is greatly affected by patient positioning. With the arm in internal rotation, the ligament may appear redundant along the anterior margin of the scapular neck and simulate a loose body or capsular stripping (**Fig. 12**). With the arm imaged in external rotation, the MGHL is under tension and more likely to blend with the anterior joint capsule.[24]

Variants

The MGHL demonstrates the largest multiplicity of normal variants. Awareness of the normal anatomic variants is critical to preventing diagnostic errors. The MGHL may be absent in a significant proportion of patients. In anatomic studies by Moseley and Overgaard,[49] the MGHL was absent in up to 30% of specimens. Subsequent arthroscopic series by Wall and O'Brien[50] confirmed this finding. The MGHL was not visualized in 12% to 21% of patients on MR arthrography.[9,14,45] Absence or attenuation of the MGHL is often associated with a prominent subscapularis recess.

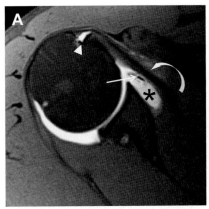

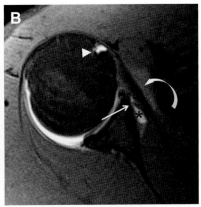

Fig. 12. MGHL deviation between neutral and internal rotation. Axial fat-suppressed T1-weighted (repetition time/echo time, 514/8.6) MR arthrographic images in neutral (*A*) and internal rotation (*B*) in a patient with a history of prior labral repair. Note medial deviation of MGHL (*arrow*) along the articular surface of the subscapularis tendon (*curved arrow*) as well as decreased volume of the subscapularis recess (*asterisk*) in internal rotation. The migrated MGHL may be potentially misinterpreted as a displaced labral fragment or scapular stripping. The position of the intertubercular grove (*arrowhead*) is used to assess rotation.

Variants involving the origin of the MGHL are also frequently identified. The most common of theses variants is a conjoint origin with either the SGHL or IGHL. Variants in which there is a common origin with the SGHL and biceps tendon or conjoined origin with the biceps tendon alone and absent SGHL may also be observed.[2]

The MGHL may be diminutive or thickened, even cordlike. A well-recognized and frequently cited normal variant is the Buford complex, which includes a cordlike thickening of the MGHL and an absent anterosuperior glenoid labrum.[20,21] Present in 1.5% of patients, this variant may be mistaken for detachment of the anterosuperior

labrum on axial images at the level of the superior glenoid.[21] Evaluation of the structure on consecutive axial images helps to demonstrate the superior origin and distal capsular merge and to differentiate it from a labral tear. A thickened cordlike MGHL can also be identified on oblique sagittal images. The MGHL more frequently appears thickened in association with a normal superior labrum or in association with a sublabral foramen.[20] Cases of longitudinal splitting or duplication of the MGHL have been reported (**Fig. 13**). In these cases, oblique sagittal images show a double parallel line along the course of the MGHL, and axial images demonstrate a U-shaped

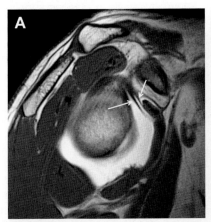

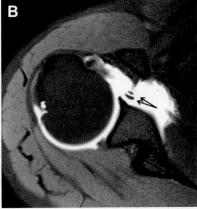

Fig. 13. Duplicated MGHL versus remote longitudinal split tear. (*A*) Oblique sagittal T1-weighted (repetition time/echo time [TR/TE], 491/9.4) MR arthrogram image shows 2 parallel low–signal intensity structures along the course of the MGHL (*arrows*). (*B*) Corresponding axial T1-weighted (TR/TE, 514/8.6) fat-saturated arthrogram in the same patient demonstrates contrast extending between the 2 distinct portions of the MGHL. A duplicated configuration of the ligament in the axial plane has also been described (*arrows*).

structure that may simulate a labral cleft or tear. Debate exists as to whether this represents a normal variant or a partially healed longitudinal split tear of the MGHL.[2]

Previous investigators have noted an association between the presence of a sublabral foramen, Buford complex, and SLAP lesions.[51,52] In the largest series to date, Ilahi and colleagues[53] prospectively analyzed 334 shoulder arthroscopies for association between anatomic variants of the anterosuperior labrum with pathology. These investigators found a significantly higher incidence of SLAP lesions in patients with variants involving partial detachment from the glenoid (sublabral foramen with or without cordlike MGHL and Buford complex), whereas in patients with more standard anatomy or only a thickened MGHL, no such association was found. The investigators hypothesized that the presence of anterosuperior labral variant anatomy may result in higher stresses on the superior BLC, predisposing to injury.

The foramen of Weitbrecht represents a normal communication between the glenohumeral joint capsule and the subscapularis bursae located between the SGHL and MGHL. Another communication, the foramen of Rouvière, exists slightly more inferior and is located between the MGHL and IGHL.[46] When the MGHL is absent, a single large communication between the glenohumeral joint and subscapularis bursa may be present, rendering the latter redundant (**Fig. 14**).[14,54] Conversely, in a recent report, Bencardino and colleagues[18] postulated that a high riding and thickened MGHL may result in constriction of the foramen of Weitbrecht, which in the presence of a sublabral foramen may render the latter as a constricted communicating pathway between the glenohumeral joint and the subscapularis recess, thus promoting the formation of a pseudoparalabral cyst about the anterosuperior quadrant.

IGHL COMPLEX

The IGHL complex is composed of an anterior and posterior band and an intervening portion, the axillary recess.[55] The complex is consistently present.[55] The anterior band arises from the anterior glenoid rim/labrum at approximately the level of the midglenoid notch, between the 2-o'clock to 4-o'clock positions, which is more cranial than the origin of the posterior band, arising at the 7-o'clock to 9-o'clock position. The posterior band also inserts more medially than the anterior band and may be identified inserting along the glenoid neck. Distally, the IGHL inserts at the surgical neck of the humerus. Two distinct patterns of humeral insertion have been described: (1) a collarlike attachment in which the entire IGHL inserts slightly inferior to the articular edge of the humeral head and (2) a V-shaped attachment in which the anterior and posterior bands of the IGHL attach adjacent to the articular edge of the humeral head, and the axillary pouch attaches at the apex of the V distal to the articular edge.[56] As discussed previously, when the arm is imaged in an ABER position, the anterior band of the IGHL becomes taut and is well visualized along its entire course.

Variants

The anterior band of the IGHL is normally thicker than the posterior band; however, the opposite may be seen. Normal slight variability in the insertion of the inferior glenohumeral ligamentous complex on the surgical neck of the humerus frequently results in a jagged appearance on axial

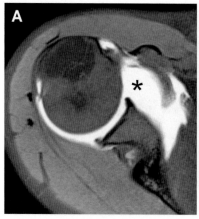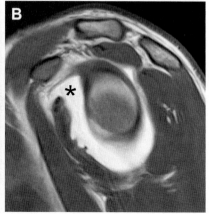

Fig. 14. Absent MGHL with large subscapularis bursa. (*A*) Axial T1-weighted (repetition time/echo time [TR/TE], 514/8.6) fat-saturated and (*B*) oblique sagittal T1-weighted (TR/TE, 420/9.4) MR arthrograms demonstrate a capacious subscapularis recess (*asterisk*) in the setting of an absent MGHL.

MR arthrographic images and should not be misinterpreted as fraying or tearing. Prominent synovial folds at the axillary recess may also be seen and can simulate debris or loose bodies.[14]

In a recent cadaveric study, Ramirez and colleagues[19] described a high origin of the anterior band of the IGHL located above the 3-o'clock position (**Fig. 15**). This high origin occurred in 4 of 10 specimens and could be mistaken for an anterior labral tear on MR arthrography. Tuoheti and colleagues[57] previously described a relationship between the long head of the biceps origin and the level of the anterior band of the IGHL origin from the anterior labrum. A variant origin of the anterior band of the IGHL from the MGHL has been previously described.[14] There have also been reports in the literature of a band of connective tissue attaching the IGHL to the SGHL termed the periarticular fiber system by Huber and Putz,[6] although there is still debate in the literature as to the nature and consistency of this structure.

A less well-known GHL of the superficial anterior capsule is the spiral GHL, named for the spiral course its fibers demonstrate when the arm is abducted and externally rotated. Originally described in classical anatomy as the fasciculus obliquus, it was revisited by Kolts and colleagues[58] in an anatomic series of 12 cadaveric specimens. The investigators reported that the ligament arises from the axillary component of the IGHL and the infraglenoid tubercle and courses laterally to fuse with the MGHL. Superiorly, the ligament blended with the superior portion of the subscapularis, inserting together with its tendon into the lesser tuberosity. In 2 other recent investigations by Merila and colleagues,[59,60] the ligament was demonstrated on MR imaging and gross dissection in 6 specimens and later confirmed to be present in 22 of 22 specimens. The investigators suggest that the spiral ligament may contribute to shoulder stability, particularly in the abducted and externally rotated position, or may affect the function of the MGHL; however, the biomechanical role of this structure is not yet fully understood.

SUMMARY

MR imaging and MR arthrography remain the primary imaging modalities for evaluation of patients with suspected internal derangement of

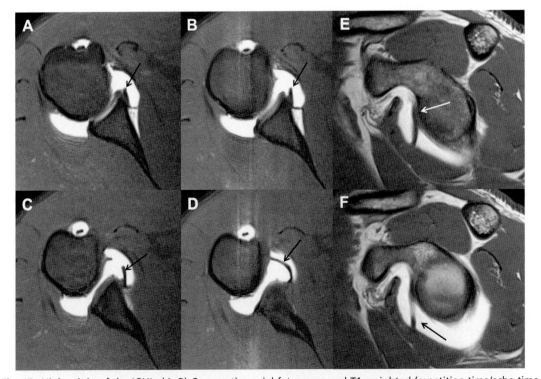

Fig. 15. High origin of the IGHL. (*A–D*) Consecutive axial fat-suppressed T1-weighted (repetition time/echo time [TR/TE], 514/8.6) MR arthrographic images demonstrate a high origin of the anterior band of the IGHL (*arrow*) from the anterior superior quadrant. (*E, F*) Oblique sagittal T1-weighted (TR/TE, 574/9.4) images from the same patient demonstrate the origin of the IGHL above the level of the anterior equator (*arrow* again denotes anterior band GHL). A high origin of the anterior band of the IGHL should not be mistaken for a displaced anterior labral fragment.

the shoulder. Accurate interpretation of these studies requires an understanding of the complex anatomy of the shoulder joint as well as the potential anatomic variants and imaging pitfalls that are routinely encountered. Although many of the variants and pitfalls have been extensively described in the radiologic and surgical literature, this body of knowledge continues to evolve.

REFERENCES

1. Massengill AD, Seeger LL, Yao L, et al. Labrocapsular ligamentous complex of the shoulder: normal anatomy, anatomic variation, and pitfalls of MR imaging and MR arthrography. Radiographics 1994;14(6):1211–23.
2. Beltran J, Bencardino J, Padron M, et al. The middle glenohumeral ligament: normal anatomy, variants and pathology. Skeletal Radiol 2002;31(5):253–62.
3. Rockwood CA, Matsen FA. The shoulder. Philadelphia: Saunders; 1990.
4. Stoller DW. Magnetic resonance imaging in orthopaedics and sports medicine. 3rd edition. Philadelphia: Lippincott Williams & Wilkins; 2007.
5. Nishida K, Hashizume H, Toda K, et al. Histologic and scanning electron microscopic study of the glenoid labrum. J Shoulder Elbow Surg 1996;5(2 Pt 1): 132–8.
6. Huber WP, Putz RV. Periarticular fiber system of the shoulder joint. Arthroscopy 1997;13(6):680–91.
7. Zanetti M, Carstensen T, Weishaupt D, et al. MR arthrographic variability of the arthroscopically normal glenoid labrum: qualitative and quantitative assessment. Eur Radiol 2001;11(4):559–66.
8. Loredo R, Longo C, Salonen D, et al. Glenoid labrum: MR imaging with histologic correlation. Radiology 1995;196(1):33–41.
9. Park YH, Lee JY, Moon SH, et al. MR arthrography of the labral capsular ligamentous complex in the shoulder: imaging variations and pitfalls. AJR Am J Roentgenol 2000;175(3):667–72.
10. Smith DK, Chopp TM, Aufdemorte TB, et al. Sublabral recess of the superior glenoid labrum: study of cadavers with conventional nonenhanced MR imaging, MR arthrography, anatomic dissection, and limited histologic examination. Radiology 1996; 201(1):251–6.
11. De Maeseneer M, Van Roy F, Lenchik L, et al. CT and MR arthrography of the normal and pathologic anterosuperior labrum and labral-bicipital complex. Radiographics 2000;20(Spec No):S67–81.
12. Tuite MJ, Orwin JF. Anterosuperior labral variants of the shoulder: appearance on gradient-recalled-echo and fast spin-echo MR images. Radiology 1996; 199(2):537–40.
13. Cooper DE, Arnoczky SP, O'Brien SJ, et al. Anatomy, histology, and vascularity of the glenoid labrum. An anatomical study. J Bone Joint Surg Am 1992; 74(1):46–52.
14. Beltran J, Bencardino J, Mellado J, et al. MR arthrography of the shoulder: variants and pitfalls. Radiographics 1997;17(6):1403–12 [discussion: 1412–5].
15. Stoller DW. MR arthrography of the glenohumeral joint. Radiol Clin North Am 1997;35(1):97–116.
16. Tuite MJ, Blankenbaker DG, Seifert M, et al. Sublabral foramen and Buford complex: inferior extent of the unattached or absent labrum in 50 patients. Radiology 2002;223(1):137–42.
17. Kaplan K, Sahajpal DT, Jazrawi L. Loose bodies in a sublabral recess: diagnosis and treatment. Bull Hosp Jt Dis 2006;63(3–4):161–5.
18. Bencardino J, Fitzpatrick D, Shepard T, et al. The sublabral foramen as a communicating pathway to the subscapularis recess. Skeletal Radiol 2011;40: 485–515.
19. Ramirez Ruiz FA, Baranski Kaniak BC, Haghighi P, et al. High origin of the anterior band of the inferior glenohumeral ligament: MR arthrography with anatomic and histologic correlation in cadavers. Skeletal Radiol 2011. [Epub ahead of print].
20. Williams MM, Snyder SJ, Buford D Jr. The Buford complex—the "cord-like" middle glenohumeral ligament and absent anterosuperior labrum complex: a normal anatomic capsulolabral variant. Arthroscopy 1994;10(3):241–7.
21. Tirman PF, Feller JF, Palmer WE, et al. The Buford complex—a variation of normal shoulder anatomy: MR arthrographic imaging features. AJR Am J Roentgenol 1996;166(4):869–73.
22. Tirman PF, Bost FW, Steinbach LS, et al. MR arthrographic depiction of tears of the rotator cuff: benefit of abduction and external rotation of the arm. Radiology 1994;192(3):851–6.
23. Cvitanic O, Tirman PF, Feller JF, et al. Using abduction and external rotation of the shoulder to increase the sensitivity of MR arthrography in revealing tears of the anterior glenoid labrum. AJR Am J Roentgenol 1997;169(3):837–44.
24. Kwak SM, Brown RR, Trudell D, et al. Glenohumeral joint: comparison of shoulder positions at MR arthrography. Radiology 1998;208(2):375–80.
25. Schreinemachers SA, van der Hulst VP, Jaap Willems W, et al. Is a single direct MR arthrography series in ABER position as accurate in detecting anteroinferior labroligamentous lesions as conventional MR arthography? Skeletal Radiol 2009;38(7):675–83.
26. Takubo Y, Horii M, Kurokawa M, et al. Magnetic resonance imaging evaluation of the inferior glenohumeral ligament: non-arthrographic imaging in abduction and external rotation. J Shoulder Elbow Surg 2005;14(5):511–5.
27. Chiavaras MM, Harish S, Burr J. MR arthrographic assessment of suspected posteroinferior labral

lesions using flexion, adduction, and internal rotation positioning of the arm: preliminary experience. Skeletal Radiol 2010;39(5):481–8.

28. Carroll KW, Helms CA. Magnetic resonance imaging of the shoulder: a review of potential sources of diagnostic errors. Skeletal Radiol 2002;31(7): 373–83.

29. Song HT, Huh YM, Kim S, et al. Anterior-inferior labral lesions of recurrent shoulder dislocation evaluated by MR arthrography in an adduction internal rotation (ADIR) position. J Magn Reson Imaging 2006;23(1):29–35.

30. Burkhart SS, Debeer JF, Tehrany AM, et al. Quantifying glenoid bone loss arthroscopically in shoulder instability. Arthroscopy 2002;18(5):488–91.

31. Kralinger F, Aigner F, Longato S, et al. Is the bare spot a consistent landmark for shoulder arthroscopy? A study of 20 embalmed glenoids with 3-dimensional computed tomographic reconstruction. Arthroscopy 2006;22(4):428–32.

32. Kim HK, Emery KH, Salisbury SR. Bare spot of the glenoid fossa in children: incidence and MRI features. Pediatr Radiol 2010;40(7):1190–6.

33. Minagawa H, Itoi E, Konno N, et al. Humeral attachment of the supraspinatus and infraspinatus tendons: an anatomic study. Arthroscopy 1998; 14(3):302–6.

34. Graichen H, Jakob J, von Eisenhart-Rothe R, et al. Validation of cartilage volume and thickness measurements in the human shoulder with quantitative magnetic resonance imaging. Osteoarthritis Cartilage 2003;11(7):475–82.

35. Dietrich TJ, Zanetti M, Saupe N, et al. Articular cartilage and labral lesions of the glenohumeral joint: diagnostic performance of 3D water-excitation true FISP MR arthrography. Skeletal Radiol 2010;39(5): 473–80.

36. Wiener E, Hodler J, Pfirrmann CW. Delayed gadolinium-enhanced MRI of cartilage (dGEMRIC) of cadaveric shoulders: comparison of contrast dynamics in hyaline and fibrous cartilage after intra-articular gadolinium injection. Acta Radiol 2009; 50(1):86–92.

37. Maizlin ZV, Clement JJ, Patola WB, et al. T2 mapping of articular cartilage of glenohumeral joint with routine MRI correlation—initial experience. HSS J 2009;5(1):61–6.

38. Matsen FA, Harryman DT, Sidles JA. Mechanics of glenohumeral instability. Clin Sports Med 1991; 10(4):783–8.

39. Caspari RB, Geissler WB. Arthroscopic manifestations of shoulder subluxation and dislocation. Clin Orthop Relat Res 1993;(291):54–66.

40. Turkel SJ, Panio MW, Marshall JL, et al. Stabilizing mechanisms preventing anterior dislocation of the glenohumeral joint. J Bone Joint Surg Am 1981; 63(8):1208–17.

41. O'Connell PW, Nuber GW, Mileski RA, et al. The contribution of the glenohumeral ligaments to anterior stability of the shoulder joint. Am J Sports Med 1990;18(6):579–84.

42. Pouliart N, Gagey OJ. The arthroscopic view of the glenohumeral ligaments compared with anatomy: fold or fact? J Shoulder Elbow Surg 2005;14(3): 324–8.

43. Moore SM, Stehle JH, Rainis EJ, et al. The current anatomical description of the inferior glenohumeral ligament does not correlate with its functional role in positions of external rotation. J Orthop Res 2008;26(12):1598–604.

44. Moore SM, Ellis B, Weiss JA, et al. The glenohumeral capsule should be evaluated as a sheet of fibrous tissue: a validated finite element model. Ann Biomed Eng 2010;38(1):66–76.

45. Palmer WE, Brown JH, Rosenthal DI. Labral-ligamentous complex of the shoulder: evaluation with MR arthrography. Radiology 1994;190(3):645–51.

46. Yeh L, Kwak S, Kim YS, et al. Anterior labroligamentous structures of the glenohumeral joint: correlation of MR arthrography and anatomic dissection in cadavers. AJR Am J Roentgenol 1998;171(5): 1229–36.

47. Pradhan RL, Itoi E, Watanabe W, et al. A rare anatomic variant of the superior glenohumeral ligament. Arthroscopy 2001;17(1):E3.

48. De Palma AF. Surgery of the shoulder. 3rd edition. Philadelphia: Lippincott; 1983.

49. Moseley HF, Övergaard B. The anterior capsular mechanism in recurrent anterior dislocation of the shoulder. J Bone Joint Surg Br 1962;44: 913–27.

50. Wall MS, O'Brien SJ. Arthroscopic evaluation of the unstable shoulder. Clin Sports Med 1995;14(4): 817–39.

51. Ilahi OA, Labbe MR, Cosculluela P. Variants of the anterosuperior glenoid labrum and associated pathology. Arthroscopy 2002;18(8):882–6.

52. Rao AG, Kim TK, Chronopoulos E, et al. Anatomical variants in the anterosuperior aspect of the glenoid labrum: a statistical analysis of seventy-three cases. J Bone Joint Surg Am 2003;85-A(4): 653–9.

53. Ilahi OA, Cosculluela PE, Ho DM. Classification of anterosuperior glenoid labrum variants and their association with shoulder pathology. Orthopedics 2008;31(3):226.

54. Palmer WE, Caslowitz PL, Chew FS. MR arthrography of the shoulder: normal intraarticular structures and common abnormalities. AJR Am J Roentgenol 1995;164(1):141–6.

55. O'Brien SJ, Neves MC, Arnoczky SP, et al. The anatomy and histology of the inferior glenohumeral ligament complex of the shoulder. Am J Sports Med 1990;18(5):449–56.

56. Bui-Mansfield LT, Taylor DC, Uhorchak JM, et al. Humeral avulsions of the glenohumeral ligament: imaging features and a review of the literature. AJR Am J Roentgenol 2002;179(3):649–55.

57. Tuoheti Y, Itoi E, Minagawa H, et al. Attachment types of the long head of the biceps tendon to the glenoid labrum and their relationships with the glenohumeral ligaments. Arthroscopy 2005;21(10): 1242–9.

58. Kolts I, Busch LC, Tomusk H, et al. Anatomical composition of the anterior shoulder joint capsule. A cadaver study on 12 glenohumeral joints. Ann Anat 2001;183(1):53–9.

59. Merila M, Helio H, Busch LC, et al. The spiral glenohumeral ligament: an open and arthroscopic anatomy study. Arthroscopy 2008;24(11): 1271–6.

60. Merila M, Leibecke T, Gehl HB, et al. The anterior glenohumeral joint capsule: macroscopic and MRI anatomy of the fasciculus obliquus or so-called ligamentum glenohumerale spirale. Eur Radiol 2004; 14(8):1421–6.

The Rotator Interval and Long Head Biceps Tendon: Anatomy, Function, Pathology, and Magnetic Resonance Imaging

Yoav Morag, MD[a],*, Asheesh Bedi, MD[b],
David A. Jamadar, MB,BS, FRCS, FRCR, DMRD[c]

KEYWORDS

- Rotator interval • Long head biceps tendon
- Glenohumeral joint instability • Tear • MR imaging

Key Points

- The rotator interval includes the superior glenohumeral ligament (SGHL) and the coracohumeral ligament (CHL), as well as the long head biceps tendon (LHBT) and the biceps tendon pulley.

- The rotator interval ligaments, LHBT, and the adjacent supraspinatus (SST) and subscapularis (SSC) tendon fibers are intimately associated in the lateral portion of the rotator interval.

- The SGHL and CHL play a role in glenohumeral joint stability while the bicipital pulley confers LHBT stability.

- Rotator interval capsuloligamentous lesions are associated with a spectrum of pathological conditions ranging from glenohumeral instability to adhesive capsulitis.

- LHBT lesions and instability are a source of anterior shoulder pain.

- LHBT instability patterns are associated with specific patterns of injury to the biceps pulley and adjacent rotator cuff tendons.

- Clinical and arthroscopic diagnosis of rotator interval and LHBT abnormality may be difficult.

- MR arthrography is well suited to depict rotator interval and LHBT lesions.

- Close inspection of the LHBT, biceps pulley, and rotator interval ligaments should be performed if tears of the leading edge of the distal SST tendon or the superior aspect of the distal SSC tendon are identified on magnetic resonance (MR) imaging.

The authors have nothing to disclose.
[a] Department of Radiology, University of Michigan Hospitals, Taubman Floor 2, Room 2910F, 1500 East Medical Center Drive, Ann Arbor, MI 48109-5326, USA
[b] Department of Orthopedic Surgery, University of Michigan Hospitals, Domino's Farms, Lobby A, 24 Frank Lloyd Wright Drive, Ann Arbor, MI 48105, USA
[c] Department of Radiology, University of Michigan Hospitals, TC 2910, 1500 East Medical Center Drive, Ann Arbor, MI 48109, USA
* Corresponding author.
E-mail address: yoavm@med.umich.edu

Magn Reson Imaging Clin N Am 20 (2012) 229–259
doi:10.1016/j.mric.2012.01.012

mri.theclinics.com

The term rotator interval was first applied by Neer[1] in 1970 when describing greater tuberosity fractures. The dictionary definition of an interval as a *space*[2] may be misleading, as it pertains to the rotator interval, because "space" implies an area devoid of structures or function. It is widely accepted that the rotator interval structures fulfill a role in biomechanics and pathology of the glenohumeral joint and long head biceps tendon (LHBT). However, there is ongoing debate regarding the biomechanical details as well as the indications for treatment. A better understanding of rotator interval anatomy and function will lead to improved treatment of rotator interval abnormalities, and guide the indications for imaging and surgical intervention.

ANATOMY

The rotator interval is an anatomically defined triangular area located between the coracoid process, the superior aspect of the subscapularis (SSC), and the anterior aspect of the supraspinatus (SST), with the coracoid process at the base and the bicipital groove at the apex (**Fig. 1**). The interval is bridged by the glenohumeral capsule, which is composed histologically of loose connective tissue in which there are thick bands of collagen fibers that form the coracohumeral ligament (CHL), superior glenohumeral ligament (SGHL), and the rotator cable.[3,4] The LHBT traverses the rotator interval as it courses toward the bicipital groove.

The constituents of the rotator interval are closely intertwined and are also associated with

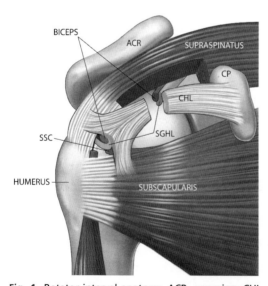

Fig. 1. Rotator interval anatomy. ACR, acromion; CHL, coracohumeral ligament; CP, coracoid process; SSC, subscapularis; SGHL, superior glenohumeral ligament. The rotator interval capsule is not depicted in this illustration.

the adjacent rotator cuff tendons. While there is a general consensus regarding the contents of the rotator interval as well as the close association between rotator interval ligaments, rotator cuff tendons, and the LHBT, there is a debate regarding their anatomic detail and function. The capsule-ligamentous layer is morphologically the most variable layer of the shoulder,[3] which may explain the variable descriptions of the rotator interval components.

The Ligaments

The CHL and SGHL run a separate course medially but are more intimately associated laterally (see **Fig. 1**). There are contradictory descriptions of the anatomy of the CHL and SGHL, which may relate to differences in study methods emphasizing the intra-articular or extra-articular portion of the ligaments, the use of fresh versus frozen cadavers, and the close association between these ligaments in the mid to lateral portion of the rotator interval.[5]

The CHL is a well-developed structure in most shoulders. This ligament is composed of relatively poorly organized dense connective tissue,[6] and although the existence of the CHL as a true ligament is not consistently supported on histologic studies,[7,8] it is a constant macroscopic network of fibers or a capsular fold noted in the anterior aspect of the glenohumeral capsule.[7] The CHL arises from the lateral aspect of the coracoid process[9]; coursing laterally it is inseparable from the capsule, spanning over the rotator interval superficial to the SGHL.[10] Distally this ligament is thought to form 2 major bands, the medial band (MCHL) and the lateral band (LCHL), which are believed to contribute to different components of the ligamentous sling encompassing the LHBT.[11,12]

The SGHL is a constant but variably expressed anatomic structure[5,10] composed of parallel bundles of collagen fibers and fibroblasts.[5] Medially, the SGHL has been described as arising from the supraglenoid tuberosity[13–15] or from the superior labrum at the 1 o'clock position,[16–18] while Turkel and colleagues[19] also described an additional proximal attachment at the base of the coracoid. The SGHL then courses laterally, parallel to the LHBT, with variable descriptions of the lateral attachment: to the lesser tuberosity,[14,15] along the bicipital groove floor and over the groove, and merging with the CHL and the humeral semicircular ligament/rotator cable.[5] In a recent cadaveric study, Kask and colleagues[5] described oblique and direct components of the SGHL. The oblique fibers typically arise from the supraglenoid tuberosity and rarely from the anterior superior labrum, fuse loosely with the overlying fibers of the CHL, course over the intra-articular LHBT, and insert on the humeral semicircular ligament/rotator cable. The direct fibers originate from the anterior superior and anterior labrum, run parallel to the LHBT, partially insert on the lesser tuberosity, then course along the floor of the bicipital groove and partially bridge over it. This description of 2 bands with a medial and lateral distal attachment is reminiscent of the 2 distal bands of the CHL. Both superior glenohumeral and CHLs are firmly attached to the outer nonarticular surface of the joint capsule.[20]

The Long Head Biceps Tendon

The proximal LHBT is an intra-articular but extrasynovial structure arising from the supraglenoid tuberosity and from the posterior or posterior and superior labrum.[21,22] The LHBT is flatter and larger in the intra-articular segment[23] with a variable morphology, especially at the origin. Accessory heads of the biceps brachii muscle have been described in approximately 9% to 20% of individuals from the greater tuberosity near the articular capsule, from the articular surface of the glenohumeral joint, from the coracoid process, or in the form of a bifurcated tendon.[24–28] Variations of the LHBT origin have also been described: LHBT confluent with the rotator cuff,[26] originating from the anterior border of the SST tendon,[29] and as of extra-articular origin.[30] Dierickx and colleagues[31] had described 12 variations of the intra-articular LHBT based on the anatomy and the dynamic behavior during arthroscopy, including variable attachment of the LHBT to the rotator cuff or capsule from a partial mesotenon (**Figs. 2** and **3**) to a complete adherence of the LHBT to the inferior surface of the capsule, as well as a split biceps tendon and complete absence of the biceps tendon. The authors are of the opinion that these variations are a result of partial detachment from the mesothelium, or synovial fusion with the inferior surface of the capsule, and that some of these variants may cause abnormalities through inferior traction on the SST tendon during abduction.

As the distal intra-articular portion of the LHBT exits the glenohumeral joint, it is enveloped by the biceps pulley, a structure formed by coalescence of rotator interval ligaments and tendon fibers.

The Biceps Pulley

Macroscopically, there is a slinglike U-shaped sheath encompassing the LHBT proximal to the

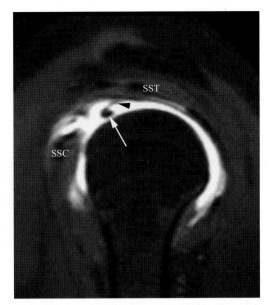

Fig. 2. Soft tissue band between LHBT and capsule. Sagittal T1-weighted MR arthrographic images with fat saturation depict a soft tissue band (*arrowhead*) attaching the LHBT (*arrow*) to the undersurface of the glenohumeral capsule. SSC, subscapularis; SST, supraspinatus.

bicipital groove, dubbed the biceps pulley. Arthroscopic/surgical observations, cadaveric dissections with histologic staining or polarized light microscopy, and biomechanical studies with dissection or imbrication of specific ligaments have been performed to elucidate the specific components of the biceps pulley and to clarify the significance of each structure in conferring stability to the LHBT.[3,10,20,32,33] Although there is a broad consensus that the pulley is predominantly ligamentous in structure, the reports differ regarding the specific ligamentous contribution to the pulley, the extent of interdigitation between the ligamentous pulley and the SSC and SST tendon fibers, and the contribution of each component, including SSC and SST tendon fibers, as it pertains to LHBT stability. Initial studies emphasized the role of the CHL and SSC in LHBT stability[34]; In 1979, Slatis and Aalto[32] identified the CHL as the "key ligament" in stabilizing the LHBT in the bicipital groove based on surgical findings and anatomic dissection, then in 1986 Petersson[35] suggested a relationship between stability of the LHBT and SSC lesions. In their extensive cadaveric study in 1992, Clark and Harryman[20] had specified that the sheath enveloping the LHBT is formed by the SSC and SST tendons, with the CHL forming a portion of the roof. More recent studies have emphasized the role of the SGHL in LHBT stability. In a cadaveric study using polarized light microscopy, Werner

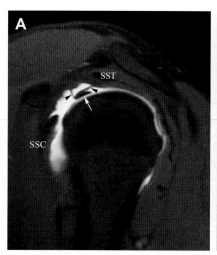
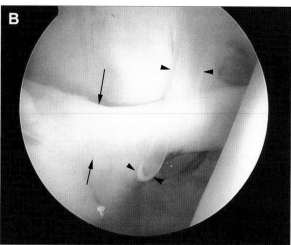

Fig. 3. Pulley-like mesotenon attachment between the LHBT and capsule. (*A*) Sagittal T1-weighted MR arthrographic images with fat saturation and (*B*) arthroscopic image depict a soft tissue pulley-like band (*arrowhead*) attaching the LHBT (*arrow*) to the undersurface of the glenohumeral capsule, consistent with a mesotenon.

and colleagues[10] described the pulley as a U-shaped fold in the lateral aspect of the rotator interval with the SGHL covering the inferior, anterior, and superior aspects of the LHBT. The roof of the pulley was formed by 3 layers: the SGHL and the CHL, with the fasciculus obliquus (spiral glenohumeral ligament) as the most superficial layer. The roof is formed by SST tendon fibers, which interdigitate with the posterior ligamentous complex while fibers from the SSC tendon intermingle with fibers of the SGHL and CHL at the level of the bicipital groove (**Fig. 4**). The pulley is divided into 2 functional ligamentous complexes; a medial pulley complex along the medial and inferior aspect of the intra-articular LHBT, and a lateral pulley

complex along the superior and lateral aspect of the intra-articular LHBT. The medial pulley complex is thought to include superficial fibers from the MCHL blending with the deeper SGHL fibers, whereas the lateral ligamentous pulley complex includes the LCHL.[22,36,37] The medial pulley complex is described as attaching to the lesser tuberosity or blending with the adjacent SSC tendon fibers[11,36,38] while the lateral pulley complex inserts on the greater tuberosity and merges with the leading edge of the SST tendon.[11,33,37]

The Transverse Ligament

The roof of the bicipital groove is formed by the transverse humeral ligament. In this case also, there is deliberation regarding the origin of this structure. In a cadaveric study by Gleason and colleagues[39] a distinct transverse ligamentous structure could not be identified, but fibers arising from the SSC tendon and from the SST tendon were determined. Macdonald and colleagues[40] claimed that the transverse ligament in most individuals is composed of fibers arising from the SSC tendon coursing through a fascia expansion arising from the pectoralis major tendon.

The Rotator Cable

In a cadaveric study of 80 shoulders, Clark and Harryman[20] had described thick fibrous bands, which appeared to be an extension of the rotator interval CHL enveloping the anterior aspect of the SST tendon. A component of this fibrous band coursing deep and perpendicular to the

Fig. 4. Histology of the LHBT pulley. Histologic slide with hematoxylin-eosin stain (×20) depicting the multilayered appearance of the biceps pulley in the sagittal plane. A, articular surface; B, bursal surface.

SST and infraspinatus tendons was described in later cadaveric and arthroscopic studies as the rotator cable or humeral semicircular ligament.[5,41]

The Superior Labrum

The superior labrum is closely associated with the LHBT and the rotator interval. LHBT fibers extending posteriorly are a major element of the posterior labrum. In addition, a sheetlike structure has been described, which arises from the rotator interval attaching to the anterior superior labrum.[22]

FUNCTION
Function of the Rotator Interval

The role of the rotator interval as a passive stabilizer of the glenohumeral joint has been a topic of long-standing research in numerous in vivo and in vitro studies. The CHL was found to be one of the factors preventing downward dislocation of the glenohumeral joint in electromyographic and cadaveric studies.[7,42] An extensive cadaveric study of the rotator interval by Harryman and colleagues[43] revealed that sectioning of the rotator interval capsule and ligaments increased passive glenohumeral flexion, extension, external rotation, and adduction, whereas imbrication caused a decrease in these motions. Their conclusion was that the rotator interval functions as a "check-rein" against excessive motion and limits posterior inferior glenohumeral translation. Jost and colleagues[12] divided the rotator interval into a medial and lateral part, based on anatomy and function. The medial part is composed of the SGHL and capsule, and a deep layer consisting of the medial fibers of the CHL. The lateral part is composed of 4 layers: the superficial layer consisting of the superficial CHL, the second layer consisting of the SST and SSC tendon fibers, the third layer consisting of the deep CHL, and the fourth layer including the lateral capsule and the SGHL. The medial part limits inferior translation, and to a lesser extent external rotation, whereas the lateral part mainly limits external rotation of the adducted arm. The CHL is a factor in external rotation and functions as a superior-inferior stabilizer.[12,44] In addition, the intra-articular pressure maintained by an intact rotator interval capsule is a stabilizer in the superior-inferior direction in neutral and internal rotation.[44]

Function of the Long Head Biceps Tendon Pulley

Anterior shearing forces are applied on the LHBT in the lateral aspect of the rotator interval.[10,14,45] Numerous anatomic and biomechanical studies have attempted to elucidate the mechanism of support and to identify the crucial supporting structures. It is generally accepted that the biceps pulley including the SGHL, CHL, and superior SSC tendon are key in conferring stability to the intra-articular long head biceps,[22,46,47] but there is still a debate regarding which are the crucial components of the pulley (**Fig. 5**). In a cadaveric biomechanical study in 1979, Slatis and Aalto[32] had demonstrated that transection of the medial part of the CHL allows the LHBT to be medially displaced, and concluded that the CHL is the key ligament in long head biceps stabilization. However, using polarized light microscopy, Werner and colleagues[10] noted that orientation of the SGHL fibers allows this ligament to resist anterior shearing stress and thus function as the primary stabilizer of the intra-articular LHBT.

Function of the Long Head Biceps Tendon

The function of the LHBT in the shoulder remains controversial. Some investigators regard this as a vestigial structure, but other studies indicate that the biceps tendon functions as a weak abductor of the shoulder[23] as well as in flexion and medial rotation of the shoulder.[48,49] Cadaveric biomechanical studies suggest that the LHBT has a stabilizing effect on the glenohumeral joint in multiple directions, diminishing stress on the inferior glenohumeral ligament,[50] while electromyographic studies are controversial. In vivo studies such as that by Warner and McMahon,[51] showing increased superior translation of the humeral head

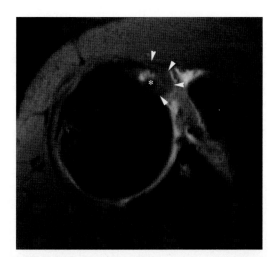

Fig. 5. Stabilizers of the LHBT. Axial T1-weighted MR arthrographic images with fat saturation depict a thickened but intact bicipital pulley (*white arrowheads*) transfixing the LHBT (*asterisk*) in the groove with an SSC tendon rupture.

relative to the glenoid associated with loss of the LHBT, suggest a role for the LHBT as a humeral depressor.[51,52] However, there are concerns regarding the accuracy of these models,[53] with the stabilizing function of the LHBT purported to be more important in rotator cuff deficient shoulders.[54]

MR IMAGING OF THE ROTATOR INTERVAL AND LONG HEAD BICEPS TENDON

MR imaging is the current imaging modality of choice in assessing the rotator interval and intra-articular LHBT (**Box 1**).[55–58] The standard MR protocol in the authors' institution for a 1.5-T scanner includes an axial intermediate weighted sequence (retention time [TR] 2500–3000, echo time [TE] 34) with fat saturation, sagittal and coronal oblique T2-weighted sequences (TR 3000–4000, TE 42) with fat saturation, and a sagittal oblique T1-weighted sequence (TR400-650, TE 10). The MR arthrogram protocol includes oblique coronal, oblique sagittal, axial, and abduction external rotation (ABER) T1-weighted (TR 450–750, TE 15) sequences with fat saturation and a coronal oblique T2-weighted sequence (TR 4000–5000, TE 50) with fat saturation (**Table 1**). These sequences follow a fluoroscopic-guided injection using an anterior approach through the SSC tendon rather than through the rotator interval, to avoid potentially confusing iatrogenic contrast extravasation through the rotator interval. However, the authors recognize that centers routinely using the rotator interval approach may be comfortable discerning iatrogenic from pathologic extravasation.[59] The authors' experience, corresponding with that of other studies,[60] indicates that the sagittal plane is best suited to depict the rotator interval as well as the long head biceps pulley while the axial plane is complementary. Whereas standard MR imaging in all 3 planes is well suited to delineate the extra-articular LHBT, it is ill suited for consistently outlining the intra-articular LHBT or the rotator interval ligaments

Table 1 Imaging protocol		
	Planes	**Sequence**
Standard MR imaging	Axial	TR 2500–3000, TE 34 FS
	Sagittal	TR 3000–4000, TE 42 FS
	Coronal oblique	TR400–650, TE 10 TR 3000–4000, TE 42 FS
MR arthrogram	Axial	TR 450–750, TE 15 FS
	Sagittal	TR 450–750, TE 15 FS
	Coronal oblique	TR 450–750, TE 15 FS TR 4000–5000, TE 50 FS
	ABER	TR 450–750, TE 15 FS

Abbreviations: ABER, abduction external rotation; FS, with fat saturation; TE, echo time; TR, retention time.

and pulley.[60] MR arthrography allows the complete delineation of the intra-articular LHBT and better delineation of the rotator interval ligaments in the intact and diseased state,[60] as well as allowing measurements of the rotator interval. Accordingly, mean measurements of the rotator interval capsule thickness of 1.8 mm and of rotator interval dimensions of 16.7 mm and 48.59 mm (height and base) have been obtained on MR arthrograms of cadaveric shoulders[60] and in patients without shoulder instability.[61] In the authors' experience, distinct rotator interval structures that can be identified on routine MR arthrography include the origin of the SGHL and the biceps pulley (**Figs. 6** and **7**), while the remaining rotator interval capsuloligamentous structures form an intermediate-signal platelike structure, which can be best delineated on MR imaging/MR arthrograms if there is coinciding intracapsular and extracapsular fluid (see **Fig. 7**; **Fig. 8**). The medial origin of the CHL ligament at the coracoid process can also be identified, especially on sequences without saturation of the fat surrounding the ligamentous origin, and focal thickening corresponding to this ligament can sometimes be appreciated on coronal oblique sequences without fat saturation (**Fig. 9**). Redundancy of the rotator interval capsuloligamentous structures on internal rotation may accentuate the ligaments, the biceps pulley and, at times, the origin of the rotator cable origin at the interval on MR arthrography (**Fig. 10**). However, even on MR arthrography, the CHL and SGHL cannot be identified as separate structures

---

Box 1
Pearls and pitfalls: MR imaging of the rotator interval and LHBT

- The sagittal plane is best suited to depict the rotator interval and the intra-articular LHBT
- MR arthrography allows better delineation of the intra-articular LHBT as well as of the rotator interval ligaments

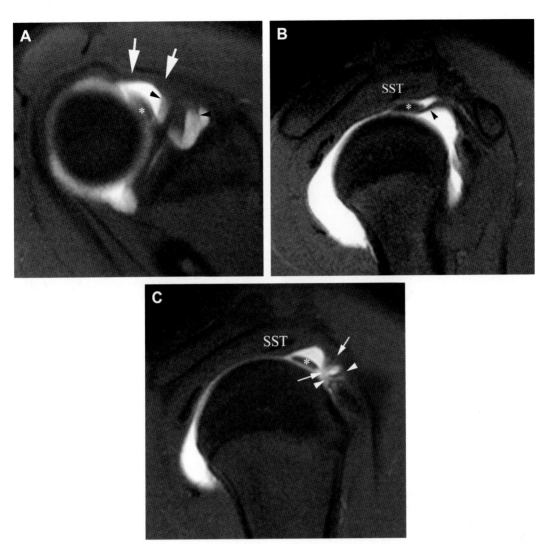

Fig. 6. Anatomy. Axial (*A*) and sagittal (*B, C*) T1-weighted MR arthrographic images with fat saturation depict the origin of the SGHL (*black arrowheads*) and the relationship between the bicipital pulley (*thin arrows*) and the SSC tendon superior fibers (*white arrowheads*). SST, supraspinatus. Asterisk indicates LHBT; thick arrows indicate fused SGHL and CHL.

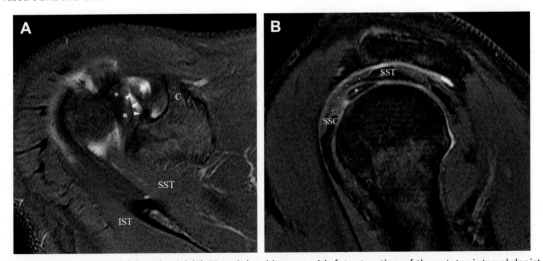

Fig. 7. Anatomy. Sagittal (*A*) and axial (*B*) T2-weighted images with fat saturation of the rotator interval depict the origin of the SGHL paralleling the LHBT (*white arrowheads*), merged capsuloligamentous structures (*dot*), and the CHL (*black arrowheads*). SSC, subscapularis; SST, supraspinatus. Asterisks indicate LHBT.

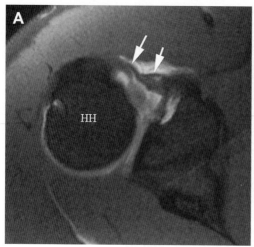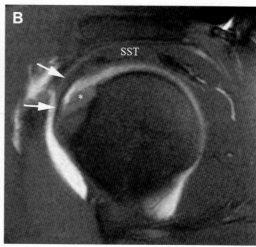

Fig. 8. Anatomy. Axial (*A*) and coronal oblique (*B*) T1-weighted MR arthrographic images with fat saturation with extracapsular extravasation of contrast depict a sheetlike structure laterally (*arrows*) in the lateral rotator interval formed by the SGHL and CHL. SST, supraspinatus. Asterisk indicates LHBT.

in the lateral rotator interval. Although high-resolution sequences (2 mm) with high image matrix have been advocated for this purpose,[11,62] the authors have not adopted this technique in routine clinical practice.

ROTATOR INTERVAL PATHOLOGY

The spectrum of pathological conditions associated with the rotator interval varies between glenohumeral instability and adhesive capsulitis, indicating the delicate balance existing between structures occupying this space. In addition to

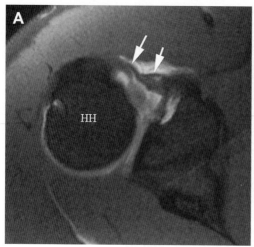

Fig. 9. Anatomy. Coronal oblique T2-weighted image depicts the CHL (*arrowheads*). Same patient as in **Fig. 7.** C, coracoid process.

lesions of the rotator interval capsule and ligaments, rotator interval abnormalities also include lesions involving the anterior aspect of the SST tendon and the superior aspect of the SSC tendon, as well as LHBT and long head biceps pulley lesions. Lesions involving different rotator interval structures occur concurrently in expected configurations, given their close proximity and interdigitation. Therefore, it is important to be familiar with common patterns of rotator interval injury and to seek out accompanying lesions when evaluating this area.

Rotator Interval Laxity and Glenohumeral Instability

Incompetence or disruption of the rotator interval components may lead to laxity. Laxity may lead to glenohumeral instability and pain.[12,43,49] In 1980, Neer and Foster[63] made the important distinction between capsular/ligamentous laxity and a Bankart lesion in the context of glenohumeral instability, and described inferior capsular shift. Rowe and Zarins[64] described a defect in the rotator interval in approximately 50% of patients assessed for dead arm syndrome, a sudden sharp pain or paralyzing pain when the shoulder is moved forcibly into maximum external rotation in elevation or following direct trauma. Rowe and Zarins believed that this syndrome is associated with transient subluxation of the shoulder, and suggested that rotator interval deficiency is probably a factor contributing to anterior subluxation of the shoulder.

The underlying etiology of rotator interval laxity, incompetence, and defects is varied, and includes

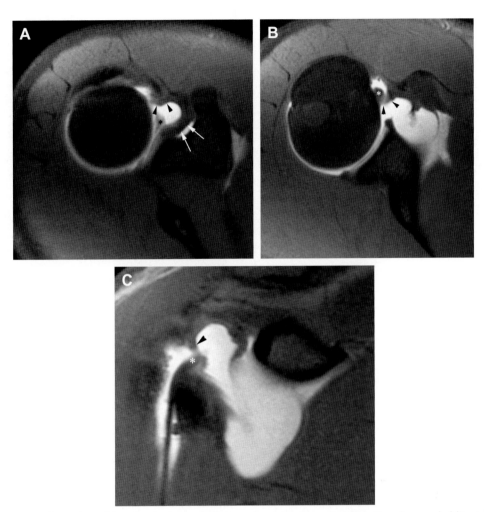

Fig. 10. Internal rotation with redundant capsule-ligamentous structures. Axial (*A, B*) and coronal oblique (*C*) T1-weighted MR arthrographic images with fat saturation reveal apparent thickening of intact and uniform SGHL (*arrows*) and bicipital pulley (*arrowheads*), likely relating to internal rotation with redundancy of these structures. Asterisk indicates LHBT.

acute posttraumatic lesions, repetitive microtrauma, and underlying ligamentous laxity with superimposed overuse injuries.[49,65] Based on cadaveric findings in 28 of 37 fetuses, Cole and colleagues[66] suggested that rotator interval defects may be congenital.

There is a spectrum of rotator interval lesions associated with rotator interval laxity and glenohumeral instability, which includes frank defects in the rotator interval as described by Rowe and Zarins[64] in athletes following trauma or excessive use of the shoulder. Nobuhara and Ikeda[67] described inflammation of the deeper tissues of the rotator interval seen in surgery in patients with instability that had responded to surgical repair. Widening of the rotator interval has been described on arthroscopy; however, this can be

difficult to identify and varies according to the surgeon's experience.[65]

Although rotator interval lesions may occur as isolated lesions,[68] they frequently occur in association with rotator cuff tendon tears.[36,69] This association is explained by the close relationship between the lateral rotator interval and the adjacent tendons, which includes reinforcement of the rotator cuff by components arising from the lateral rotator interval such as the rotator cable, and reinforcement of the lateral rotator interval by fibers from the SST and SSC tendons.[7]

Patients may describe pain and instability while instability is noted and a sulcus sign may be present on clinical examination. In the setting of a rotator interval lesion and laxity, the sulcus sign may persist on external rotation because of the

Table 2
MR imaging findings associated with rotator interval laxity

Morphologic changes	Ligamentous thickening Ligamentous attenuation Ligamentous irregularity
Secondary imaging findings	Subcoracoid bursal fluid
Extracapsular contrast extravasation	Subacromial subdeltoid bursa Subcoracoid bursa Along the subcoracoid process Along the lesser tuberosity
Dimensions of the rotator interval	Increased[a]

[a] Controversial.

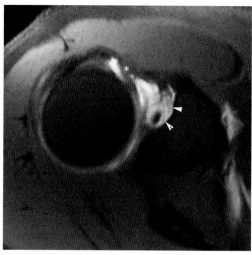

Fig. 12. SGHL injury. Axial T1-weighted MR arthrographic image with fat saturation depicts an irregular and attenuated SGHL (*arrowheads*) following acute injury. C, coracoid process. Asterisk indicates LHBT.

loss of the tightening effect of the rotator interval ligaments and capsule.[49] This finding is important in distinguishing a pathologic sulcus sign secondary to rotator interval insufficiency from a sulcus sign attributable to generalized ligamentous laxity.

Closure of the rotator interval to address glenohumeral instability remains controversial. Although most patients with rotator interval insufficiency require a standard capsulolabral repair and/or advancement as a supplement to closure of the defect, isolated approximation or imbrication of the defect may confer adequate stability in selected patients. Field and colleagues[68] reported on 15 patients with rotator interval defects and instability in the absence of other pathologic glenohumeral lesions. With follow-up of a mean of 3.3 years, all patients achieved either a good or excellent result using the American Shoulder and Elbow Surgeons evaluation scale and the Rowe

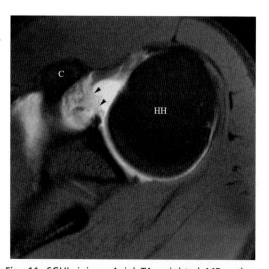

Fig. 11. SGHL injury. Axial T1-weighted MR arthrographic images with fat saturation reveal a thick irregular SGHL (*arrowheads*) in a patient with glenohumeral instability. C, coracoid process; HH, humeral head.

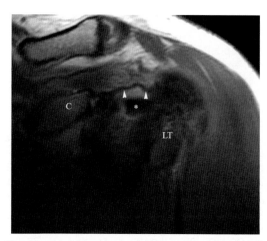

Fig. 13. CHL injury. Coronal oblique T2-weighted MR arthrogram image depicts a wavy CHL (*arrowheads*) following subacute injury. C, coracoid process; LT, lesser tuberosity. Asterisk indicates LHBT.

rating scale. In this regard, surgical closure may have a role in cases with a persistent sulcus sign despite external rotation, or in cases where instability persists despite an appropriate capsulolabral advancement and retensioning of the inferior glenohumeral ligament complex.[49]

MR Imaging of Rotator Interval Lesions in the Unstable Shoulder

MR imaging including MR arthrography is relatively insensitive for diagnosing instability patterns, with a low prevalence of labral tears such as atraumatic multidirectional instability.[70] Therefore, defining MR imaging criteria for rotator interval pathology in the context of instability is desirable (Table 2).

Changes in ligamentous morphology and signal have been described on MR imaging and MR arthrography, including thickening or attenuation of the rotator interval ligaments (Figs. 11–13).[55,71] Subcoracoid bursal fluid may be associated with rotator cuff and interval tears,[72] and identifying fluid in this area should prompt a thorough investigation of the rotator interval (Fig. 14). Extracapsular extension of contrast is the hallmark of rotator interval defects or tears on MR arthrography. The extracapsular contrast may undergo a variable course and has been described as filling the subcoracoid bursa, subacromial/subdeltoid bursa (Figs. 15 and 16), tracking along the undersurface of the coracoid process or along the lesser tuberosity (Fig. 17). In addition, distention of the joint on MR arthrography facilitates identification of

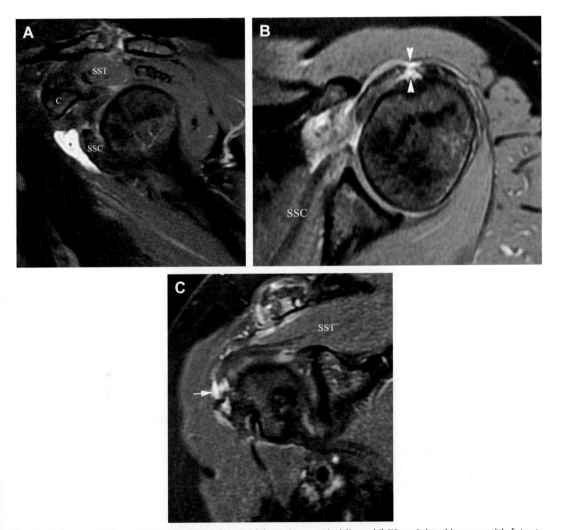

Fig. 14. Subcoracoid bursal fluid. Sagittal (A), axial (B), and coronal oblique (C) T2-weighted images with fat saturation depict (A) fluid in the subcoracoid bursa (asterisk), (B) a lesion in the lateral rotator interval (arrowhead), and (C) an SST tendon tear (arrow). C, coracoid process; SSC, subscapularis.

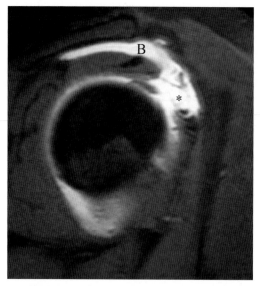

Fig. 15. Rotator interval tear. Sagittal T1-weighted MR image with fat saturation depicts a rotator interval tear (*asterisk*) following prolotherapy with contrast extending to the subacromial bursa (B). H, humeral head; SSC, subscapularis; SST, supraspinatus. Asterisk indicates LHBT.

capsular irregularity (**Fig. 18**) and thinning.[36,71–74] The medial origin of the SGHL and the CHL may be irregular, attenuated, thickened, or discontinuous on consecutive images on MR arthrography, accordingly suggesting a ligamentous lesion or complete tear.[55,75] However, assessment of diffuse caliber changes involving the ligaments is subjective[71] and may not be straightforward.

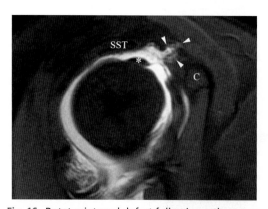

Fig. 16. Rotator interval defect following arthroscopy. Sagittal T1-weighted MR arthrographic image with fat saturation depicts contrast outpouching (*arrowheads*) through the rotator interval following arthroscopy. C, coracoid process; SST, supraspinatus. Asterisk indicates LHBT.

Identifying rotator interval capsuloligamentous laxity without frank discontinuity on imaging may be difficult. In some studies, measurements of rotator interval dimensions have revealed significant differences between patients with and without glenohumeral instability, including significantly greater measurements of the triangular rotator interval base, height, surface area, and depth in patients with instability.[61,76] In a retrospective study by Kim and colleagues,[61] the distance between the superior aspect of the SSC and the anterior aspect of the SST tendons just anterior to the coracoid base was measured on sagittal MR arthrographic images. The distance was significantly greater in patients with recurrent anterior instability (mean 21.87 mm) than in patients without instability (mean 16.73 mm) (**Fig. 19**). However, measurements may vary based on injection and scanning technique, types of glenohumeral instability, and differences in patient size, with some contradictory results reported in the literature.[61,77,78] In an MR arthrographic study by Provencher and colleagues,[77] a statistically significant difference in rotator interval dimensions was not identified between patients with or without instability, emphasizing the potential difficulty in these measurements. Therefore, qualitative criteria may be more easily applied. Along those lines, this same study by Provencher and colleagues[77] described the position of the intra-articular long head biceps as more anterior relative to the leading edge of the SST tendon in posterior instability compared with anterior instability or in cases without instability, suggesting a widened and incompetent rotator interval.

Adhesive Capsulitis and Contractures of the Rotator Interval

Adhesive capsulitis is characterized by pain and is typically accompanied by limitations in passive and active range of motion.[49] Adhesive capsulitis occurs in 2% to 3% of the general population, and may be idiopathic or associated with prior trauma, diabetes mellitus, hypothyroidism, and other disorders such as hemodialysis or surgery.[49,57,79]

Rotator interval contractures vary from a mild form accompanying mild rotator cuff impingement to severe forms associated with adhesive capsulitis. Ozaki and colleagues[80] described contracture of the CHL and rotator interval in 17 operated patients with adhesive capsulitis. These investigators described fibrosis and hyalinization and fibrinoid degeneration in the contracted connective tissues, with relief of the symptoms following resection of these structures. Based on corresponding

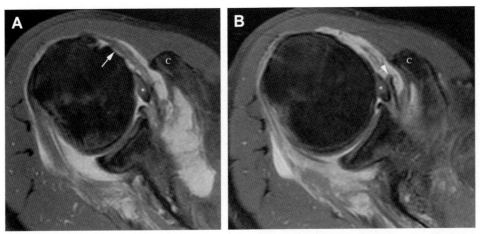

Fig. 17. Tear of the rotator interval with associated SSC tendon tear. Axial T2-weighted images with fat saturation depict a rotator interval tear and distal SSC tendon tear with (*A*) an uncovered superior aspect of the lesser tuberosity (*arrow*), intra-articular dislocation of the LHBT (*asterisk*), and (*B*) a medially retracted stump of the rotator interval capsuloligamentous structures (*arrowhead*). C, coracoid process.

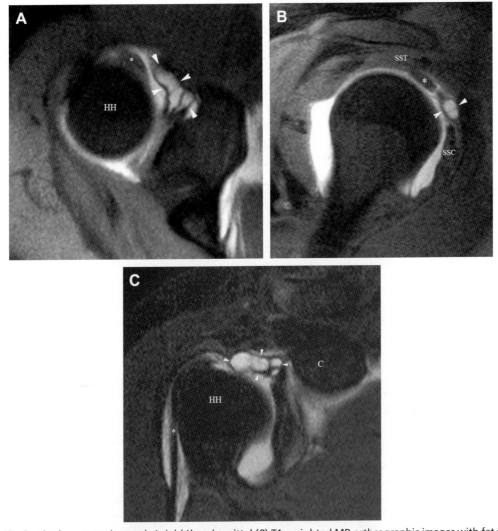

Fig. 18. Cyst in the rotator interval. Axial (*A*) and sagittal (*B*) T1-weighted MR arthrographic images with fat saturation and coronal oblique (*C*) sagittal T2-weighted MR arthrographic image with fat saturation depict cysts (*arrowheads*) involving the SGHL and the lateral rotator interval capsule-ligamentous structures. C, coracoid process; HH, humeral head; SST, supraspinatus. Asterisk indicates LHBT.

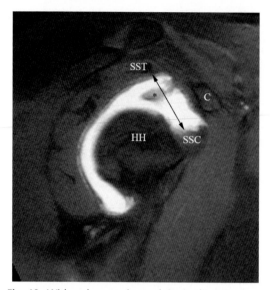

Fig. 19. Widened rotator interval. Sagittal T1-weighted MR image with fat saturation depict a widened rotator interval (*double-headed arrow*). C, coracoid process; HH, humeral head; SSC, subscapularis; SST, supraspinatus. Asterisk indicates LHBT.

Table 3 MR imaging findings associated with adhesive capsulitis	
Morphologic changes	Capsular, rotator interval, axillary thickening Capsular increased intermediate weighted signal Obliteration of the fat signal in the rotator interval
Intravenous contrast administration	Rapid enhancement of the rotator interval, synovium, axillary recess, capsule
Intra-articular contrast	Decreased axillary recess volumes Decreased rotator interval dimensions Thickening of the axillary recess capsule-synovium

findings in a cadaveric study, Neer and colleagues[9] suggested that the contracture of the CHL may be associated with limited external rotation in patients with adhesive capsulitis.

Staging of adhesive capsulitis is based on clinical parameters including duration, pain, limited range of motion, examination under anesthesia, and arthroscopic and pathologic histologic findings.[81] Stage 1 includes a hypertrophic, hypervascular synovitis with underlying normal capsule. In stage 2, in addition to the hypervascular synovitis there is accompanying thickening of the underlying capsule and perivascular scar formation, and in stage 3 there is atrophic synovitis and dense capsular scar.[56]

Imaging had not played a major role in the diagnosis of adhesive capsulitis before the advent of MR imaging, with radiographs typically unrevealing and arthrograms possibly showing decreased capsular volume. However, MR imaging is showing promise in identifying adhesive capsulitis and excluding other causes for shoulder pain and limited range of motion (**Table 3**). Various MR imaging protocols target different histologic stages of adhesive capsulitis including hyperplastic synovitis, capsuloligamentous thickening, hypervascularity, and changes related to scarring. Sofka and colleagues[56] had found variable capsular thickening and increased signal on intermediate weighted sequences, which corresponds to the hypertrophic, hypervascular synovitis and

inflammatory changes seen in stages 1 and 2 (**Fig. 20**). Studies following intravenous contrast administration show relatively rapid glenohumeral joint enhancement in cases with adhesive capsulitis compared with cases without adhesive capsulitis,[82] with enhancement involving the rotator interval capsule, synovium, axillary recess, anterior and posterior capsules, fibrovascular tissue encasing the CHL and SGHL, and the LHBT.[58,83,84] MR imaging and MR arthrographic studies have demonstrated thickening of the axillary pouch,[79,83] thickening of the CHL and rotator interval capsule,[57,79,85] synovitis-like changes along the cranial SSC tendon and at the opening of the SSC recess, and decreased axillary recess volumes (**Fig. 21**).[57,85] Mengiardi and colleagues[57] described obliteration of the fat signal in a triangular area defined by the coracoid process, CHL, and rotator interval capsule as a specific but insensitive sign of adhesive capsulitis (see **Fig. 20**). On an MR arthrographic study, Kim and colleagues[86] found a significantly decreased distance between the superior aspect of the SSC and the anterior aspect of the SST tendons on sagittal images, and a decreased distance between the coracoid base and the lateral ridge of the bicipital groove on axial images. Numerous studies[79,85,86] have attempted to quantify the structural changes accompanying adhesive capsulitis. Although a significant difference was often found in these quantitative studies between adhesive capsulitis

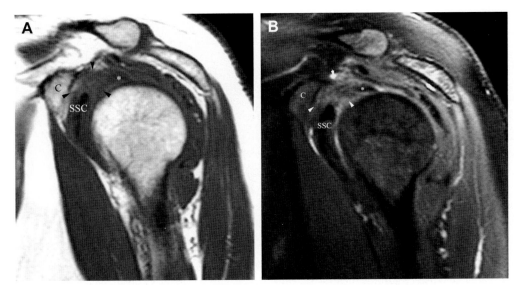

Fig. 20. Arthroscopically confirmed adhesive capsulitis. Sagittal T1-weighted image (*A*) and sagittal T2-weighted image with fat saturation (*B*) depict replacement of the expected fatty signal in the medial rotator interval with decreased T1-weighted signal and increased T2-weighted signal (*arrowheads*) in a patient with surgically proven adhesive capsulitis described on arthroscopy as injected and thickened. C, coracoid; SSC, subscapularis. Asterisk indicates LHBT.

and controls, identifying a reproducible cutoff measurement is difficult because the imaging technique (noncontrast, intravenous contrast, intra-articular contrast studies) and measurement techniques differ between studies. In a meta-analysis performed by Petchprapa and colleagues,[11] no significant difference in measurement was found between adhesive capsulitis and control cases with regard to axillary recess width; however, the thickness of the capsule-synovium in the axillary

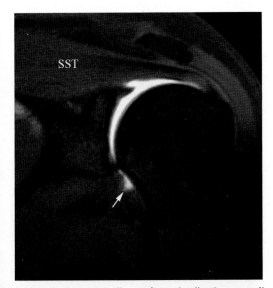

Fig. 21. Arthroscopically confirmed adhesive capsulitis. Coronal oblique T1-weighted MR arthrographic image with fat saturation depicts a contracted axillary recess (*arrow*) in arthroscopically confirmed adhesive capsulitis. SST, supraspinatus.

Box 2
Pearls and pitfalls: MR imaging of rotator interval pathology

- Contrast extravasation through the rotator interval on MR arthrography indicates a rotator interval defect/tear unless contrast injection has been performed through the rotator interval

- Contrast extravasation through the rotator interval may occur following arthroscopy

- Capsule and ligamentous thickening and decreased T1 signal involving the fat anterior to the rotator interval capsule have been associated with adhesive capsulitis

- Rotator interval dimensions and measurements of rotator interval ligaments may be influenced by multiple factors, including injection and scanning techniques as well as patient size

- There is controversy regarding the coraco-humeral interval measurement that would indicate subcoracoid impingement

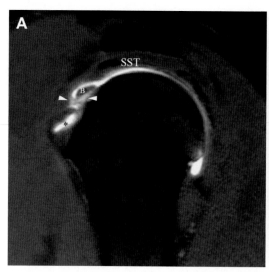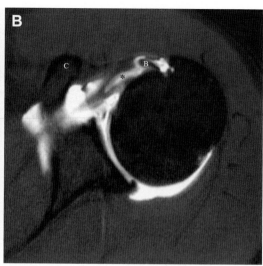

Fig. 22. Partial-thickness tear of the superior SSC with intact medial biceps pulley on an MR arthrogram. Sagittal (*A*) and axial (*B*) T1-weighted MR arthrographic images with fat saturation depict (*A*) a partial-thickness SSC tendon tear (*asterisk*), intact medial biceps pulley (*arrowheads*), and (*B*) a medially subluxed LHBT (B). C, coracoid process; SST, supraspinatus.

recess was significantly greater in adhesive capsulitis cases.

Conservative management including nonsteroidal agents, gentle physiotherapy, and steroid injections are typically satisfactory in most cases. Cases unresponsive to conservative management may undergo surgical rotator interval release followed by manipulation under anesthesia.[49]

Subcoracoid Impingement

Subcoracoid impingement describes entrapment of the SSC tendon and muscle between the coracoid process and the lesser tuberosity,[87] and is primarily a clinical diagnosis of exclusion.[88] Subcoracoid impingement may be idiopathic, posttraumatic, associated with instability, iatrogenic in nature, or may be associated with chronic overuse with the shoulder forward flexed, adducted, and internally rotated.[89,90] Patients typically complain of dull anterior shoulder pain when the lesser tuberosity comes into contact with the coracoid process, accompanied by tenderness in the soft tissues surrounding the lesser tuberosity and coracoid process. Numerous imaging studies have attempted to define a coracohumeral interval distance that would indicate subcoracoid impingement. A reproducible cutoff measurement was not identified in some cadaveric[91] and static imaging studies,[92,93] whereas in other studies the measurements vary between 5.5 and 11 mm.[94–96] A dynamic mechanism with anterior instability being a contributing factor has been

suggested,[92,94] with ongoing debate regarding the optimal scanning position of the humerus.[97]

Injection of the subcoracoid region may serve for both diagnostic confirmation and therapeutic purposes.[49]

Some investigators have described subcoracoid impingement as a cause of rotator interval injury, including rotator interval tears.[69,98] Therefore, this diagnosis should be considered in patients with rotator interval tears, anterior superior rotator cuff injury, or biceps injury (**Box 2**).[49]

Biceps Pulley Lesions

The lateral aspect of the rotator interval is occupied by structures comprising the biceps pulley, therefore injury to this area is tantamount to a biceps pulley injury. The etiology and spectrum

---

Box 3
Pearls and pitfalls: MR imaging of LHBT pulley lesions

- Contrast extension from the joint over the lesser tuberosity indicates an LHBT pulley tear
- Tears of the leading edge of the SST tendon may involve the lateral component of the LHBT pulley
- Tears of the superior SSC tendon may be associated with tears of the medial component of the LHBT pulley

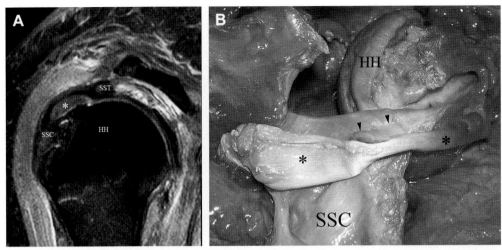

Fig. 23. Long head biceps tendinopathy proximal to the bicipital groove. Sagittal T2-weighted MR image with fat saturation (*A*) of a cadaveric shoulder specimen depicts (*A*) a thick LHBT (*asterisk*) with increased signal in the rotator interval with corresponding anatomic dissection (*B*) illustrating the focal LHBT thickening proximal to the bicipital pulley (*arrowheads*), which has been dissected and reflected with the SSC tendon off the humeral attachment. HH, humeral head; SSC, subscapularis; SST, supraspinatus. Asterisks indicate LHBT.

of injuries to this structure are similar to lesions in the rotator interval in general; however, it is often accompanied by LHBT abnormality and instability as well as rotator cuff tendon injury.[33,69] The clinical presentation is nonspecific, with prevailing symptoms typically a result of the accompanying LHBT and rotator cuff tendon lesions.[99]

Pulley lesions are not uncommon. In a large retrospective arthroscopic study of 1007 shoulders, Baumann and colleagues[100] reported a 7.1% incidence of pulley lesions. A strong association exists between pulley lesions and SST and SSC tendon tears,[36,37] named "anterior superior tears" by Bennett,[37] with rotator cuff tendon tears identified in 26.4% of cases with arthroscopically proven pulley tears.[100] This association is due to the close structural and functional relationship between structures in the anterior shoulder, and is best illustrated in the setting of anterior superior impingement syndrome.

Surgical repair of the LHBT pulley remains controversial. This approach has been largely abandoned, as the vast majority of symptomatic pulley lesions and biceps abnormalities have been addressed effectively with biceps tenodesis.[49] McClelland and colleagues[75] recently reported on 16 patients with a displaced LHBT in the setting of associated subscapularis tendon abnormality, and reported that long head biceps reduction and reconstruction of the biceps pulley offered no advantage over tenotomy or tenodesis alone.

Imaging of Biceps Pulley Lesions

Injury to the lateral rotator interval/biceps pulley may be difficult to identify at surgery and had been dubbed accordingly "hidden lesions" by Walch and colleagues,[36] highlighting the role of preoperative imaging. MR imaging characteristics

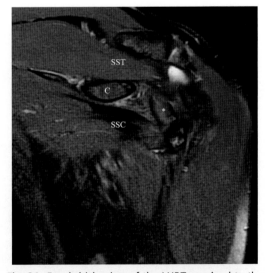

Fig. 24. Focal thickening of the LHBT proximal to the bicipital groove. Coronal oblique T2-weighted image with fat saturation depicts prominent focal thickening of the LHBT (*asterisk*) proximal to the bicipital groove.

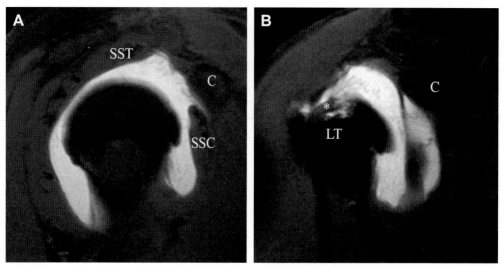

Fig. 25. Ruptured LHBT. Sagittal and coronal oblique T1-weighted MR arthrographic images with fat saturation depict an empty medial rotator interval (A) with the LHBT stump (asterisk) in the lateral rotator interval (B). C, coracoid process; LT, lesser tuberosity; SSC, subscapularis; SST, supraspinatus.

of biceps pulley lesions are similar to those of rotator interval lesions in general, and include contrast extravasation and abnormal signal on T2-weighted sequences.[101] More specific to pulley lesions is involvement of the superior SSC and anterior SST tendons adjacent to the lateral rotator interval as well as associated LHBT subluxation/dislocation.[37,101] MR arthrography is especially beneficial in identifying injury to the supporting structures of the biceps tendon, with contrast extending beyond the confines of the anterior joint capsule or along an exposed lesser tuberosity.[36,55,71] However, localizing discrete lesions to specific ligamentous components of the pulley is difficult even on MR arthrography,[11,99] especially in discerning a combined lesion to the medial pulley and SSC tendon from an isolated SSC (**Fig. 22**) or isolated medial pulley lesion (**Box 3**).

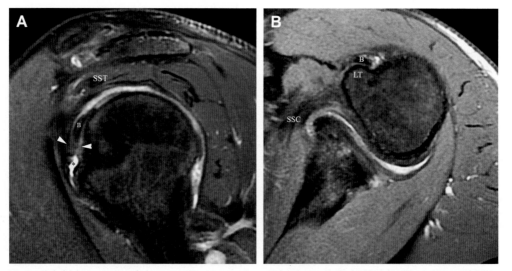

Fig. 26. Partial-thickness tear of the superior SSC tendon with intact medial biceps pulley on conventional MR imaging. Sagittal (A) and axial (B) T2-weighted images with fat saturation depict (A) a partial-thickness SSC tendon tear (asterisk), intact medial bicipital pulley (arrowheads), and (B) a medially subluxed LHBT (B). SSC, subscapularis; SST, supraspinatus.

Labral Tears, Rotator Interval Lesions, and Biceps Pulley Lesions

In a retrospective arthroscopic study by Bennett,[102] an association was noted between superior labrum anterior-posterior (SLAP) tears and medial biceps pulley injury. Forty-three percent of patients with SLAP tears had injury to the medial biceps pulley. Bennett hypothesized that the forces injuring the biceps anchor at the labral attachment may also injure the biceps pulley. This association was also noted in a separate retrospective arthroscopic study by Braun and colleagues,[103] who had also found a significant association between SLAP tears and posterolateral pulley tears. In anterior-inferior instability, rotator interval lesions may accompany Bankart lesions, whereas in posterior instability, reverse Bankart lesions and capsular laxity are a concern.[65] Although these associations have been contested,[104] it is important to seek out accompanying labral abnormality on imaging, as all these lesions should be addressed at surgery.[65]

LONG HEAD BICEPS TENDON PATHOLOGY

The LHBT has been shown to slide up to 18 mm in and out of the glenohumeral joint during forward

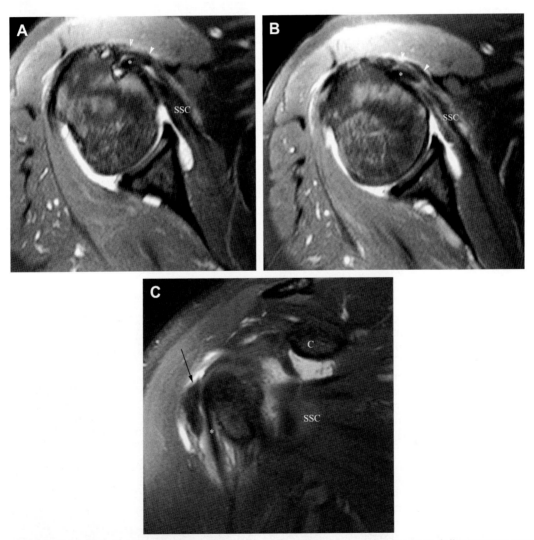

Fig. 27. Medial subluxation of the LHBT between the SSC tendon and the overlying capsuloligamentous structures. Axial T1-weighted MR arthrographic images with fat saturation (*A, B*) and coronal oblique T1-weighted MR arthrographic image with fat saturation depict (*A* inferior to *B*) a medially subluxed LHBT (*asterisk*) between the SSC tendon (SSC) and the overlying CHL and capsule (*arrowheads*), with (*C*) an associated tear (*arrow*) of the anterior aspect of the SST tendon. C, coracoid process.

flexion and internal rotation, and turns 30° to 40° as it exits the joint and thus is subjected to mechanical stress in the groove, at the pulley, and by rotator cuff abnormality.[33,105] These mechanical stresses coupled with a netlike pattern of sensory and sympathetic innervation of the LHBT, concentrated at the biceps tendon anchor, may explain why the LHBT is well recognized as a pain generator in the anterior shoulder.[106,107] The morphology of the bicipital groove may play a role in long head biceps pathology. Higher medial walls with smaller opening angles were found in patients with long head biceps abnormality in a radiographic and ultrasonographic study by Pfahler and colleagues[108]; however, this association was not confirmed in a later MR imaging study by Abboud and colleagues.[109]

Grauer and colleagues[45] described a continuum of the intra-articular long head biceps abnormality from the labrum to the rotator interval including tendinosis, rupture, instability, and pulley and SLAP lesions, a combination of these not being uncommon. There is a significant association between long head biceps tendinopathy, biceps pulley lesions, rotator cuff abnormality, and SLAP lesions.[53]

Intrinsic Tendon Degeneration

Tenosynovitis, tendinosis, delamination, prerupture, and rupture may represent the natural history of progressive degeneration of biceps.[23] Intratendinous ganglion cyst of the LHBT is an additional tendon lesion that has rarely been reported.[110] The mechanism of injury has been classified into 3 categories[111]: (1) impingement tendinopathy, described as impingement of the LHBT between the humeral head, acromion, and greater tuberosity; (2) tendinopathy with subluxation, which occurs with injury to the biceps pulley and supporting structures; and (3) attrition tendinopathy, also called primary tendinopathy, occurring because of new bone formation and adhesions in the bicipital groove, with resultant stenosis. The constrained path in the groove is also the underlying cause of long head biceps tenosynovitis, which is associated with fluid, adhesions, and hyperemia on arthroscopy.[108,112,113] Focal LHBT lesions may occur proximal to the groove (**Fig. 23**) or within the groove, as well as in a diffuse form involving both intra-articular and extra-articular tendon segments,[114] with the variable distribution likely relating to differences in the underlying mechanism.

There is a significant association between LHBT abnormality, impingement, and tears of the SSC and SST tendons. Macroscopic changes with an

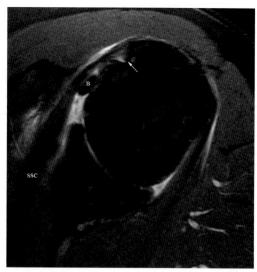

Fig. 28. Intra-articular LHBT dislocation. Axial T2-weighted image with fat saturation depicts an intra-articular dislocation of the LHBT (B). C, coracoid process; SSC, subscapularis. Arrow indicates bicipital groove.

increase in LHBT diameter have been noted on arthroscopic and cadaveric studies of rotator cuff tendon tears.[115–118] This increase in tendon diameter has been noted primarily at the entrance to the bicipital groove (**Fig. 24**)[117] and has been considered a compensatory mechanism against a degenerative process of the LHBT.[119,120] In some cases,

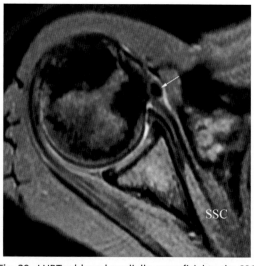

Fig. 29. LHBT subluxed medially, superficial to the SSC tendon. Axial T2-weighted image with fat saturation depicts dislocation of the LHBT (*arrow*) superficial to the SSC tendon.

a specific clinical syndrome named the hourglass biceps occurs. This syndrome includes pain and locking of the shoulder on elevation of the arm, and has been associated with focal thickening of the intra-articular LHBT in an hourglass configuration. The thickened LHBT is unable to slide into the bicipital groove on elevation, and causes pain and locking.[121]

Histologic examination of the intra-articular LHBT associated with rotator cuff tears reveals degeneration with disorganization of the fibrillar structures and proliferation of mucoid ground substance.[122] As the abnormality progresses, LHBT fibrillation, splits, hypertrophy, attenuation, and circumferential or longitudinal partial tendon tears may occur.[114] Often, hypertrophic tendons become encased in scar and adhere to the bicipital groove.[23]

Tendon Rupture

LHBT ruptures account for 96% of all biceps brachii injuries.[123] Spontaneous tendon ruptures are typically seen in patients older than 50 years and are associated with tendon degeneration (**Fig. 25**).[23,53,124]

Isolated Lesions of the Long Head Biceps Tendon

Isolated LHBT lesions are more common in a younger athletic population. The LHBT is subject to significant forces of acceleration and deceleration

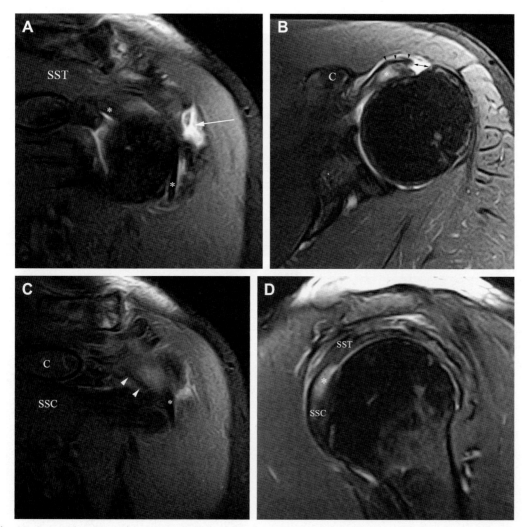

Fig. 30. Supraspinatus tendon tear extending to the lateral aspect of the LHBT pulley. Coronal oblique (*A, C*), axial (*B*), and sagittal (*D*) T2-weighted images with fat saturation depict (*A*) an SST tendon tear (*arrow*) extending (*B*) to the lateral aspect of the LHBT pulley (*double-headed arrow*), with (*C*) an intact medial LHBT pulley (*white arrowheads*) and a (*D*) surgically proven partial tear of the LHBT (*asterisk*). C, coracoid process; SSC, subscapularis; SST, supraspinatus. Black arrowheads indicate superior biceps pulley. Asterisks indicate LHBT.

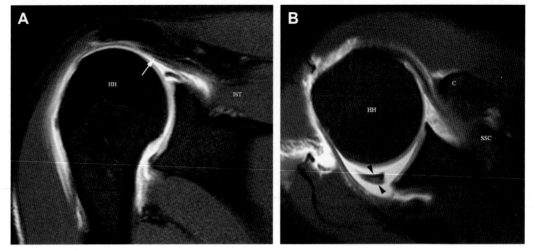

Fig. 31. Posterior dislocation of the LHBT with superior and posterior rotator cuff tendon tears. Coronal oblique (*A*) and axial (*B*) T1-weighted MR arthrographic images with fat saturation reveal an infraspinatus tendon tear (*arrow*) (supraspinatus tendon tear not shown) with posterior dislocation of the LHBT (*arrowheads*). C, coracoid process; HH, humeral head; IST, infraspinatus; SSC, subscapularis.

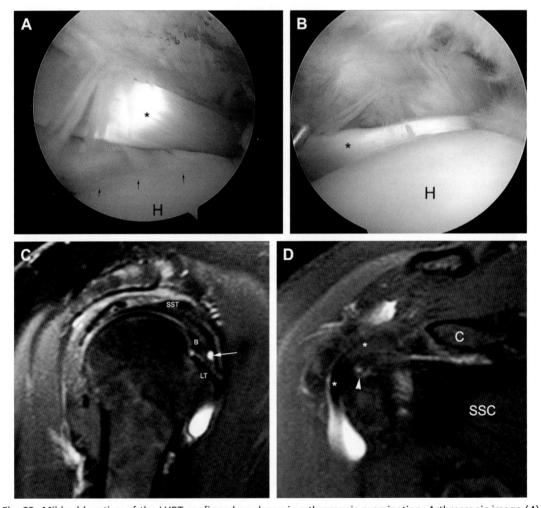

Fig. 32. Mild subluxation of the LHBT confirmed on dynamic arthroscopic examination. Arthroscopic image (*A*) depicts subtle chondral imprint (*arrows*) with mild medial subluxation of the LHBT (*asterisk*) on traction (*B*). Sagittal (*C*) and coronal oblique (*D*) T2-weighted images with fat saturation depict (*C*) a rotator interval lesion (*arrow*) and (*D*) a subchondral high T2 signal (*arrowhead*) in the area of the chondral imprint. LT, lesser tuberosity; H, humeral head. Asterisks indicate LHBT.

in throwing. Tenosynovitis, tears, instability, and SLAP lesions are all a potential consequence of these forces. Type 2 SLAP tears affect the long head biceps anchor, whereas type 4 SLAP tears extend into the tendon.[23]

Long Head Biceps Tendon Instability

Lesions involving the supporting structures of the intra-articular LHBT including the bicipital pulley and the adjacent rotator cuff tendons are associated with long head biceps instability. There are several classifications regarding patterns of LHBT instability based on the various patterns of injury to these supporting structures. Based on arthroscopic observations, Bennett[37] classified long head biceps instability into 5 types. Type 1 lesions have tears of the distal SSC tendon and an intact medial biceps pulley, with resultant increased motion of the LHBT within the sheath caused by deformity of the medial bicipital sheath wall (**Fig. 26**). Type 2 lesions have a tear involving the medial biceps pulley without a tear of the SSC tendon. These lesions result in medial subluxation of the LHBT between the SSC and the CHL/capsule (**Fig. 27**). Type 3 lesions have a combined tear of the medial biceps pulley and distal SSC tendon, resulting in medial dislocation of the LHBT including intra-articular dislocation (**Fig. 28**). Type 4 lesions have tears of the LCHL in the lateralmost part of the rotator interval, with resultant biceps dislocation superficial to the SSC tendon (**Fig. 29**). LCHL tears are often a consequence of tear propagation from the anterior aspect of the distal SST tendon (**Fig. 30**). Type 5 lesions include a complete tear of both the medial and lateral bicipital sheath with associated SSC and SST tendon tears.[125] Braun and colleagues[103] defined LHBT instability as anterior, posterior, or combined, and described associated biceps pulley tears as isolated anteromedial/medial tears, posterolateral/lateral tears, or combined tears. Anterior instability is associated with SSC tendon tears,[126] and posterior dislocation rarely occurs as a complication of glenohumeral dislocation when there is injury to the supporting lateral structures. This spectrum includes greater tuberosity fractures, disruption of the SST and infraspinatus tendons or subperiosteal stripping of the SST, and infraspinatus tendons from the bony attachment (**Fig. 31**).[127]

Long head biceps pulley lesions and instability are associated with variable intrinsic LHBT abnormality, and long-standing dislocations of the LHBT may scar to the SSC tendon and will not relocate spontaneously.[23,36,126,128]

DIAGNOSIS AND IMAGING OF LONG HEAD BICEPS TENDON LESIONS AND INSTABILITY

LHBT lesions or LHBT instability may be a difficult clinical diagnosis, as the symptoms are often nonspecific and include snapping, weakness, and anterior shoulder pain. On physical examination, LHBT pain is typically elicited by palpation over the bicipital groove or through provocation by performing a Speed or Yergason test.[65,107] A presumptive diagnosis of biceps tendon abnormality based on clinical examination is not infrequently made despite a lack of noticeable abnormality on arthroscopy.[107] Along similar lines, only 49% of macroscopically abnormal LHBT on histology was considered abnormal on arthroscopy.[129] Subtle long head biceps instability may also represent a diagnostic challenge on arthroscopy, and has been associated with focal chondromalacia near the bicipital groove. This type of chondromalacia has been named the biceps tendon footprint, which is also associated with rotator cuff tendon tears and long head biceps tenosynovitis (**Fig. 32**). This focal chondromalacia may be an indicator of subtle long head biceps chronic subluxation,[130,131] and potentially is the only arthroscopic sign of instability in cases where there is an injury to the deep fibers arising from the SSC tendon with overlying intact ligamentous components of the pulley.[131]

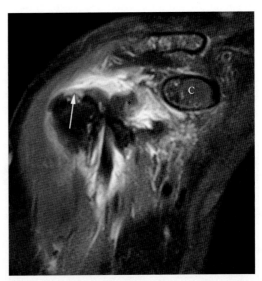

Fig. 33. Partial-thickness tears of the LHBT. Coronal oblique T2-weighted image with fat saturation depicts a thickened LHBT (*asterisk*) with an arthroscopically confirmed partial-thickness tendon tear and associated SST tendon tear (*arrow*). C, coracoid process.

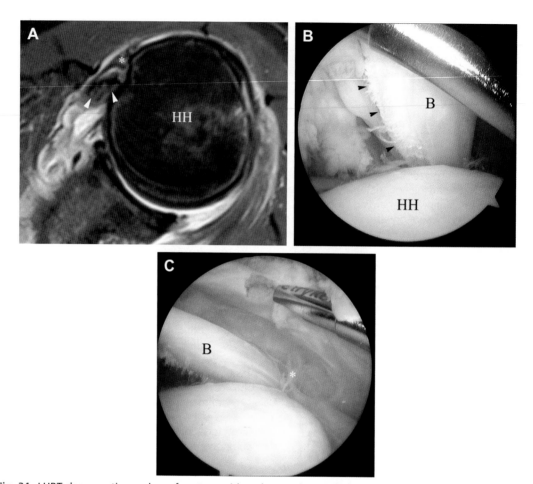

Fig. 34. LHBT degenerative undersurface tear with arthroscopic correlation. Axial T2-weighted image with fat saturation (*A*) and arthroscopic images (*B, C*) depict LHBT undersurface degenerative tear (*arrowheads*) with components of the lateral biceps pulley still intact (*asterisk*). B, LHBT; C, coracoid process; HH, humeral head; SSC, subscapularis.

At present, anterior shoulder pain with rotator cuff tear is a relative indication to remove the LHBT, with an effective treatment algorithm yet to be developed. Tenodesis and tenotomy are considered a simple and efficient treatment for both isolated long head biceps abnormality and combined lesions of the biceps labral complex and rotator cuff tendons; however, there is

Table 4	
MR imaging findings associated with long head biceps tendon abnormality	
Tendinosis and partial-thickness tendon tears	Tendon thickening, attenuation, contour irregularity, focal signal changes
Circumferential and longitudinal partial-thickness tears	Tendon caliber changes and intrasubstance high T2-weighted clefts
Complete LHBT rupture	Complete absence of the LHBT
LHBT dislocation	Empty bicipital groove
LHBT subluxation	LHBT medially perched on the lesser tuberosity Associated injury to the superior SSC and/or anterior SST tendons and the LHBT pulley Morphologic changes associated with tendinopathy

concern in this regard given the potential contribution of the LHBT to glenohumeral stability.[53]

The inconsistency between the clinical findings, histology and arthroscopic findings highlights the potential role of diagnostic imaging in diagnosing LHBT and concomitant lesions before surgical intervention.[36,55,71,107] The diagnostic challenge is compounded by a well-described complication of residual pain following biceps tenodesis that has been attributed to multiple factors,[132] understating the clinical difficulty in dealing with LHBT abnormality.

On MR imaging, sagittal and axial planes are the primary planes for visualizing the intra-articular and extra-articular LHBT while the coronal plane may be of value in cases of focal tendon changes proximal to the groove.[120] Tendon thickening or attenuation, contour irregularity, and focal signal changes have been described on MR imaging in association with tendinosis and partial tendon tears (**Figs. 33** and **34, Table 4**),[101,120] while abrupt changes in tendon caliber and intrasubstance high T2-weighted signal clefts indicate circumferential or longitudinal partial-thickness LHBT tears (**Figs. 35** and **36**).[114] Some of these changes may be subtle, posing a diagnostic imaging challenge.[101,120] Zanetti and colleagues[101] reported only moderate specificity and almost moderate interobserver agreement in assessing for long head biceps tendinopathy on MR arthrograms. This study used a 1.0-T scanner without fat saturation and, while acknowledging that their diagnostic capabilities have improved with the advance of MR technology, identifying subtle LHBT tendinosis and partial tendon tears remains a diagnostic challenge to the authors. A similar sentiment was

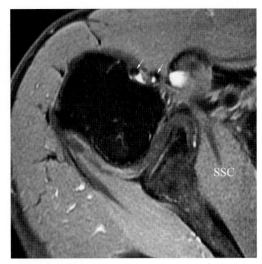

Fig. 36. LHBT longitudinal tear. Axial T2-weighted image with fat saturation depicts a longitudinal tear of the LHBT with one of the components subluxed medially (*arrows*). SSC, subscapularis.

conveyed in a more recent study by Gaskin and colleagues,[120] who had described focal tendon enlargement and signal abnormalities involving the LHBT just proximal to the groove, dubbed bicipital groove entrance lesions.

A complete absence of the LHBT is considered diagnostic of a complete rupture (see **Fig. 28**).[133] However, scar or debris formation have been shown to be a potential confounding factor in making this diagnosis on MR imaging.[101,114]

The imaging diagnosis of frank dislocation of the LHBT with permanent loss of contact between the LHBT and the bicipital groove[134] and with an empty bicipital groove is typically a straightforward diagnosis usually made on axial sequences. However, LHBT subluxation may prove more challenging; axial, coronal, and sagittal planes are contributory to the diagnosis,[55] with an LHBT medially perched on the lesser tuberosity, biceps pulley lesions, and adjacent rotator cuff tendon lesions suggestive of LHBT instability (see **Fig. 32; Fig. 37**).[55,135] Additional imaging findings associated with LHBT instability may include changes related to tendinopathy such as changes in tendon morphology and signal and fluid surrounding the tendon.[136] The authors' standard protocol does not include imaging of the shoulder in internal rotation. Although their clinical impression is that the modified Crass position used in ultrasonography may detect subtle LHBT instability, the authors believe that this position would be too difficult to maintain during the MR scan. However, the authors have found that subtle

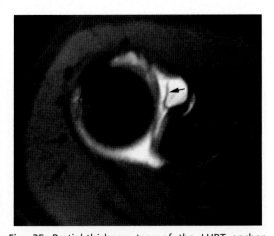

Fig. 35. Partial-thickness tear of the LHBT anchor. Axial T1-weighted MR arthrogram with fat saturation depict a longitudinal tear of the proximal LHBT (*arrow*).

254

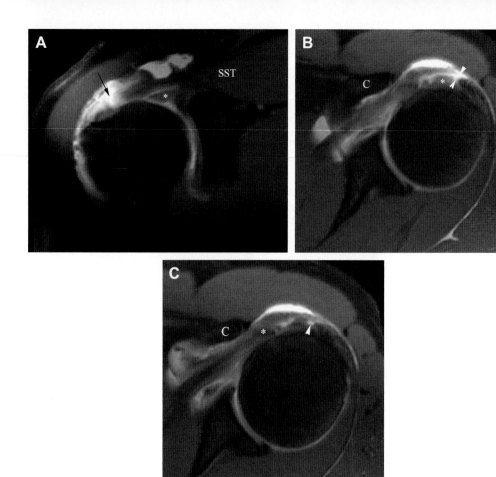

Fig. 37. SST tendon tear extending to involve the lateral portion of the pulley. Coronal oblique (*A*) and axial (*B, C*) T1-weighted MR arthrographic images with fat saturation depict a (*A*) focal full-thickness tear involving the anterior aspect of the SST tendon (*arrow*) extending (*B* superior to *C*) to the lateral aspect of the LHBT pulley (*arrowheads*) without frank LHBT (*asterisk*) dislocation. C, coracoid process; SST, supraspinatus.

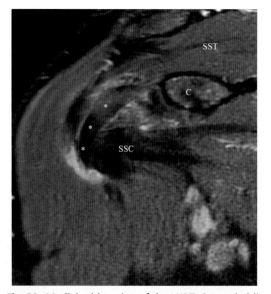

Fig. 38. Medial subluxation of the LHBT. Coronal oblique T2-weighted images with fat saturation depict a medially subluxed LHBT (*asterisks*). C, coracoid process; SSC, subscapularis; SST, supraspinatus.

delamination of the superior SSC tendon by a medially subluxed LHB tendon can be identified on sagittal sequences, and on coronal oblique images subtle subluxation may be identified by a change in the angle formed by the biceps as it enters the bicipital groove. This angle is typically abrupt, while in subluxation may assume a subtle curving course (**Fig. 38**). Subtle LHBT subluxation

Box 4
Pearls and pitfalls: MR imaging of LHBT lesions and instability

- LHBT tendinosis and partial-thickness tendon tears may be subtle and difficult to diagnose on MR imaging
- LHBT tendinosis and partial tears should be suspected in the context of LHBT subluxation or dislocation
- LHBT subluxation should be sought out in the presence of tears involving the superior SSC tendon or the leading edge of the SST tendon

Box 5
What the clinician needs to know

- Tenosynovitis or partial-thickness injury of the LHBT, particularly lesions or distal to the groove, which may not be immediately apparent on arthroscopy
- LHBT instability with associated injury to the subscapularis tendon
- Evidence of LHBT pulley injury suggesting LHBT instability
- Extension of rotator cuff tendon tears into the rotator interval
- SGHL or CHL injury or rotator interval lesions as an isolated finding or accompanying other capsulolabral insufficiency in the context of shoulder instability

may not be appreciated on the axial sequences because of volume averaging (**Box 4**).

SUMMARY

The rotator interval and LHBT have become the focus of much research and discussion as their role in shoulder dysfunction is revealed and optimal treatment options are debated. The role of diagnostic imaging, such as MR imaging, in the context of rotator interval lesions has grown accordingly, in an attempt to provide anatomic detail that may go undetected on clinical evaluation and arthroscopy. Rotator interval and LHBT lesions may be subtle on MR imaging, and require comprehension of rotator interval anatomy and familiarity with injury patterns. As the therapeutic approach advances, imaging may need to evolve as well, to provide more structural detail and possibly provide dynamic information as well (**Box 5**).

REFERENCES

1. Neer CS 2nd. Displaced proximal humeral fractures. I. Classification and evaluation. J Bone Joint Surg Am 1970;52(6):1077–89.
2. Merriam-Webster Inc. The Merriam-Webster dictionary. Springfield (MA): Merriam-Webster; 2005.
3. Cooper DE, O'Brien SJ, Warren RF. Supporting layers of the glenohumeral joint. An anatomic study. Clin Orthop Relat Res 1993;(289):144–55.
4. Fallon J, Blevins FT, Vogel K, et al. Functional morphology of the supraspinatus tendon. J Orthop Res 2002;20(5):920–6.
5. Kask K, Poldoja E, Lont T, et al. Anatomy of the superior glenohumeral ligament. J Shoulder Elbow Surg 2010;19(6):908–16.
6. Kolts I, Busch LC, Tomusk H, et al. Anatomy of the coracohumeral and coracoglenoidal ligaments. Ann Anat 2000;182(6):563–6.
7. Clark J, Sidles JA, Matsen FA. The relationship of the glenohumeral joint capsule to the rotator cuff. Clin Orthop Relat Res 1990;(254):29–34.
8. Cooper DE, O'Brien SJ, Arnoczky SP, et al. The structure and function of the coracohumeral ligament: an anatomic and microscopic study. J Shoulder Elbow Surg 1993;2(2):70–7.
9. Neer CS 2nd, Satterlee CC, Dalsey RM, et al. The anatomy and potential effects of contracture of the coracohumeral ligament. Clin Orthop Relat Res 1992;(280):182–5.
10. Werner A, Mueller T, Boehm D, et al. The stabilizing sling for the long head of the biceps tendon in the rotator cuff interval. A histoanatomic study. Am J Sports Med 2000;28(1):28–31.
11. Petchprapa CN, Beltran LS, Jazrawi LM, et al. The rotator interval: a review of anatomy, function, and normal and abnormal MRI appearance. AJR Am J Roentgenol 2010;195(3):567–76.
12. Jost B, Koch PP, Gerber C. Anatomy and functional aspects of the rotator interval. J Shoulder Elbow Surg 2000;9(4):336–41.
13. Burkart AC, Debski RE. Anatomy and function of the glenohumeral ligaments in anterior shoulder instability. Clin Orthop Relat Res 2002;(400):32–9.
14. Ferrari DA. Capsular ligaments of the shoulder. Anatomical and functional study of the anterior superior capsule. Am J Sports Med 1990;18(1):20–4.
15. Kolts I, Busch LC, Tomusk H, et al. Anatomical composition of the anterior shoulder joint capsule. A cadaver study on 12 glenohumeral joints. Ann Anat 2001;183(1):53–9.
16. Hunt SA, Kwon YW, Zuckerman JD. The rotator interval: anatomy, pathology, and strategies for treatment. J Am Acad Orthop Surg 2007;15(4):218–27.
17. Ide J, Maeda S, Takagi K. Normal variations of the glenohumeral ligament complex: an anatomic study for arthroscopic Bankart repair. Arthroscopy 2004;20(2):164–8.
18. Palmer WE, Brown JH, Rosenthal DI. Labral-ligamentous complex of the shoulder: evaluation with MR arthrography. Radiology 1994;190(3):645–51.
19. Turkel SJ, Panio MW, Marshall JL, et al. Stabilizing mechanisms preventing anterior dislocation of the glenohumeral joint. J Bone Joint Surg Am 1981;63(8):1208–17.
20. Clark JM, Harryman DT 2nd. Tendons, ligaments, and capsule of the rotator cuff. Gross and microscopic anatomy. J Bone Joint Surg Am 1992;74(5):713–25.
21. Vangsness CT Jr, Jorgenson SS, Watson T, et al. The origin of the long head of the biceps from the scapula and glenoid labrum. An anatomical study of 100 shoulders. J Bone Joint Surg Br 1994;76(6):951–4.

22. Arai R, Kobayashi M, Toda Y, et al. Fiber components of the shoulder superior labrum. Surg Radiol Anat 2012;34(1):49–56.

23. Ahrens PM, Boileau P. The long head of biceps and associated tendinopathy. J Bone Joint Surg Br 2007;89(8):1001–9.

24. Gheno R, Zoner CS, Buck FM, et al. Accessory head of biceps brachii muscle: anatomy, histology, and MRI in cadavers. AJR Am J Roentgenol 2010; 194(1):W80–3.

25. Warner JJ, Paletta GA, Warren RF. Accessory head of the biceps brachii. Case report demonstrating clinical relevance. Clin Orthop Relat Res 1992;(280):179–81.

26. Kim KC, Rhee KJ, Shin HD. A long head of the biceps tendon confluent with the intra-articular rotator cuff: arthroscopic and MR arthrographic findings. Arch Orthop Trauma Surg 2009;129(3):311–4.

27. Kim KC, Rhee KJ, Shin HD, et al. Biceps long head tendon revisited: a case report of split tendon arising from single origin. Arch Orthop Trauma Surg 2008;128(5):495–8.

28. Nakatani T, Tanaka S, Mizukami S. Bilateral four-headed biceps brachii muscles: the median nerve and brachial artery passing through a tunnel formed by a muscle slip from the accessory head. Clin Anat 1998;11(3):209–12.

29. Richards DP, Schwartz M. Anomalous intraarticular origin of the long head of biceps brachii. Clin J Sport Med 2003;13(2):122–4.

30. Hyman JL, Warren RF. Extra-articular origin of biceps brachii. Arthroscopy 2001;17(7):E29.

31. Dierickx C, Ceccarelli E, Conti M, et al. Variations of the intra-articular portion of the long head of the biceps tendon: a classification of embryologically explained variations. J Shoulder Elbow Surg 2009;18(4):556–65.

32. Slatis P, Aalto K. Medial dislocation of the tendon of the long head of the biceps brachii. Acta Orthop Scand 1979;50(1):73–7.

33. Habermeyer P, Magosch P, Pritsch M, et al. Antero-superior impingement of the shoulder as a result of pulley lesions: a prospective arthroscopic study. J Shoulder Elbow Surg 2004;13(1):5–12.

34. Schofield PM, Bowes RJ, Brooks N, et al. Exercise capacity and spontaneous heart rhythm after trans-venous fulguration of atrioventricular conduction. Br Heart J 1986;56(4):358–65.

35. Petersson CJ. Spontaneous medial dislocation of the tendon of the long biceps brachii. An anatomic study of prevalence and pathomechanics. Clin Orthop Relat Res 1986;(211):224–7.

36. Walch G, Nove-Josserand L, Levigne C, et al. Tears of the supraspinatus tendon associated with "hidden" lesions of the rotator interval. J Shoulder Elbow Surg 1994;3(6):353–60.

37. Bennett WF. Subscapularis, medial, and lateral head coracohumeral ligament insertion anatomy. Arthroscopic appearance and incidence of "hidden" rotator interval lesions. Arthroscopy 2001;17(2):173–80.

38. Arai R, Mochizuki T, Yamaguchi K, et al. Functional anatomy of the superior glenohumeral and coracohumeral ligaments and the subscapularis tendon in view of stabilization of the long head of the biceps tendon. J Shoulder Elbow Surg 2010;19(1):58–64.

39. Gleason PD, Beall DP, Sanders TG, et al. The transverse humeral ligament: a separate anatomical structure or a continuation of the osseous attachment of the rotator cuff? Am J Sports Med 2006; 34(1):72–7.

40. MacDonald K, Bridger J, Cash C, et al. Transverse humeral ligament: does it exist? Clin Anat 2007; 20(6):663–7.

41. Burkhart SS. Fluoroscopic comparison of kinematic patterns in massive rotator cuff tears. A suspension bridge model. Clin Orthop Relat Res 1992;(284): 144–52.

42. Basmajian JV, Bazant FJ. Factors preventing downward dislocation of the adducted shoulder joint. An electromyographic and morphological study. J Bone Joint Surg Am 1959;41:1182–6.

43. Harryman DT 2nd, Sidles JA, Harris SL, et al. The role of the rotator interval capsule in passive motion and stability of the shoulder. J Bone Joint Surg Am 1992;74(1):53–66.

44. Itoi E, Berglund LJ, Grabowski JJ, et al. Superior-inferior stability of the shoulder: role of the coracohumeral ligament and the rotator interval capsule. Mayo Clin Proc 1998;73(6):508–15.

45. Grauer JD, Paulos LE, Smutz WP. Biceps tendon and superior labral injuries. Arthroscopy 1992; 8(4):488–97.

46. Arai R, Sugaya H, Mochizuki T, et al. Subscapularis tendon tear: an anatomic and clinical investigation. Arthroscopy 2008;24(9):997–1004.

47. Kwon YW, Hurd J, Yeager K, et al. Proximal biceps tendon—a biomechanical analysis of the stability at the bicipital groove. Bull NYU Hosp Jt Dis 2009; 67(4):337–40.

48. Glousman R, Jobe F, Tibone J, et al. Dynamic electromyographic analysis of the throwing shoulder with glenohumeral instability. J Bone Joint Surg Am 1988;70(2):220–6.

49. Gaskill TR, Braun S, Millett PJ. The rotator interval: pathology and management. Arthroscopy 2011; 27(4):556–67.

50. Rodosky MW, Harner CD, Fu FH. The role of the long head of the biceps muscle and superior glenoid labrum in anterior stability of the shoulder. Am J Sports Med 1994;22(1):121–30.

51. Warner JJ, McMahon PJ. The role of the long head of the biceps brachii in superior stability of the glenohumeral joint. J Bone Joint Surg Am 1995;77(3): 366–72.

52. Kido T, Itoi E, Konno N, et al. The depressor function of biceps on the head of the humerus in shoulders with tears of the rotator cuff. J Bone Joint Surg Br 2000;82(3):416–9.

53. Elser F, Braun S, Dewing CB, et al. Anatomy, function, injuries, and treatment of the long head of the biceps brachii tendon. Arthroscopy 2011;27(4):581–92.

54. Bigliani LU, Kelkar R, Flatow EL, et al. Glenohumeral stability. Biomechanical properties of passive and active stabilizers. Clin Orthop Relat Res 1996;(330):13–30.

55. Morag Y, Jacobson JA, Shields G, et al. MR arthrography of rotator interval, long head of the biceps brachii, and biceps pulley of the shoulder. Radiology 2005;235(1):21–30.

56. Sofka CM, Ciavarra GA, Hannafin JA, et al. Magnetic resonance imaging of adhesive capsulitis: correlation with clinical staging. HSS J 2008; 4(2):164–9.

57. Mengiardi B, Pfirrmann CW, Gerber C, et al. Frozen shoulder: MR arthrographic findings. Radiology 2004;233(2):486–92.

58. Carrillon Y, Noel E, Fantino O, et al. Magnetic resonance imaging findings in idiopathic adhesive capsulitis of the shoulder. Rev Rhum Engl Ed 1999; 66(4):201–6.

59. Depelteau H, Bureau NJ, Cardinal E, et al. Arthrography of the shoulder: a simple fluoroscopically guided approach for targeting the rotator cuff interval. AJR Am J Roentgenol 2004;182(2):329–32.

60. Chung CB, Dwek JR, Cho GJ, et al. Rotator cuff interval: evaluation with MR imaging and MR arthrography of the shoulder in 32 cadavers. J Comput Assist Tomogr 2000;24(5):738–43.

61. Kim KC, Rhee KJ, Shin HD, et al. Estimating the dimensions of the rotator interval with use of magnetic resonance arthrography. J Bone Joint Surg Am 2007;89(11):2450–5.

62. Lee JC, Guy S, Connell D, et al. MRI of the rotator interval of the shoulder. Clin Radiol 2007;62(5): 416–23.

63. Neer CS 2nd, Foster CR. Inferior capsular shift for involuntary inferior and multidirectional instability of the shoulder. A preliminary report. J Bone Joint Surg Am 1980;62(6):897–908.

64. Rowe CR, Zarins B. Recurrent transient subluxation of the shoulder. J Bone Joint Surg Am 1981;63(6): 863–72.

65. Fitzpatrick MJ, Powell SE, Tibone JE, et al. The anatomy, pathology, and definitive treatment of rotator interval lesions: current concepts. Arthroscopy 2003;19(Suppl 1):70–9.

66. Cole BJ, Rodeo SA, O'Brien SJ, et al. The anatomy and histology of the rotator interval capsule of the shoulder. Clin Orthop Relat Res 2001;(390):129–37.

67. Nobuhara K, Ikeda H. Rotator interval lesion. Clin Orthop Relat Res 1987;(223):44–50.

68. Field LD, Warren RF, O'Brien SJ, et al. Isolated closure of rotator interval defects for shoulder instability. Am J Sports Med 1995;23(5):557–63.

69. Le Huec JC, Schaeverbeke T, Moinard M, et al. Traumatic tear of the rotator interval. J Shoulder Elbow Surg 1996;5(1):41–6.

70. Tung GA, Hou DD. MR arthrography of the posterior labrocapsular complex: relationship with glenohumeral joint alignment and clinical posterior instability. AJR Am J Roentgenol 2003;180(2):369–75.

71. Vinson EN, Major NM, Higgins LD. Magnetic resonance imaging findings associated with surgically proven rotator interval lesions. Skeletal Radiol 2007;36(5):405–10.

72. Grainger AJ, Tirman PF, Elliott JM, et al. MR anatomy of the subcoracoid bursa and the association of subcoracoid effusion with tears of the anterior rotator cuff and the rotator interval. AJR Am J Roentgenol 2000;174(5):1377–80.

73. Bigoni BJ, Chung CB. MR imaging of the rotator cuff interval. Magn Reson Imaging Clin N Am 2004;12(1):61–73, vi.

74. Ho CP. MR imaging of rotator interval, long biceps, and associated injuries in the overhead-throwing athlete. Magn Reson Imaging Clin N Am 1999; 7(1):23–37.

75. McClelland D, Bell SN, O'Leary S. Relocation of a dislocated long head of biceps tendon is no better than biceps tenodesis. Acta Orthop Belg 2009;75(5):595–8.

76. Hsu YC, Pan RY, Shih YY, et al. Superior-capsular elongation and its significance in atraumatic posteroinferior multidirectional shoulder instability in magnetic resonance arthrography. Acta Radiol 2010;51(3):302–8.

77. Provencher MT, Dewing CB, Bell SJ, et al. An analysis of the rotator interval in patients with anterior, posterior, and multidirectional shoulder instability. Arthroscopy 2008;24(8):921–9.

78. Tetro AM, Bauer G, Hollstien SB, et al. Arthroscopic release of the rotator interval and coracohumeral ligament: an anatomic study in cadavers. Arthroscopy 2002;18(2):145–50.

79. Lefevre-Colau MM, Drape JL, Fayad F, et al. Magnetic resonance imaging of shoulders with idiopathic adhesive capsulitis: reliability of measures. Eur Radiol 2005;15(12):2415–22.

80. Ozaki J, Nakagawa Y, Sakurai G, et al. Recalcitrant chronic adhesive capsulitis of the shoulder. Role of contracture of the coracohumeral ligament and rotator interval in pathogenesis and treatment. J Bone Joint Surg Am 1989;71(10):1511–5.

81. Hannafin JA, Chiaia TA. Adhesive capsulitis. A treatment approach. Clin Orthop Relat Res 2000;(372):95–109.

82. Tamai K, Yamato M. Abnormal synovium in the frozen shoulder: a preliminary report with dynamic

magnetic resonance imaging. J Shoulder Elbow Surg 1997;6(6):534–43.

83. Gokalp G, Algin O, Yildirim N, et al. Adhesive capsulitis: contrast-enhanced shoulder MRI findings. J Med Imaging Radiat Oncol 2011;55(2):119–25.

84. Connell D, Padmanabhan R, Buchbinder R. Adhesive capsulitis: role of MR imaging in differential diagnosis. Eur Radiol 2002;12(8):2100–6.

85. Lee MH, Ahn JM, Muhle C, et al. Adhesive capsulitis of the shoulder: diagnosis using magnetic resonance arthrography, with arthroscopic findings as the standard. J Comput Assist Tomogr 2003;27(6):901–6.

86. Kim KC, Rhee KJ, Shin HD. Adhesive capsulitis of the shoulder: dimensions of the rotator interval measured with magnetic resonance arthrography. J Shoulder Elbow Surg 2009;18(3):437–42.

87. Lo IK, Parten PM, Burkhart SS. Combined subcoracoid and subacromial impingement in association with anterosuperior rotator cuff tears: an arthroscopic approach. Arthroscopy 2003;19(10):1068–78.

88. Dines DM, Warren RF, Inglis AE, et al. The coracoid impingement syndrome. J Bone Joint Surg Br 1990;72(2):314–6.

89. Gerber C, Terrier F, Ganz R. The role of the coracoid process in the chronic impingement syndrome. J Bone Joint Surg Br 1985;67(5):703–8.

90. Renoux S, Monet J, Pupin P, et al. Preliminary note on biometric data relating to the human coracoacromial arch. Surg Radiol Anat 1986;8(3):189–95.

91. Radas CB, Pieper HG. The coracoid impingement of the subscapularis tendon: a cadaver study. J Shoulder Elbow Surg 2004;13(2):154–9.

92. MacMahon PJ, Taylor DH, Duke D, et al. Contribution of full-thickness supraspinatus tendon tears to acquired subcoracoid impingement. Clin Radiol 2007;62(6):556–63.

93. Bergin D, Parker L, Zoga A, et al. Abnormalities on MRI of the subscapularis tendon in the presence of a full-thickness supraspinatus tendon tear. AJR Am J Roentgenol 2006;186(2):454–9.

94. Bonutti PM, Norfray JF, Friedman RJ, et al. Kinematic MRI of the shoulder. J Comput Assist Tomogr 1993;17(4):666–9.

95. Friedman RJ, Bonutti PM, Genez B. Cine magnetic resonance imaging of the subcoracoid region. Orthopedics 1998;21(5):545–8.

96. Giaroli EL, Major NM, Lemley DE, et al. Coracohumeral interval imaging in subcoracoid impingement syndrome on MRI. AJR Am J Roentgenol 2006;186(1):242–6.

97. Beall DP, Morag Y, Ly JQ, et al. Magnetic resonance imaging of the rotator cuff interval. Semin Musculoskelet Radiol 2006;10(3):187–96.

98. Dumontier C, Sautet A, Gagey O, et al. Rotator interval lesions and their relation to coracoid impingement syndrome. J Shoulder Elbow Surg 1999;8(2):130–5.

99. Weishaupt D, Zanetti M, Tanner A, et al. Lesions of the reflection pulley of the long biceps tendon. MR arthrographic findings. Invest Radiol 1999;34(7):463–9.

100. Baumann B, Genning K, Bohm D, et al. Arthroscopic prevalence of pulley lesions in 1007 consecutive patients. J Shoulder Elbow Surg 2008;17(1):14–20.

101. Zanetti M, Weishaupt D, Gerber C, et al. Tendinopathy and rupture of the tendon of the long head of the biceps brachii muscle: evaluation with MR arthrography. AJR Am J Roentgenol 1998;170(6):1557–61.

102. Bennett WF. Correlation of the SLAP lesion with lesions of the medial sheath of the biceps tendon and intra-articular subscapularis tendon. Indian J Orthop 2009;43(4):342–6.

103. Braun S, Horan MP, Elser F, et al. Lesions of the biceps pulley. Am J Sports Med 2011;39(4):790–5.

104. Patzer T, Kircher J, Lichtenberg S, et al. Is there an association between SLAP lesions and biceps pulley lesions? Arthroscopy 2011;27(5):611–8.

105. Braun S, Millett PJ, Yongpravat C, et al. Biomechanical evaluation of shear force vectors leading to injury of the biceps reflection pulley: a biplane fluoroscopy study on cadaveric shoulders. Am J Sports Med 2010;38(5):1015–24.

106. Alpantaki K, McLaughlin D, Karagogeos D, et al. Sympathetic and sensory neural elements in the tendon of the long head of the biceps. J Bone Joint Surg Am 2005;87(7):1580–3.

107. Singaraju VM, Kang RW, Yanke AB, et al. Biceps tendinitis in chronic rotator cuff tears: a histologic perspective. J Shoulder Elbow Surg 2008;17(6):898–904.

108. Pfahler M, Branner S, Refior HJ. The role of the bicipital groove in tendinopathy of the long biceps tendon. J Shoulder Elbow Surg 1999;8(5):419–24.

109. Abboud JA, Bartolozzi AR, Widmer BJ, et al. Bicipital groove morphology on MRI has no correlation to intra-articular biceps tendon pathology. J Shoulder Elbow Surg 2010;19(6):790–4.

110. Rutten MJ, de Jong MD, van Loon T, et al. Intratendinous ganglion of the long head of the biceps tendon: US and MRI features (2010: 9b). Intratendinous ganglion. Eur Radiol 2010;20(12):2997–3001.

111. Burkhead WZ Jr. The biceps tendon. In: Matsen FA, editor. The shoulder. 3rd edition. Philadelphia: Saunders; 1990. p. 791–836.

112. Post M, Benca P. Primary tendinitis of the long head of the biceps. Clin Orthop Relat Res 1989;(246):117–25.

113. Neviaser TJ. Arthroscopy of the shoulder. Orthop Clin North Am 1987;18(3):361–72.

114. Tuckman GA. Abnormalities of the long head of the biceps tendon of the shoulder: MR imaging findings. AJR Am J Roentgenol 1994;163(5):1183–8.

115. Neer CS 2nd. Anterior acromioplasty for the chronic impingement syndrome in the shoulder: a preliminary report. J Bone Joint Surg Am 1972; 54(1):41–50.

116. Chen CH, Hsu KY, Chen WJ, et al. Incidence and severity of biceps long head tendon lesion in patients with complete rotator cuff tears. J Trauma 2005;58(6):1189–93.

117. Toshiaki A, Itoi E, Minagawa H, et al. Cross-sectional area of the tendon and the muscle of the biceps brachii in shoulders with rotator cuff tears: a study of 14 cadaveric shoulders. Acta Orthop 2005;76(4):509–12.

118. Beall DP, Williamson EE, Ly JQ, et al. Association of biceps tendon tears with rotator cuff abnormalities: degree of correlation with tears of the anterior and superior portions of the rotator cuff. AJR Am J Roentgenol 2003;180(3):633–9.

119. Sakurai G, Ozaki J, Tomita Y, et al. Morphologic changes in long head of biceps brachii in rotator cuff dysfunction. J Orthop Sci 1998;3(3): 137–42.

120. Gaskin CM, Anderson MW, Choudhri A, et al. Focal partial tears of the long head of the biceps brachii tendon at the entrance to the bicipital groove: MR imaging findings, surgical correlation, and clinical significance. Skeletal Radiol 2009; 38(10):959–65.

121. Boileau P, Ahrens PM, Hatzidakis AM. Entrapment of the long head of the biceps tendon: the hourglass biceps—a cause of pain and locking of the shoulder. J Shoulder Elbow Surg 2004;13(3): 249–57.

122. Joseph M, Maresh CM, McCarthy MB, et al. Histological and molecular analysis of the biceps tendon long head post-tenotomy. J Orthop Res 2009; 27(10):1379–85.

123. Carter AN, Erickson SM. Proximal biceps tendon rupture: primarily an injury of middle age. Phys Sportsmed 1999;27(6):95–101.

124. Warren RF. Lesions of the long head of the biceps tendon. Instr Course Lect 1985;34:204–9.

125. Bennett WF. Arthroscopic bicipital sheath repair: two-year follow-up with pulley lesions. Arthroscopy 2004;20(9):964–73.

126. Lafosse L, Reiland Y, Baier GP, et al. Anterior and posterior instability of the long head of the biceps tendon in rotator cuff tears: a new classification based on arthroscopic observations. Arthroscopy 2007;23(1):73–80.

127. Mullaney PJ, Bleakney R, Tuchscherer P, et al. Posterior dislocation of the long head of biceps tendon: case report and review of the literature. Skeletal Radiol 2007;36(8):779–83.

128. Werner A, Ilg A, Schmitz H, et al. Tendinitis of the long head of biceps tendon associated with lesions of the "biceps reflection pulley". Sportverletz Sportschaden 2003;17(2):75–9 [in German].

129. Murthi AM, Vosburgh CL, Neviaser TJ. The incidence of pathologic changes of the long head of the biceps tendon. J Shoulder Elbow Surg 2000;9(5):382–5.

130. Sistermann R. The biceps tendon footprint. Acta Orthop 2005;76(2):237–40.

131. Castagna A, Mouhsine E, Conti M, et al. Chondral print on humeral head: an indirect sign of long head biceps tendon instability. Knee Surg Sports Traumatol Arthrosc 2007;15(5):645–8.

132. Sanders B, Lavery KP, Pennington S, et al. Clinical success of biceps tenodesis with and without release of the transverse humeral ligament. J Shoulder Elbow Surg 2012;21(1):66–71.

133. van Leersum M, Schweitzer ME. Magnetic resonance imaging of the biceps complex. Magn Reson Imaging Clin N Am 1993;1(1):77–86.

134. Walch G, Nove-Josserand L, Boileau P, et al. Subluxations and dislocations of the tendon of the long head of the biceps. J Shoulder Elbow Surg 1998;7(2):100–8.

135. Spritzer CE, Collins AJ, Cooperman A, et al. Assessment of instability of the long head of the biceps tendon by MRI. Skeletal Radiol 2001;30(4):199–207.

136. Nakata W, Katou S, Fujita A, et al. Biceps pulley: normal anatomy and associated lesions at MR arthrography. Radiographics 2011;31(3):791–810.

The Throwing Shoulder: the Orthopedist Perspective

Randy M. Cohn, MD[a], Laith M. Jazrawi, MD[b],*

KEYWORDS

- Throwing • Overhead athlete • Shoulder • SLAP tears
- Rotator cuff

The throwing athlete provides a unique challenge to the orthopedic surgeon. A repetitive overhead throwing motion places high forces on the shoulder, predisposing these athletes to injuries in the glenohumeral region. Although the baseball pitcher is often thought of as the prototypical throwing athlete, the pathologic conditions of the throwing shoulder can be seen in football quarterbacks, javelin throwers, handball players, and many other athletes who are involved in repetitive overhead throwing, as well as in athletes who participate in nonthrowing sports that include repetitive overhead motion, such as tennis and swimming. In the United States, there are almost 2.3 million participants in Little League baseball,[1] approximately 500,000 student athletes playing high school baseball,[2] more than 27,000 collegiate baseball players,[3] and millions of adults playing recreational baseball annually. As a result, pathology of the throwing shoulder is common in orthopedic practice and not just limited to high-level professional athletes.

KINEMATICS AND BIOMECHANICS OF THROWING

The act of throwing involves coordination of motion that begins in the toes and ends in the fingertips, a sequence of events described as the kinetic chain.[4] Coordinated sequential muscle activation is essential for energy transfer from the lower extremities and trunk to the upper extremity resulting in projectile release.[5] Any disruption or physical condition that alters the kinetic chain can affect the shoulder and predispose a throwing athlete to shoulder dysfunction.[4]

The throwing motion, as typified by the baseball pitcher, can be divided into 6 phases: windup, early cocking, late cocking, acceleration, deceleration, and follow-through (**Fig. 1**).[6,7] During windup, minimal stress is placed on the shoulder as the arm is brought into a position of slight abduction and minimal internal rotation.[8] In early cocking, the shoulder is brought into a position of 90° abduction. This phase is marked by deltoid activation at the initiation of early cocking and activation of the supraspinatus, infraspinatus, and teres minor late in the phase. In the late cocking phase, the shoulder is brought into a position of maximal external rotation. Shoulder abduction is maintained at approximately 90°, and the scapula retracts to facilitate this position. This combination of abduction and external rotation causes a posterior translation of the humeral head on the glenoid.[9] Supraspinatus, infraspinatus, and teres minor activation reaches maximum at the

The authors received no funding to support this article.

The authors have nothing to disclose.

[a] Orthopaedic Surgery, New York University Hospital for Joint Diseases, 301 East 17th Street, Suite 1402, New York, NY 10016, USA

[b] Division of Sports Medicine, New York University Hospital for Joint Diseases, 301 East 17th Street, Suite 1402, New York, NY 10016, USA

* Corresponding author.

E-mail address: laith.jazrawi@nyumc.org

Magn Reson Imaging Clin N Am 20 (2012) 261–275

doi:10.1016/j.mric.2012.01.001

A

B

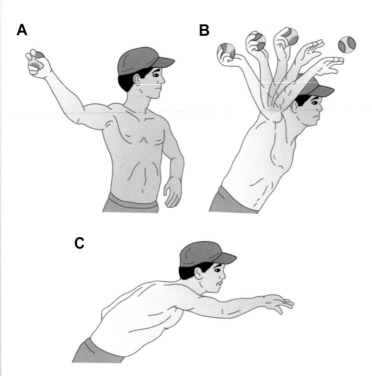

C

Fig. 1. The phases of the pitching cycle include (A) wind-up/cocking phases, (B) acceleration phase, and (C) follow-through phase. (*From* Delee JC, Drez D Jr, Miller MD. Orthopaedic sports medicine: practices and principles. 3rd edition. Philadelphia: Elsevier; 2010; with permission.)

midportion of this phase, followed by activation of the subscapularis muscle toward the end of late cocking. Rotation of the torso results in a shear force across the anterior shoulder of 400 N and a compressive force of 650 N.[8] In the acceleration phase, the shoulder internally rotates at velocities greater than 7000 degrees per second, culminating in release of the projectile. Deceleration is the most violent phase of the throwing cycle because contraction of all muscle groups is necessary to slow arm rotation. Loads on the shoulder joint are highest in this phase, with posterior sheer forces of 400 N, inferior shear forces of 300 N, and compression greater than 1000 N.[8,9] In the follow-through phase, muscle firing returns to resting levels and loads at the shoulder joint decrease.[10,11] This entire process is completed in less than 2 seconds.[8]

Similar motions and stresses occur in the shoulder of other overhead athletes. For the football quarterback, the phases of throwing are similar, but the added weight of the football seems to affect the shoulder position and stresses in all phases. Quarterbacks achieve maximal external rotation earlier in the throwing cycle to allow for more time for acceleration during internal rotation. In addition, the quarterback has increased elbow flexion and horizontal abduction of the arm during late cocking to decrease the length of the lever arm, decreasing the impact of the heavier football.

This position lessens the loads placed on the shoulder and may account for the lower incidence of shoulder injuries in this population compared with baseball pitchers.[8] In contrast to baseball pitchers, most shoulder injuries in football quarterbacks are due to direct trauma, as opposed to overuse injuries from the throwing motion.[12] The tennis serve also uses a motion pattern and muscle function that are very similar to the baseball pitch. In the overhead serve, there is similar cocking, acceleration, and follow-through phases, which place maximum stress on the soft tissues about the shoulder.[13] In swimming, the arm provides a sustained drive for propulsion through the water. The pull phase is equivalent to the acceleration phase of throwing; however, the pull is slower and less stressful. The recovery phase is a period of rapid repositioning, which is equivalent to the cocking phase in the throwing athlete.[14]

SHOULDER ANATOMY AND ADAPTATIONS IN THROWERS

The repetitive throwing motion may result in bony and soft tissue adaptations that affect the stability and mobility of the glenohumeral joint.[4] In the non-thrower, the combined internal and external rotation with the arm in 90° of abduction approaches 180°.[15] In repetitive throwing athletes, this arc of motion is shifted posteriorly, with an increase in the external rotation of 9° to 16° with a subsequent decrease in internal rotation with the arm in 90° abduction.[8,16,17] This alteration in mobility may be due to increased humeral head retroversion in the throwing athlete, defined as the acute angle in a medial and posterior direction between the axis of the elbow joint and the axis through the center of the humeral head.[18] Increases in humeral retroversion allow the articulating surfaces of the humeral head and glenoid to remain in contact as the shoulder externally rotates during the cocking phases of the throwing motion, allowing a greater degree of external rotation before the shoulder is constrained by the anterior capsule.[19] An increase in the bone mineral density in the throwing arm of athletes has also been described.[20]

Soft tissue changes also occur about the throwing shoulder in overhead athletes. Increased laxity, as shown by the presence of a sulcus sign, has been seen in overhead throwing athletes.[8] The sulcus sign is defined as a dimpling of the skin underneath the acromion with inferior traction on the arm.[4,21] A positive sulcus sign may be due to laxity of coracohumeral ligament and rotator interval structures, which restrain external rotation.[4,16] Increased external rotation may also result from microtears in the anteroinferior glenohumeral ligament, resulting in increased capsular laxity.[4] This can be seen by an increase in anterior glenohumeral translation with the shoulder in abducted and externally rotated position.[8] In addition, increased posterior laxity has been seen in the shoulders of throwing athletes.[18] Generalized hypertrophy of the shoulder girdle musculature, including the anterior and posterior chest wall muscles, is also seen in high-level throwing athletes.[8] Adaptations in rotator cuff strength also occur, including greater internal rotation strength in the throwing arm compared with the contralateral upper extremity.[18,22] External rotation strength has been found to be equivalent between the throwing and nonthrowing arm in most studies,[18,22] although 2 studies have found a decrease in external rotation strength in the throwing arm.[23,24] According to clinical recommendations, the strength of external rotators should be between 66% and 75% of internal rotators to minimize injury to the glenohumeral joint.[24,25]

EVALUATION OF THE THROWING SHOULDER

Evaluation of the throwing athlete begins with a comprehensive history taking, starting with the onset of symptoms and the inciting event. Location, quality, and duration of pain and symptoms are essential in determining the cause of the injury process. The physician should ask at what point in the throwing cycle does pain occur and what type of pitches exacerbate symptoms (velocity, number of pitches). Equally important is a comprehensive history of prior shoulder problems and treatments, as well as other injuries along the kinetic chain. In addition, the physician should ask about other activities that exacerbate pain as well as interventions that improve symptoms.[26]

A thorough physical examination is essential when evaluating the injured throwing athlete. Examination should begin with observation of the athlete for posture and symmetry in the standing position. The neck should be assessed for range of motion and strength because pain from neck and cervical spinal problems can radiate to the shoulder. Significant bony landmarks should be palpated, including the cervical spine, acromioclavicular joint, coracoid process, biceps tendon, greater tuberosity, and glenohumeral joint. Range of motion should be assessed with the athlete in the sitting and standing positions, including forward elevation in the plane of the scapula as well as internal and external rotation at 0° and 90° abduction. Scapulothoracic motion should be also observed because this is an important contributor to glenohumeral motion. Manual strength testing of internal rotation, external rotation, and abduction should be compared with the contralateral shoulder to assess for weakness.[26]

Stability testing is essential to assess for anterior, posterior, inferior, and multidirectional laxity. Various tests have been described to assess for anteroposterior glenohumeral translation, with the shoulder in varying positions of abduction and rotation. Classification of anteroposterior translation is based on the scale proposed by Altchek and colleagues[27,28]: 1+, increased translation compared with the contralateral shoulder but inability to bring the humeral head passed the glenoid rim; 2+, translation occurs when the humeral head can be subluxed over the glenoid rim; 3+, translation is the ability to lock the humeral head over the glenoid rim. During stability testing, it is essential to assess for a reproduction of symptoms and pain in addition to the humeral head translation.

Specialized tests to assess for various pathophysiologic entities should be performed to narrow the differential diagnosis and direct radiologic evaluation.[26,29–31] The tests by Hawkins and Kennedy[29] and Neer[30] should be performed to assess for subacromial impingement. Anterior, posterior, and multidirectional instability should be graded with tests such as the anterior drawer, Jobe relocation test, and sulcus sign.[25] The O'Brien active compression test should be performed to evaluate for possible superior labral anterior posterior (SLAP) lesions, although this test result can also be positive with biceps tendonitis and acromioclavicular problems. The Speed and Yergason tests are performed to identify possible biceps tendonitis, and the cross-arm adduction test is used to assess acromioclavicular joint pathology.[32] Plain radiographs routinely obtained to assess the shoulder of the throwing athlete include anteroposterior views in internal and external rotation, axillary view, Stryker notch view, and an outlet view. Higher-level imaging, including computed tomographic (CT) scan, magnetic resonance (MR) imaging, and MR arthrography, are recommended to assess for specific pathologic entities and are subsequently discussed.

PATHOLOGIC CONDITIONS COMMON IN THROWING ATHLETES
Anterior Instability

Laxity is defined as the passive motion of a joint in a given direction, and excessive laxity can be physiologic or pathologic in the throwing athlete.[4] The term shoulder instability refers to the sensation of the humeral head moving excessively in relation to the glenoid. Although frank instability is less common in the throwing athlete, throwing athletes may have acquired laxity as a result of the repetitive throwing motion. Although some laxity is necessary for throwing athletes to perform at the highest levels, excessive laxity can lead to pathologic conditions in the shoulder.[4] However, the term instability is often used to describe the acquired laxity that occurs in throwing athletes.

During the throwing motion, the position of abduction and maximal external rotation during late cocking places stress on the anterior shoulder structures. Repetitive microtrauma can result in stretching of the capsule and ligamentous structures, resulting in anterior translation of the humeral head on the glenoid. In addition, stretch and eccentric muscle contraction during the throwing motion can cause microtears that can destabilize the anterior shoulder muscles, compounding anterior instability.[7,8] As the anterior capsule fails, there is further anterior translation of the humeral head during the most stressful phases of the throwing cycle.[8] As the humeral head translates anteriorly, the greater tuberosity of the humeral head can contact the posterosuperior glenoid rim, pinching the rotator cuff and labrum between these 2 structures, a process referred to as internal impingement.[33] Increased anterior laxity can thus lead to rotator cuff tendonitis, subacromial impingement, SLAP lesions, and other pathologic entities. Acute trauma is a less common cause of instability in the throwing athlete.

Throwing athletes with shoulder instability often present with a vague complaint of shoulder pain. The throwing shoulder should be compared with the contralateral extremity in assessing glenohumeral laxity. It is essential for the treating physician to differentiate between lesions that occur due to chronic laxity or instability from those that occur as an acute pathologic condition. The Jobe relocation test is helpful in distinguishing structures that fail due to primary overload from those that fail due to anterior instability.[8,34] The patient is placed supine with the arm in 90° abduction and maximal external rotation. The physician then applies a posteriorly directed force on the humeral head. The pain and apprehension that is alleviated with a posteriorly directed force provides evidence for instability.[8]

Standard radiographs usually add little information to the evaluation of the throwing athlete with chronic anterior laxity, in comparison with instability from an acute traumatic episode because a humeral head impaction fracture or glenoid rim fracture is less likely. MR arthrography is the modality of choice for assessing glenohumeral instability and diagnosing labroligamentous injuries (**Fig. 2**).[35]

Treatment is aimed at relieving pain, restoring motion, and increasing strength to improve the dynamic stability of the shoulder, with most throwing athletes responding well to an appropriate nonoperative protocol. Because the capsulolabral complex has no contractile elements, there is no effective noninvasive means to restore tension in these structures. However, capsular stretch can often be compensated for by improving dynamic stabilization while avoiding positions of abduction and external rotation.[6,28] When a trial of nonoperative management fails to relieve symptoms, surgical intervention is often warranted. Diagnostic arthroscopy can reveal anteroinferior capsular lesions, anterior labral damage, humeral head subluxation, or undersurface tears of the supraspinatus or infraspinatus tendons. The drive-through sign is positive when the arthroscope can be easily passed between the humeral head and anterior glenoid with the arm in external rotation, resulting from a lax anterior capsule.[6] With gross laxity of the capsular or ligamentous structures, a stabilization procedure may be indicated, to reinforce the anterior capsule. Anterior capsulolabral reconstruction, as described by Altchek and colleagues,[36] involves making a T-shaped incision in the anterior capsule, with advancement of the inferior flap superiorly

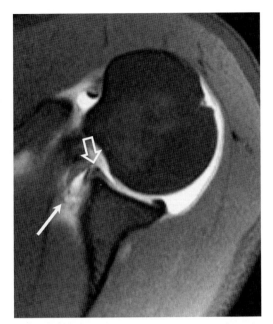

Fig. 2. Anterior capsulolabral injuries in the throwing athlete are more likely to result from repetitive injury than a single traumatic event. Axial fat-suppressed T1-weighted MR arthrogram demonstrates tear of the anterior labrum (*arrow*) as well as contrast extravasation consistent with an anterior capsular injury (*open arrow*).

and the superior flap medially to reduce capsular laxity both anteriorly and inferiorly. Anterior capsulorrhaphy can also be accomplished arthroscopically with the use of sutures and suture anchors. The treating surgeon must be cognizant to not overtighten the anterior capsule, resulting in a restricted range of motion. In current orthopedic practice, arthroscopic stabilization procedures are much more commonly performed than open procedures in throwing athletes because they are associated with better outcomes in this population.[28,37]

SLAP Lesions

SLAP lesions can present in the throwing athlete as a dead arm or as inability of the athlete to throw at the preinjury velocity because of pain and subjective feelings of discomfort in the shoulder.[38] It is postulated that SLAP tears can occur as a result of the peel-back mechanism with the arm in the cocked position of abduction and external rotation. In late cocking, the vector of the biceps tendon shifts posteriorly, which transmits a torsional force to the posterior superior labrum. If the superior labrum is not well fixed to the glenoid, this force will cause the labrum to rotate medially over the glenoid rim onto the posterosuperior scapular neck.[39,40] In throwing athletes, SLAP lesions may be attributed to repetitive traction from overuse.[6,41]

Four types of SLAP lesions are described (**Fig. 3**).[42] Type I lesions involve fraying and degeneration of the superior labrum, with the labrum and biceps anchor remaining fixed to the glenoid rim. Type II lesions include detachment of the superior labrum and biceps anchor from their insertion. In Type III lesions, a bucket-handle tear occurs in the superior labrum, while the periphery of the superior labrum and biceps anchor remain attached to the glenoid rim. In Type IV tears the bucket-handle tear extends into the biceps anchor. Type II SLAP tears can be subdivided based on anatomic location of the tear: anterior to the biceps insertion, posterior, and combined anterior and posterior.[43] In a study by Burkhart and coworkers,[44] 44 pitchers with Type II SLAP lesions were all found to have tight posteroinferior capsules evident on physical examination as a marked decrease in internal rotation with the arm in 90° abduction. It is postulated that, as the arm abducts and externally rotates during late cocking, a tight posteroinferior capsule pushes the humeral head superiorly, causing a posterosuperior shift in the glenohumeral fulcrum. The end result is an increased force at the biceps-labral attachment, further contributing to the peel-back mechanism.[6,44]

The throwing athlete with an SLAP lesion often reports sharp pain in the shoulder during late cocking, as the arm is abducted and brought into a position of maximal external rotation. On physical examination, an audible popping or snapping is often heard with shoulder motion.[6] In addition, dynamic scapular winging can often be observed, caused by periscapular muscle weakness and a tight posteroinferior capsule.[38] Various tests can help the examiner determine the location of the SLAP lesion, including the Speed test, O'Brien cross-arm test, and Jobe relocation test.[38]

Radiographic evaluation is usually normal in patients with isolated SLAP tears. If an SLAP tear is suspected on clinical examination, the orthopedist usually turns to MR imaging, although MR arthrography is gaining more widespread use because of reported increased sensitivity (**Fig. 4**).[45] Specific questions the shoulder surgeon would want to know from MR imaging have been presented by Jost and Gerber,[46] including the following: is the biceps insertion normal; is there an SLAP lesion; what type of SLAP; and is there tendinopathy (of the biceps tendon). However, it is essential to examine the entire shoulder region because associated injuries are common with SLAP tears. With MR arthrography, Bencardino and colleagues[47] found

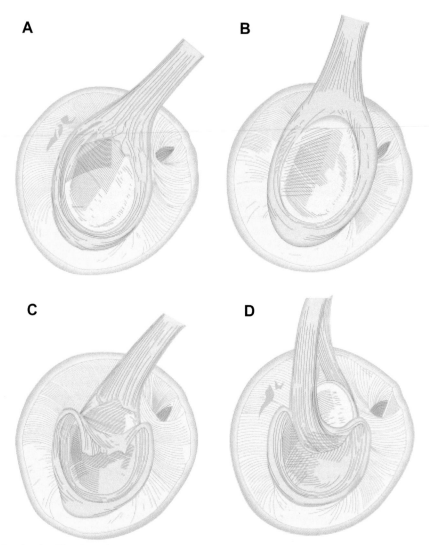

Fig. 3. The Snyder classification of superior labrum anterior posterior (SLAP) lesions. (*A*) Type I has degenerative tearing, but the biceps tendon remains attached. (*B*) Type II has detachment of the superior labrum–biceps tendon complex from the superior glenoid and is most common in overhead athletes. (*C*) Type III has a bucket-handle tear of the superior labrum. (*D*) Type IV has tearing of the superior labrum and biceps tendon. (*From* Delee JC, Drez D Jr, Miller MD. Orthopaedic sports medicine: practices and principles. 3rd edition. Philadelphia: Elsevier; 2010; with permission.)

that SLAP lesions were associated with partial rotator cuff tears in 42% of patients, frayed or lax inferior glenohumeral ligaments in 26%, Bankart lesions in 16%, Hill-Sachs lesions in 16%, chondral lesions in 16%, loose bodies in 10%, complete rotator cuff tears in 5%, and posterior labral tears in 5%.

Definitive diagnosis of SLAP lesions can only be made with diagnostic arthroscopy.[38] Arthroscopic evaluation may reveal hemorrhage or granulation tissue on the undersurface of the biceps tendon, a space between the articular cartilage margin of the glenoid and the attachment of the labrum and biceps tendon, or a separation of the labrum from the glenoid with traction on the biceps tendon.[6,48] The treating surgeon must be aware of normal anatomic variants, such as a meniscoid labrum.[49] SLAP tears of types I and III can often be treated with debridement. Type II SLAP tears are treated with arthroscopic fixation, usually with a suture anchor technique. Treatment of type IV SLAP tears depends on the extent of tearing of the biceps tendon and can range from resection from the torn portion to suture repair of the tendon with fixation of the labrum.[44,48] It is essential for the orthopedist to perform a thorough diagnostic

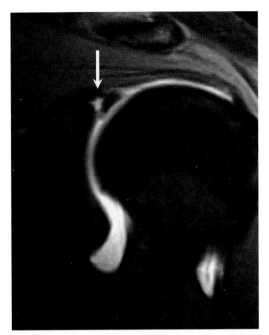

Fig. 4. Coronal fat-suppressed T1-weighted MR arthrogram in a 23-year-old baseball pitcher with vague shoulder pain. There is abnormal contrast between the superior surface of the glenoid and superior labrum, consistent with a type II SLAP tear (*arrow*).

arthroscopy examination to diagnose and treat SLAP tears and associated injuries.

As SLAP tears can occur from the peel-back mechanism with the shoulder in abduction and external rotation, the surgical repair is protected from these positions for several weeks.[50] Postoperative rehabilitation should emphasize stretching of the tight posteroinferior capsule because tightness may place the repair at risk in the throwing athlete.[38,51] The throwing athlete can usually

return to light throwing activity by 6 months after surgical repair.

Rotator Cuff Tears

In the throwing athlete, rotator cuff tears are usually the result of degeneration over several years of repeated stress, with repetitive microtraumatic injuries of the rotator cuff tendons. Injury to the rotator cuff can occur throughout the throwing motion. During cocking, the rotator cuff must resist compression and anterior shear forces, resulting in tensile stresses on the cuff tissue.[14] In the fully cocked position (90° abduction and maximal external rotation), the posterosuperior rotator cuff tendons, including the posterior aspect of the supraspinatus and anterior aspect of the infraspinatus, are pinched between the humerus and glenoid rim, a finding termed internal impingement.[33] As the arm accelerates, impingement can occur between the rotator cuff and undersurface of the acromion. With compression against the coracoacromial arch, termed external impingement, the anteroinferior aspect of the acromion presses on the bursal side of the rotator cuff.[30,33] Injury to the rotator cuff can also occur during deceleration, as it resists horizontal adduction, internal rotation, anterior translation, and distraction forces.[6] With weakness in the rotator cuff muscles, fatigue, or improper mechanics, superior migration of the humeral head can accentuate subacromial impingement, resulting in further injury to the rotator cuff tendons.[8] In the throwing athlete, most rotator cuff tears are partial and articular sided, implying internal impingement as the likely mechanism (**Fig. 5**).[26,33] Full-thickness tears of the rotator cuff and acute traumatic rotator cuff

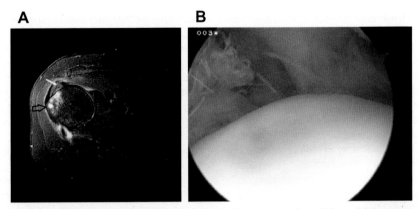

Fig. 5. Articular-sided partial rotator cuff tears are common in the throwing athlete. (*A*) Fat-suppressed coronal T2-weighted MR image and (*B*) an intra-articular arthroscopic view in a throwing athlete demonstrate an articular-sided partial rotator tear of the supraspinatus tendon superimposed on tendinosis (*arrow*) with associated subcortical changes of the greater tuberosity (*open arrow*).

tears are less common in the young throwing athlete.[26,52]

Patients with rotator cuff injury typically present with pain in throwing shoulder that can be poorly localized. The shoulder should be inspected to assess for supraspinatus or infraspinatus atrophy, seen with chronic rotator cuff injury. Tenderness in either muscle belly may be elicited on palpation. With partial rotator cuff tears, gross weakness is usually not present. Pain occurs as the arm is brought into a position of abduction and maximal external rotation, as the rotator cuff is compressed between the greater tuberosity and the posterior superior glenoid rim.[33] Pain may also be elicited by having the patient accelerate the arm from an abducted and externally rotated position to internal rotation.[6] The drop arm test is assessed by having the patient slowly lower the arm from a position of maximal forward elevation. The test result is positive if the patient is unable to resist gravity and lower the arm slowly, as it drops suddenly to the side. Although a positive drop arm test result usually indicates a rotator cuff tear, a negative test result does not preclude the diagnosis.[53]

Although plain radiographs often add little to the diagnosis of rotator cuff tears, they should be obtained to assess for associated conditions or alternative pathology, such as calcific tendonitis. If a rotator cuff tear is suspected based on history taking and physical examination, MR imaging is indicated. Some questions the shoulder surgeon intends to answer with MR imaging include the following: is there a partial or complete tear; is a partial tear bursal sided, articular sided, or intrasubstance; which tendons are involved; are they retracted and how far; are there associated muscular changes such as atrophy or fatty infiltration.[46] However, it is essential to correlate MR imaging findings with clinical examination, because partial-thickness rotator cuff tears have been found in approximately 20% of asymptomatic patients on MR imaging.[54,55] It is unknown if these changes can represent a normal variant or a subclinical finding that may lead to future problems.[55] MR arthrography has been shown to be more sensitive and specific in detecting partial articular-sided rotator cuff tears (**Fig. 6**).[56]

Physical therapy along with antiinflammatory medications is the mainstay of initial management for throwing athletes with rotator cuff tears. Physical therapy should focus on tissue-specific stretching and strengthening of the rotator cuff muscles.[4] Corticosteroid injections can be used judiciously for refractory pain and inflammation. Because of the failure of conservative management, arthroscopy is used to definitively diagnose and treat rotator cuff tears. In nonathletic patients, simple debridement has shown a success rate of 80% to 90%; however, results are more variable in throwing athletes.[26] In a population of elite baseball pitchers, Reynolds and colleagues[57] report that only 55% of throwing athletes were able to return to the same or higher level of competition after debridement of small partial-thickness rotator cuff tears. Full-thickness rotator cuff tears are an indication for repair of the tendon back to bone. Postoperatively, the patient's arm is placed in a sling for pain control. Rehabilitation is begun on the first postoperative day with passive abduction and rotation exercises. The throwing athlete should have a return of rotational strength of 85% to 90% of the contralateral extremity before resuming functional activities, usually around 6 months, with a full year often needed for return to competitive throwing.[6,51] Communication between the treating surgeon and throwing athlete is essential to manage expectations and the recovery process because return to prior abilities is less consistent in this athletic population.

Biceps Tendonitis

Biceps tendonitis is a common cause of shoulder pain in the throwing athlete. With the arm in external rotation, the biceps muscle resists internal rotation of the humerus and distraction of the humeral head from the glenoid.[58] In the position of abduction and external rotation, the long head of the biceps can override the lesser tuberosity, resulting in inflammation and damage to the tendon.[7] In addition, with poor throwing mechanics, biceps muscle load may increase, further potentiating the risk for injury.[8]

Throwing athletes with biceps tendonitis often complain of pain over the anterior aspect of the shoulder, pain localized to the bicipital groove, radiating distally into the biceps muscle belly or proximally into the shoulder and neck. Patients with symptoms related to biceps instability may report a clicking or popping sensation in the anterior shoulder with throwing motions.[32] Clinical diagnosis of symptomatic biceps tendinopathy can be difficult because the physical examination may mimic that of other pathologic entities about the shoulder. Tenderness may be elicited with palpation of the long head of the biceps tendon in the bicipital groove. Several tests have been described to identify biceps tendonitis; however, no specific test has been found to have a reliable positive predictive value.[32] The Speed test result is positive with pain in the bicipital groove with resisted forward flexion of the arm with the forearm supinated, the elbow extended, and the arm in

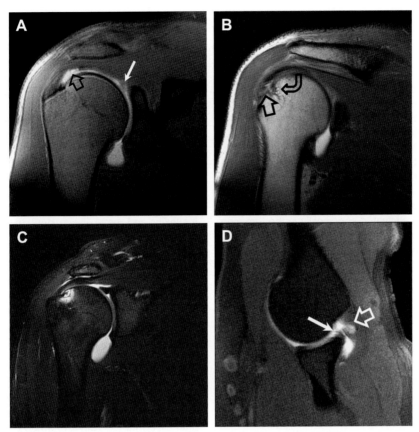

Fig. 6. A 35-year-old, male, baseball and soft ball player with posterior shoulder pain. (*A*) Coronal fat-suppressed T1-weighted MR arthrogram demonstrates a broad-based partial articular-sided tear of the posterior supraspinatus tendon (*open arrow*) and a tear of the posterosuperior labrum (*white arrow*) outlined by contrast solution. (*B*) Coronal fast-spin echo T2-weighted image demonstrates articular-sided fraying and tear of the infraspinatus tendon (*open arrow*) associated with subcortical cystic changes of the greater tuberosity (*curved arrow*). (*C*) Coronal fat-suppressed T2-weighted image demonstrates to a better extent associated cystic changes and marrow edema involving the greater tuberosity. (*D*) Fat-suppressed abduction external rotation T1-weighted MR arthrogram demonstrates a posterosuperior labral tear (*white arrow*) and undersurface rotator cuff tear (*open arrow*).

90° of forward flexion. The Yergason test may elicit pain on resisted supination of the forearm with the elbow flexed to 90°. These tests are specific but not sensitive in detecting biceps tendonitis and SLAP lesions.[59] Rupture of the long head of the biceps tendon, as identified by the gross deformity, Popeye sign, is uncommon in the young throwing athlete.

Radiographs are routinely obtained with suspected biceps pathologic conditions, but they are seldom helpful in the diagnosis of biceps tendonitis. Although MR imaging allows visualization of the biceps tendon, bicipital groove, bony osteophytes, and fluid, it has demonstrated poor concordance with arthroscopic findings in the detection of pathologic conditions of biceps and poor to moderate sensitivity for inflammation, partial-thickness tear, and rupture.[32,60] MR arthrography

is more sensitive and specific for the diagnosis of biceps tendonitis and associated pathologic conditions such as rotator cuff tears and SLAP lesions.[61] In addition, close inspection of MR imaging is warranted in the axial and sagittal oblique planes as subluxation and dislocation of the long head of the biceps tendon is associated with tears of the subscapularis tendon.[32]

A trial of nonoperative management for tendonitis of the long head of the biceps includes rest, activity modification, and nonsteroidal antiinflammatory medications. Selective corticosteroid injections may aid in the diagnosis of biceps tendonitis when the cause of shoulder pain is in doubt. A corticosteroid injection into the glenohumeral joint can reduce inflammation in the biceps tendon because its sheath is contiguous with the synovium of the glenohumeral joint.[32] An injection into the bicipital groove may help differentiate biceps tendonitis from other causes of anterior shoulder pain.[62] When conservative management fails to provide relief of symptoms, surgical management may be indicated. Debridement of the intra-articular portion of the biceps tendon has been proposed by some investigators when there is fraying of the tendon without instability.[32,63] The most commonly performed procedures for pathologic conditions of the long head of the biceps tendon are tenotomy and tenodesis. Biceps tenotomy involves releasing the long head of the biceps from its proximal origin without refixation. Patients report high levels of pain-free recovery and satisfaction with this procedure, but it has not been evaluated specifically in the throwing athlete.[64] Biceps tenodesis, open or arthroscopic, involves releasing the long head of the biceps tendon from its attachment on the posterosuperior glenoid and refixating the tendon in the intertubercular groove of the humerus. Gentle active-assisted exercises are begun approximately 1 week after surgery and continued for several months. Muscle resistance and isokinetic exercises are begun about 2 months after surgery, with 8 months typically needed for full recovery.[7] In one study of 53 young athletes, 77% resumed sports and could throw satisfactorily after biceps tenodesis.[65] Other investigators report similar findings with high-level athletes.[63]

Bennett Lesion

The Bennett lesion is an extra-articular ossification of the posteroinferior capsule at its insertion on the glenoid and is seemingly unique to throwing athletes.[6] The exostosis likely occurs from traction of the posterior band of the inferior glenohumeral ligament during the deceleration phase of the throwing cycle.[66] Alternatively, the lesion may be due to subluxation and impingement of the humeral head on the posterior capsule, leading to calcification. In symptomatic throwers, the lesion is often associated with tearing of the posterior labrum and the undersurface of the posterior rotator cuff.[67] However, a large enough lesion or a fractured lesion may itself be symptomatic.[6,26]

Athletes typically present with posterior shoulder pain during the late cocking or deceleration phase. On physical examination, pain may be elicited with abduction and external rotation of the arm, as during the late cocking phase, or adduction and internal rotation of the arm, as in the deceleration phase. The throwing shoulder should be evaluated for laxity and instability in both the anterior and posterior directions.

The Stryker notch view is used to assess the size of the Bennett lesion.[66] CT arthrography may demonstrate the extra-articular calcification originating from the posteroinferior glenoid.[67] Although MR imaging is not necessary to visualize the Bennett lesion itself, it can be useful to assess associated damage to the labrum and rotator cuff (**Fig. 7**).[66,67]

Nonoperative management consisting of rest and nonsteroidal antiinflammatory medications is usually effective if symptoms are due to the lesion alone. Debridement of the exostosis is indicated after failed conservative treatment with posterior shoulder pain, tenderness localized to the posterior glenoid and capsule, and the presence of a large osteophyte on radiographic examination. Frayed labral tissue and partial-thickness rotator cuff tears should be debrided at the time of arthroscopic examination.[66] Physical therapy consists of a program to increase motion and strengthen the shoulder girdle. The athlete may return to a throwing program when isokinetic testing reveals a strength deficit of less than 10% compared

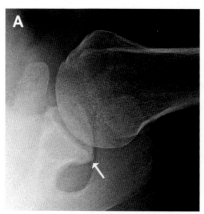 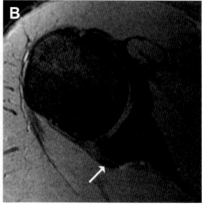

Fig. 7. (*A*) Axillary radiograph in a throwing athlete with ossification of the posterior glenoid rim (*arrow*). (*B*) Gradient-echo T2-weighted axial MR image with low–signal intensity focus in the posterior capsular periosteal junction consistent with a Bennett lesion (*arrow*).

with the contralateral shoulder.[66] However, some investigators believe that operative removal of the exostosis is unnecessary if associated pathologic conditions to the labrum, capsule, and rotator cuff are addressed.[67]

Acromioclavicular Pathology

Pain in the throwing shoulder may be because of pathologic conditions outside the glenohumeral joint. Degeneration and instability of the acromioclavicular joint is uncommon in the throwing athlete, although repetitive horizontal adduction during follow-through may result in abnormal loading of the joint. In the throwing athlete, isolated acromioclavicular pathology is more likely because of overzealous upper body training or a prior low-grade acromioclavicular sprain than the repetitive throwing motion itself.[26]

Throwing athletes with acromioclavicular pathologic conditions typically complain of pain in the superior aspect of the shoulder, which may be exacerbated during the follow-through stage, as the arm is brought into horizontal adduction. Tenderness is elicited on palpation of the acromioclavicular joint, and pain is reproduced with cross-arm adduction. Instability should be assessed by grasping the distal end of the clavicle and applying a directed force anteriorly, posteriorly, superiorly, and inferiorly.

Radiographs show degeneration with loss of subchondral bone detail, translucency, and cystic changes.[26,68] The Zanca view should be obtained, as well as comparison images of the contralateral shoulder.[69] MR imaging may show diffuse bone marrow edema in the clavicle end and opposing acromion as well as capsular thickening and associated joint effusion (**Fig. 8**).[70]

A trial of nonoperative management consists of rest and nonsteroidal antiinflammatory medications. Corticosteroid injections can be used selectively; however, accuracy of injection into the acromioclavicular joint is poor without image guidance.[71] With persistent symptoms, surgical excision of the distal clavicle, either open or arthroscopic, is indicated. Treatment of acute grade III acromioclavicular sprains remains controversial. Although nonoperative treatment is usually successful in the general population, some investigators believe that surgical reconstruction may be beneficial in throwing athletes to prevent alterations in throwing mechanics.[26,69]

Scapulothoracic Pathology

The scapula is of critical importance in evaluating a throwing athlete with shoulder complaints. The scapula provides for a stable base in the glenohumeral articulation, retraction, and protraction of the shoulder complex along the scapular wall; elevation of the acromion; a base for muscle attachment; and a link to the transfer of forces from the trunk to the arm during the throwing motion.[8,72] Scapular dysfunction occurs from abnormal function and imbalance of the periscapular musculature and from repetitive microtrauma associated with the throwing motion.[8] Less commonly, injury to the long thoracic nerve or spinal accessory nerve can result in scapular dysfunction. In the throwing athlete, tightness in the posterior capsule and musculature can lead to increased protraction of the scapula in cocking and follow-through phases. This can result in a closing down

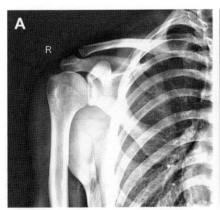 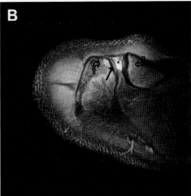

Fig. 8. An 18 year-old throwing athlete presented with shoulder pain and tenderness on palpation of the acromioclavicular joint. (*A*) Anteroposterior radiograph with borderline widening of the acromioclavicular interval, measuring 9 mm at its widest point and (*B*) T2-weighted axial MR image with mild subchondral edema in the distal clavicle and acromial process (*curved arrows*) as well as mild edema in the acromioclavicular joint capsule (*arrow*) with a small joint effusion (*asterisk*). These findings are consistent with a grade I acromioclavicular joint sprain.

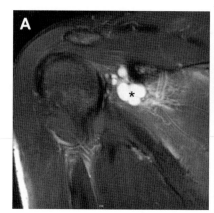 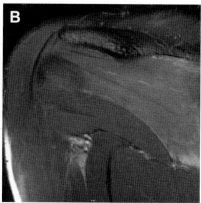

Fig. 9. Coronal T2-weighted MR images in a throwing athlete with vague shoulder pain. (A) A paralabral ganglion cyst is present at the level of the spinoglenoid notch (asterisk). (B) Compression of the infraspinatus branch of the suprascapular nerve resulting in isolated denervation edemalike changes of the infraspinatus muscle.

of the subacromial arch, further exacerbating subacromial impingement.[72] In addition, loss or coordinated retraction and protraction can result in relative glenoid anteversion, decreasing the ability to resist anterior translation of the humeral head, thus increasing the shear forces on the anterior soft tissue structures.[8]

Entrapment of the suprascapular nerve is a cause of rotator cuff dysfunction in the throwing athlete. The nerve can be compressed at the suprascapular notch as it crosses under the transverse scapular ligament. The suprascapular nerve can also be compressed at the lateral edge of the scapular spine, at the spinoglenoid notch.[26] With proximal entrapment, athletes often complain of weakness and posterolateral shoulder pain. Wasting of the supraspinatus and infraspinatus muscle bellies may be observed. Distal suprascapular nerve entrapment seems to be unique to throwing athletes and is characterized by isolated wasting of the infraspinatus muscle belly (Fig. 9).[26,73] As the shoulder is brought into a position of maximal abduction and external rotation, the medial tendinous margin between the infraspinatus and supraspinatus muscles impinges against the scapular spine, compressing the infraspinatus branch of the suprascapular nerve. Other proposed mechanisms of injury include direct trauma, compression by a mass, traction injury, and hypertrophied spinoglenoid ligament.[74] Surgical intervention with widening of the spinoglenoid notch resulted in complete resolution of symptoms in a group of elite volleyball players.[75] Successful treatment in a professional baseball pitcher has also been reported with resection of the spinoglenoid ligament.[74]

Scapulothoracic bursitis or a snapping scapula in the throwing athlete is likely due to changes in the soft tissue between the anterior border of the scapula and the posterior chest wall. Increasing inflammation can lead to pain and crepitus during the throwing motion. On physical examination, the athlete may be able to reproduce the snapping sensation and a small mass may be palpable at the superior or inferomedial angle of the scapula. Imaging may be helpful to rule out a bony cause of the snapping sensation, such as an osteochondroma.[26] Conservative treatment involves rest, nonsteroidal antiinflammatory medications, corticosteroid injections, and scapular strengthening exercises. If pain persists, open or arthroscopic bursal excision can be successful at reducing symptoms.[26,76,77]

SUMMARY

The extreme range of motion at the shoulder, high velocities and stresses, and repetitive nature of the throwing motion place the throwing athlete at risk for a wide range of pathologic entities. The treating orthopedist must fully understand the biomechanics of the throwing cycle and how it contributes to the potential injuries in the throwing shoulder during each phase of the throwing motion. The throwing athlete complaining of shoulder pain or instability should undergo a complete evaluation, including a thorough history taking and physical examination and appropriate radiographic studies, to identify the causes of the symptoms. Nonoperative treatment consisting of a period of rest and antiinflammatory medications followed by physical therapy and a gradual return to activity is often successful at bringing the throwing athlete back to competition. When symptoms persist, surgical intervention may be necessary to address the underlying pathologic condition. The goal of orthopedic care and rehabilitation is to allow the throwing athlete to return symptom free to the preinjury level of competition.

REFERENCES

1. Available at: http://www.littleleague.org/media/news-archive/03_2006/06participation.htm. Accessed July 8, 2011.
2. Available at: http://www.nfhs.org/WorkArea/Download Asset.aspx?id=4198. Accessed July 8, 2011.
3. Dick R, Sauers EL, Agel J, et al. Descriptive epidemiology of collegiate men's baseball injuries: National Collegiate Athletic Association Injury Surveillance System, 1988-1989 through 2003-2004. J Athl Train 2007;42(2):183–93.
4. Braun S, Kokmeyer D, Millett PJ. Shoulder injuries in the throwing athlete. J Bone Joint Surg Am 2009; 91(4):966–78.
5. Hirashima M, Kadota H, Sakurai S, et al. Sequential muscle activity and its functional role in the upper extremity and trunk during overarm throwing. J Sports Sci 2002;20(4):301–10.
6. Park SS, Loebenberg ML, Rokito AS, et al. The shoulder in baseball pitching: biomechanics and related injuries—part 2. Bull Hosp Jt Dis 2002; 61(1–2):80–8.
7. Park SS, Loebenberg ML, Rokito AS, et al. The shoulder in baseball pitching: biomechanics and related injuries—part 1. Bull Hosp Jt Dis 2002;61(1–2):68–79.
8. Meister K. Injuries to the shoulder in the throwing athlete. Part one: biomechanics/pathophysiology/classification of injury. Am J Sports Med 2000; 28(2):265–75.
9. Harryman DT 2nd, Sidles JA, Clark JM, et al. Translation of the humeral head on the glenoid with passive glenohumeral motion. J Bone Joint Surg Am 1990;72(9):1334–43.
10. Fleisig GS, Andrews JR, Dillman CJ, et al. Kinetics of baseball pitching with implications about injury mechanisms. Am J Sports Med 1995;23(2):233–9.
11. Dillman CJ, Fleisig GS, Andrews JR. Biomechanics of pitching with emphasis upon shoulder kinematics. J Orthop Sports Phys Ther 1993;18(2):402–8.
12. Kelly BT, Barnes RP, Powell JW, et al. Shoulder injuries to quarterbacks in the national football league. Am J Sports Med 2004;32(2):328–31.
13. Perry J. Anatomy and biomechanics of the shoulder in throwing, swimming, gymnastics, and tennis. Clin Sports Med 1983;2(2):247–70.
14. Meister K, Andrews JR. Classification and treatment of rotator cuff injuries in the overhand athlete. J Orthop Sports Phys Ther 1993;18(2):413–21.
15. Wilk KE, Meister K, Andrews JR. Current concepts in the rehabilitation of the overhead throwing athlete. Am J Sports Med 2002;30(1):136–51.
16. Bigliani LU, Codd TP, Connor PM, et al. Shoulder motion and laxity in the professional baseball player. Am J Sports Med 1997;25(5):609–13.
17. Crockett HC, Gross LB, Wilk KE, et al. Osseous adaptation and range of motion at the glenohumeral joint in professional baseball pitchers. Am J Sports Med 2002;30(1):20–6.
18. Kaplan KM, Elattrache NS, Jobe FW, et al. Comparison of shoulder range of motion, strength, and playing time in uninjured high school baseball pitchers who reside in warm- and cold-weather climates. Am J Sports Med 2011;39(2):320–8.
19. Osbahr DC, Cannon DL, Speer KP. Retroversion of the humerus in the throwing shoulder of college baseball pitchers. Am J Sports Med 2002;30(3):347–53.
20. McClanahan BS, Harmon-Clayton K, Ward KD, et al. Side-to-side comparisons of bone mineral density in upper and lower limbs of collegiate athletes. J Strength Cond Res 2002;16(4):586–90.
21. Neer CS 2nd, Foster CR. Inferior capsular shift for involuntary inferior and multidirectional instability of the shoulder. A preliminary report. J Bone Joint Surg Am 1980;62(6):897–908.
22. Brown LP, Niehues SL, Harrah A, et al. Upper extremity range of motion and isokinetic strength of the internal and external shoulder rotators in major league baseball players. Am J Sports Med 1988;16(6):577–85.
23. Hinton RY. Isokinetic evaluation of shoulder rotational strength in high school baseball pitchers. Am J Sports Med 1988;16(3):274–9.
24. Wilk KE, Andrews JR, Arrigo CA, et al. The strength characteristics of internal and external rotator muscles in professional baseball pitchers. Am J Sports Med 1993;21(1):61–6.
25. Wilk KE, Obma P, Simpson CD, et al. Shoulder injuries in the overhead athlete. J Orthop Sports Phys Ther 2009;39(2):38–54.
26. Meister K. Injuries to the shoulder in the throwing athlete. Part two: evaluation/treatment. Am J Sports Med 2000;28(4):587–601.
27. Altchek DW, Warren RF, Wickiewicz TL, et al. Arthroscopic labral debridement. A three-year follow-up study. Am J Sports Med 1992;20(6):702–6.
28. Altchek DW, Dines DM. Shoulder injuries in the throwing athlete. J Am Acad Orthop Surg 1995; 3(3):159–65.
29. Hawkins RJ, Kennedy JC. Impingement syndrome in athletes. Am J Sports Med 1980;8(3):151–8.
30. Neer CS 2nd. Impingement lesions. Clin Orthop Relat Res 1983;(173):70–7.
31. O'Brien SJ, Pagnani MJ, Fealy S, et al. The active compression test: a new and effective test for diagnosing labral tears and acromioclavicular joint abnormality. Am J Sports Med 1998;26(5):610–3.
32. Nho SJ, Strauss EJ, Lenart BA, et al. Long head of the biceps tendinopathy: diagnosis and management. J Am Acad Orthop Surg 2010;18(11):645–56.
33. Davidson PA, Elattrache NS, Jobe CM, et al. Rotator cuff and posterior-superior glenoid labrum injury associated with increased glenohumeral motion: a new site of impingement. J Shoulder Elbow Surg 1995;4(5):384–90.

34. Jobe FW, Kvitne RS, Giangarra CE. Shoulder pain in the overhand or throwing athlete. The relationship of anterior instability and rotator cuff impingement. Orthop Rev 1989;18(9):963–75.

35. Bergin D. Imaging shoulder instability in the athlete. Magn Reson Imaging Clin N Am 2009;17(4): 595–615, v.

36. Altchek DW, Warren RF, Skyhar MJ, et al. T-plasty modification of the Bankart procedure for multidirectional instability of the anterior and inferior types. J Bone Joint Surg Am 1991;73(1):105–12.

37. Montgomery WH 3rd, Jobe FW. Functional outcomes in athletes after modified anterior capsulolabral reconstruction. Am J Sports Med 1994;22(3): 352–8.

38. Burkhart SS, Morgan C. SLAP lesions in the overhead athlete. Orthop Clin North Am 2001;32(3): 431–41, viii.

39. Burkhart SS, Morgan CD, Kibler WB. The disabled throwing shoulder: spectrum of pathology Part I: pathoanatomy and biomechanics. Arthroscopy 2003;19(4):404–20.

40. Burkhart SS, Morgan CD. The peel-back mechanism: its role in producing and extending posterior type II SLAP lesions and its effect on SLAP repair rehabilitation. Arthroscopy 1998;14(6):637–40.

41. Andrews JR, Carson WG Jr, McLeod WD. Glenoid labrum tears related to the long head of the biceps. Am J Sports Med 1985;13(5):337–41.

42. Snyder SJ, Karzel RP, Del Pizzo W, et al. SLAP lesions of the shoulder. Arthroscopy 1990;6(4):274–9.

43. Morgan CD, Burkhart SS, Palmeri M, et al. Type II SLAP lesions: three subtypes and their relationships to superior instability and rotator cuff tears. Arthroscopy 1998;14(6):553–65.

44. Burkhart SS, Morgan CD, Kibler WB. Shoulder injuries in overhead athletes. The "dead arm" revisited. Clin Sports Med 2000;19(1):125–58.

45. Chandnani VP, Yeager TD, DeBerardino T, et al. Glenoid labral tears: prospective evaluation with MRI imaging, MR arthrography, and CT arthrography. AJR Am J Roentgenol 1993;161(6):1229–35.

46. Jost B, Gerber C. What the shoulder surgeon would like to know from MR imaging. Magn Reson Imaging Clin N Am 2004;12(1):161–8, vii.

47. Bencardino JT, Beltran J, Rosenberg ZS, et al. Superior labrum anterior-posterior lesions: diagnosis with MR arthrography of the shoulder. Radiology 2000; 214(1):267–71.

48. Mileski RA, Snyder SJ. Superior labral lesions in the shoulder: pathoanatomy and surgical management. J Am Acad Orthop Surg 1998;6(2):121–31.

49. Tischer T, Vogt S, Kreuz PC, et al. Arthroscopic anatomy, variants, and pathologic findings in shoulder instability. Arthroscopy 2011;27(10):1434–43.

50. Wilk KE, Reinold MM, Dugas JR, et al. Current concepts in the recognition and treatment of superior labral (SLAP) lesions. J Orthop Sports Phys Ther 2005;35(5):273–91.

51. Ellenbecker TS, Reinold MM. Rehabilitation principles following rotator cuff and superior labral repair. In: Kibler WB, editor. OKU sports medicine 4. Rosemont (IL): American Academy of Orthopaedic Surgeons; 2009. p. 217–25.

52. Tibone JE, Elrod B, Jobe FW, et al. Surgical treatment of tears of the rotator cuff in athletes. J Bone Joint Surg Am 1986;68(6):887–91.

53. Zuckerman JD, Mirabello SC, Newman D, et al. The painful shoulder: part II. Intrinsic disorders and impingement syndrome. Am Fam Physician 1991; 43(2):497–512.

54. Miniaci A, Dowdy PA, Willits KR, et al. Magnetic resonance imaging evaluation of the rotator cuff tendons in the asymptomatic shoulder. Am J Sports Med 1995;23(2):142–5.

55. Miniaci A, Mascia AT, Salonen DC, et al. Magnetic resonance imaging of the shoulder in asymptomatic professional baseball pitchers. Am J Sports Med 2002;30(1):66–73.

56. Meister K, Thesing J, Montgomery WJ, et al. MR arthrography of partial thickness tears of the undersurface of the rotator cuff: an arthroscopic correlation. Skeletal Radiol 2004;33(3):136–41.

57. Reynolds SB, Dugas JR, Cain EL, et al. Debridement of small partial-thickness rotator cuff tears in elite overhead throwers. Clin Orthop Relat Res 2008;466(3):614–21.

58. Rodosky MW, Harner CD, Fu FH. The role of the long head of the biceps muscle and superior glenoid labrum in anterior stability of the shoulder. Am J Sports Med 1994;22(1):121–30.

59. Holtby R, Razmjou H. Accuracy of the Speed's and Yergason's tests in detecting biceps pathology and SLAP lesions: comparison with arthroscopic findings. Arthroscopy 2004;20(3):231–6.

60. Mohtadi NG, Vellet AD, Clark ML, et al. A prospective, double-blind comparison of magnetic resonance imaging and arthroscopy in the evaluation of patients presenting with shoulder pain. J Shoulder Elbow Surg 2004;13(3):258–65.

61. Zanetti M, Hodler J. MR imaging of the shoulder after surgery. Magn Reson Imaging Clin N Am 2004;12(1):169–83, viii.

62. Tallia AF, Cardone DA. Diagnostic and therapeutic injection of the shoulder region. Am Fam Physician 2003;67(6):1271–8.

63. Ahrens PM, Boileau P. The long head of biceps and associated tendinopathy. J Bone Joint Surg Br 2007; 89(8):1001–9.

64. Gill TJ, McIrvin E, Mair SD, et al. Results of biceps tenotomy for treatment of pathology of the long head of the biceps brachii. J Shoulder Elbow Surg 2001;10(3):247–9.

65. O'Donoghue DH. Subluxing biceps tendon in the athlete. Clin Orthop Relat Res 1982;(164):26–9.

66. Meister K, Andrews JR, Batts J, et al. Symptomatic thrower's exostosis. Arthroscopic evaluation and treatment. Am J Sports Med 1999;27(2):133–6.

67. Ferrari JD, Ferrari DA, Coumas J, et al. Posterior ossification of the shoulder: the Bennett lesion. Etiology, diagnosis, and treatment. Am J Sports Med 1994;22(2):171–5 [discussion: 175–6].

68. Scavenius M, Iversen BF. Nontraumatic clavicular osteolysis in weight lifters. Am J Sports Med 1992;20(4):463–7.

69. Simovitch R, Sanders B, Ozbaydar M, et al. Acromioclavicular joint injuries: diagnosis and management. J Am Acad Orthop Surg 2009;17(4):207–19.

70. Patten RM. Atraumatic osteolysis of the distal clavicle: MR findings. J Comput Assist Tomogr 1995;19(1):92–5.

71. Daley EL, Bajaj S, Bisson LJ, et al. Improving injection accuracy of the elbow, knee, and shoulder: does injection site and imaging make a difference? A systematic review. Am J Sports Med 2011;39(3):656–62.

72. Kibler WB. The role of the scapula in athletic shoulder function. Am J Sports Med 1998;26(2):325–37.

73. Ringel SP, Treihaft M, Carry M, et al. Suprascapular neuropathy in pitchers. Am J Sports Med 1990;18(1):80–6.

74. Cummins CA, Bowen M, Anderson K, et al. Suprascapular nerve entrapment at the spinoglenoid notch in a professional baseball pitcher. Am J Sports Med 1999;27(6):810–2.

75. Sandow MJ, Ilic J. Suprascapular nerve rotator cuff compression syndrome in volleyball players. J Shoulder Elbow Surg 1998;7(5):516–21.

76. Sisto DJ, Jobe FW. The operative treatment of scapulothoracic bursitis in professional pitchers. Am J Sports Med 1986;14(3):192–4.

77. Kuhn JE, Plancher KD, Hawkins RJ. Symptomatic scapulothoracic crepitus and bursitis. J Am Acad Orthop Surg 1998;6(5):267–73.

Superior Labrum Anterior and Posterior Lesions and Microinstability

Eric Y. Chang, MD[a,b,*], Evelyne Fliszar, MD[b],
Christine B. Chung, MD[a,b]

KEYWORDS

- SLAP • Microinstability • Superior labrum
- Periarticular fiber system

The glenohumeral joint provides the greatest range of motion of any joint in the human body. To achieve this mobility, complex interactions between several static and dynamic stabilizers must occur. Any injury that disturbs these interactions can lead to altered movement between the humeral head and the glenoid.

Over the past several decades, histologic studies, in vivo and in vitro biomechanical studies, and improved arthroscopic techniques have contributed to improved knowledge and treatment of abnormalities of the glenohumeral joint, including the labrum. In particular, continuing advances in magnetic resonance (MR) technology have allowed for improved noninvasive visualization of the stabilizers of the shoulder. In this article, the authors review the concept of glenohumeral joint microinstability and its relationship with superior labrum anterior and posterior (SLAP) lesions, review the role of the labrum as a stabilizer of the shoulder, and focus on the diagnosis and classification of SLAP lesions.

MICROINSTABILITY OF THE GLENOHUMERAL JOINT
Definition and Pathoetiology

The concept of microinstability is challenging from a clinical standpoint as well as in its description in the literature. There is no universally accepted definition. Furthermore, the literature describes microinstability in markedly different patient groups with multiple mechanisms of injury to different structures. At the most basic level, some use the term macroinstability interchangeably with dislocation and define microinstability as any rotational or directional pathologic laxity that leads to abnormal mechanics within the shoulder without frank dislocation.[1] A more specific and generally agreed definition of microinstability has been used to describe the pathology in the superior half of the glenohumeral joint with resultant abnormal translation of the humeral head on the glenoid.[2,3] This condition leads to subluxation without dislocation because of the limits to translation imposed by the coracoid, acromion, coracoacromial ligament, and rotator cuff.[2,4] A review of the literature yields 2 viewpoints of microinstability, a clinical classification group and a structural abnormality group, which are not mutually exclusive and demonstrate shared concepts.

In the clinical classification group, microinstability lies between the spectrum of TUBS (Traumatic instability, Unidirectional in nature, with a Bankart lesion typically responding to Surgery) and AMBRII (Atraumatic instability, Multidirectional in nature with Bilateral shoulder findings, which may respond

The authors have nothing to disclose.
[a] Department of Radiology, VA San Diego Healthcare System, 3350 La Jolla Village Drive, MC 114, San Diego, CA 92161, USA
[b] Department of Radiology, University of California San Diego Medical Center, 200 West Arbor Drive, San Diego, CA 92126, USA
* Corresponding author. Department of Radiology, VA San Diego Healthcare System, 3350 La Jolla Village Drive, MC 114, San Diego, CA 92161.
E-mail address: ericchangmd@gmail.com

Magn Reson Imaging Clin N Am 20 (2012) 277–294
doi:10.1016/j.mric.2012.01.002
1064-9689/12/$ – see front matter Published by Elsevier Inc.

to a Rehabilitation program or require an Inferior capsular shift or Interval closure). Two distinct cohorts have been described classically: young individuals with chronic repetitive microtrauma from overhead motions (also referred to by some as AIOS, Acquired Instability in Overstressed Shoulder)[5–12] and those without chronic overhead motions.[10,13–15]

With regard to overhead athletes, and specifically in the throwing shoulder of baseball pitchers, some have classified internal impingement as microinstability.[2,16] Although abnormal function in overhead athletes may be a spectrum with some overlap of impingement and instability,[17] most of the literature on this topic delineates the 2 entities.[18,19] In 1991, Walch and colleagues[18,19] described internal impingement as an intra-articular impingement that occurs in all shoulders in the abducted externally rotated position. In this position, the undersurface of the posterosuperior rotator cuff may become pinched between the labrum and greater tuberosity. Some consider that this phenomenon of impingement leads to abnormality of the throwing shoulder,[20,21] whereas others do not.[22] Those that do not consider impingement to be a pathologic entity describe a separate pathologic cascade leading to the dead shoulder of throwing, which involves the SLAP lesion.[22] In this group, repair of the SLAP lesion with physical therapy is usually curative.[23]

Regarding the group of patients who do not use chronic forceful overhead motions, there are 2 additional subsets: those with trauma and those without trauma. The more common subset in this group is traumatic and includes most patients with SLAP lesions as described by Snyder and colleagues[13] (a total of 23 patients, 13 of whom had a compression force to the shoulder and 6 of whom had a sudden pull on the arm). This subgroup would also include most of the patients described by Savoie and colleagues[14] with superior labrum anterior cuff (SLAC) lesions (a total of 40 patients, 6 of whom were in motor vehicle accidents and 15 of whom had traumatic falls onto the shoulder). A much rarer subset of this second group of patients who do not use overhead motions is atraumatic with typical complaints of shoulder pain after a period of inactivity such as pregnancy or immobilization, classified as AMSI (Atraumatic Minor Shoulder Instability).[10] AMSI patients may have static anatomic variants of the middle glenohumeral ligament (MGHL) (absence, hypoplasia, or a Buford complex).[10,15] In the literature, the term minor instability has been used to encompass both AIOS and AMSI.[10]

Microinstability: Structural Abnormality Group of Literature

From the diagnostic radiologist's perspective, the structural abnormality class of microinstability is the more useful one. In the literature, this class of microinstability includes patients of varying ages with multiple mechanisms of injury. One article estimates that the incidence of microinstability is 5% in those with shoulder pain.[4] This group shares the etiology of acute trauma or repetitive stress, leading to injury of one or more supporting structures of the superior half of the glenohumeral joint, including injury to the labrum, MGHL, rotator interval structures, and rotator cuff. Injuries to any of these supporting structures can lead to predictable pathologic translation of the humeral head relative to the glenoid.

Labral injuries constitute the largest portion of this group (discussed in detail in the following sections). The MGHL has been shown to be an important secondary restraint to both inferior and anterior translation (**Fig. 1**).[24,25] Savoie and colleagues[9] reported on isolated MGHL avulsions in 33 patients with anterior instability, who were treated with improvement in pain and function.

The rotator interval includes the superior glenohumeral ligament (SGHL), coracohumeral ligament, glenohumeral[26] joint capsule, and biceps tendon, all of which contribute to stability.[27] The SGHL has been shown to be an important secondary restraint to anterior and superior translation of the humeral head in shoulder flexion and lesser degrees of abduction.[24,25] Injury to the SGHL can lead to anterosuperior instability (**Fig. 2**) and secondary impingement of the rotator cuff tendon.[9,28,29] With regard to this specific association, the term SLAC was introduced by Savoie and colleagues[14] to describe anterosuperior labral lesions, SGHL avulsion or injury, and anterior cuff pathology. Studies have shown that injury to the rotator interval or other containing structures can result in increased posterior and inferior translation with the arm in neutral position and increased anterior translation with the arm flexed 60°.[28,30–32]

LABRAL ANATOMY AND BIOMECHANICAL CONSIDERATIONS

The glenoid labrum is a vascularized ring of fibrous tissue that surrounds the bony glenoid.[33–35] The labrum serves numerous functions, including providing nutrition to the glenoid cavity and maintaining joint lubrication.[36] Biomechanically the labrum stabilizes the joint by deepening the glenoid fossa and increasing articular surface area

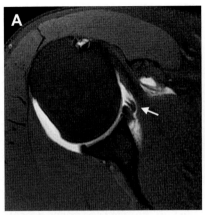
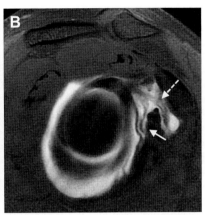

Fig. 1. A 44-year-old baseball player with pain and clinical instability. Axial (*A*) and coronal (*B*) T1-weighted (T1) fat-suppressed (FS) MR arthrogram images using a posterior approach demonstrate thick and irregular superior glenohumeral ligament (SGHL) (*dashed arrow*) with longitudinal split tearing of the middle glenohumeral ligament (*arrows*).

by approximately one-third.[37] The labrum also acts to protect the chondral surface from compression and sheer damage,[35] and serves as an attachment for capsuloligamentous structures, biceps, and triceps.[37,38] In addition, it acts as a valve that maintains negative intra-articular pressure and stability.[39]

For localization purposes, the labrum can be divided into 4 (superior, anterior, inferior, posterior or anterosuperior, anteroinferior, posteroinferior, posterosuperior) or more circular sectors. Alternatively, the labrum can be divided into a clock face with the most common designation using 12 o'clock to represent superior and 3 o'clock to represent anterior.[40] The initial descriptions of SLAP extended between 10 and 2 o'clock.[13,41] However, designation of the precise 12 o'clock location can be difficult depending on which structure is used. A study on the biceps anchor showed

that if the supraglenoid tubercle is used to represent 12 o'clock, the biceps anchor was situated at 12 o'clock 44% of the time and posterior to this 51% of the time (11 o'clock with reference to the supraglenoid tubercle).[42]

From a functional point of view, the labrum, biceps tendon, and glenohumeral ligaments can be considered as a single functional unit. Huber and Putz[43] performed macroscopic and microscopic analyses, which showed bundles of parallel collagen fibers that run around the entire circumference of the glenoid and into the surrounding structures, termed the periarticular fiber system (PAFS). In their study, the bulk of the substance at the posterosuperior aspect of the labrum actually consisted of extended periarticular fiber bundles from the biceps tendon. Huber and Putz[43] concluded that the labrum is not to be regarded as an isolated structure. These results

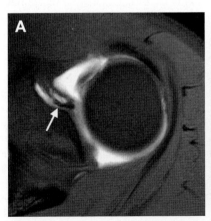
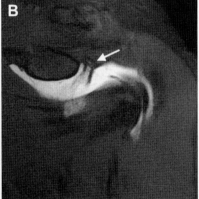

Fig. 2. A 34-year-old man with clinical instability. Axial (*A*) and coronal (*B*) T1 FS MR arthrogram images using a posterior approach demonstrate an arthroscopically confirmed isolated proximal SGHL split tear (*arrows*).

were most recently confirmed by Arai and colleagues,[26] who additionally described a histologically distinct structure that they termed the sheetlike structure, coursing from the glenoid neck and labrum with extension into the rotator interval. This distinct membranous structure courses differently from the SGHL and contains numerous elastic fibers in a crimp pattern, suggesting that it is subject to constant tensile stress.

In some individuals, however, the PAFS demonstrates variability. Pal and colleagues[44] found that in approximately 25% of their 24 specimens, the long head of the biceps tendon originated principally from the supraglenoid tubercle, not the labrum. Others have reported that the long head of the biceps tendon was seen to originate from the undersurface of the rotator cuff[45] or even extra-articularly without attachment to either the superior labrum or supraglenoid tubercle.[46,47] The glenohumeral ligaments also demonstrate considerable variability. The MGHL has been described to be the most variable of the glenohumeral ligaments, being present between 70% and 85% of the time in anatomic[48] and MR studies,[49,50] with a variable origin.[51] Less variable is the SGHL, the anatomy of which was more recently elucidated by Kask and colleagues[52] as being composed of oblique and direct fibers. The direct fibers were seen to invariably originate from the glenoid labrum whereas the oblique fibers originated from the supraglenoid tubercle except for those few specimens with absence of the MGHL, with both oblique and direct fibers originating from the labrum in these cases. Patient variability likely influences predisposition to certain patterns of injury, given an identical mechanism.

LABRAL VARIANTS

In addition to variability of the perilabral structures, there is a wide range of variability of the labrum itself. This range includes labral morphology and signal intensity as well as common anatomic variations that have been described in the superior and anterosuperior glenoid region, including the sublabral sulcus, sublabral foramen or hole, and the Buford complex. Multiple variations can occur in the same individual, for instance a sublabral foramen with a cordlike MGHL.[53]

Labral morphology varies depending on the region. The inferior half of the labrum is usually rounded and firmly continuous with the articular cartilage, with detachment considered an abnormal finding.[54] By contrast, the superior and anterosuperior labrum can be rounded or meniscal in shape (roughly triangular) and can be normally mobile.[54] The superior labrum can be categorized into a triangular type, bumper type, or meniscoid type depending on shape and extent onto the articular surface.[55] In one study of 52 shoulders in young asymptomatic patients, there was extensive variability in morphology regarding the dominant features of the anterior and posterior labra, respectively: triangular (45%, 73%), round (19%, 12%), cleaved (15%, 0%), notched (8%, 0%), flat (7%, 6%), and absent (6%, 8%).[56] These studies show that labral morphology is widely varied, more so anteriorly than posteriorly and much more so superiorly than inferiorly.

Increased signal intensity in the labrum may be caused by a magic angle phenomenon, particularly in the posterosuperior aspect.[57] The magic angle phenomenon is a well-recognized nuclear MR artifact seen in clinical imaging of tissues containing well-ordered collagen fibers.[58] In these tissues, dipolar interactions between water hydrogen protons occur along the long axis of the collagen fibers.[59] This restricted motion causes rapid T2 relaxation and essentially no signal on typical spin-echo images.[60] However, when the long axis of collagen bundles is oriented approximately 55° to the main magnetic field (B0), dipolar interactions are minimized and T2 relaxation time lengthens approximately 100-fold, causing increased signal.[59] This artifact can be avoided by confirming abnormal signal intensity on longer echo-time images. However, even in regions of the labrum not typically demonstrating a magic angle, increased signal intensity does not necessarily indicate a tear. Some reports indicate that this can be seen as a normal finding or be caused by degeneration.[61]

Numerous anatomic variations occur in the superior and anterosuperior portions of the glenoid region, which poses a diagnostic challenge because it is also a common location for abnormalities. In 1992, Cooper and colleagues[54] first described the sublabral recess, which occurs beneath the superior labrum and long head of the biceps origin and is covered by a synovial lining. Only at this region does the hyaline articular cartilage of the glenoid extend over the edge of the glenoid rim and onto the superior neck of the scapula.[54] Multiple studies using cadavers and imaging have found the incidence of the sublabral recess to be up to 75%.[62–64] The sublabral recess can extend posterior to the biceps anchor, particularly when the biceps anchor is primarily to the anterior labrum.[42,65] In the radiologic literature, the appearance of this recess has been designated as the single Oreo cookie sign, whereby on the coronal images the recess (white cream) is interposed between the labrum and glenoid (black cookies).[63] Numerous studies have shown that the most common cause of interpretation errors lies in the difficulty of differentiation of SLAP type II lesions from sublabral recesses.[66,67]

Although not without exceptions, several signs have been described to help in delineating sublabral recesses from SLAP lesions. Characteristics of the high-signal region interposed between the superior labrum and adjacent glenoid rim that have been shown to support a SLAP lesion include extension laterally as it extends superiorly (in contradistinction to extension medially with superior extension, which would point toward the patient's head), irregular borders (**Fig. 3**), width on transverse images greater than 2 mm on conventional MR and 2.5 mm on MR arthrography, an uneven width anterosuperiorly and posterosuperiorly (**Fig. 4**), and extension posterior to the long head of the biceps tendon.[62,68,69] Although all of these signs have some support in the literature, additional reports have indicated low to moderate accuracy with some, particularly with increased width between the glenoid and labrum and posterior extension beyond the biceps anchor.[68,70] In cases where the ancillary finding of a perilabral ganglion cyst is present, diagnosis of a labral tear can be made with confidence (**Fig. 5**).[71]

Nearby, but distinct from the sublabral recess, is the sublabral foramen, located in the superior aspect of the anterior labrum.[72] The sublabral foramen, otherwise referred to as the sublabral hole, refers to the absence of labral attachment in the anterosuperior glenoid quadrant, and has been reported to be seen in approximately 12% of patients.[53] In distinction from the sublabral recess, which is located at the site of attachment of the biceps tendon, a sublabral foramen is anterior to the biceps anchor.[73] The term Buford

complex was coined to describe a cordlike MGHL continuous with the superior labrum and an absence of anterosuperior labral tissue, found in up to approximately 7% of patients.[53,74,75]

True incidence of these variations in the general population is not known because studies are not based on a population of healthy shoulders in randomly selected individuals. It is also not known whether these variants represent normal development or are acquired. Some studies have shown that these variants are not present in very early development[76] but occur after the third trimester of life.[77,78] It has been hypothesized that these variants are a consequence of physiologic mobility and are not a sign of instability.[54,64]

However, numerous studies have demonstrated that certain variant superior and anterosuperior labral anatomy predisposes to abnormality. Rao and colleagues[79] prospectively evaluated 546 patients who underwent arthroscopy, and after multivariate analysis discovered that the presence of a sublabral foramen with or without a cordlike MGHL and those with Buford complexes were significantly associated with labral fraying and SGHL abnormality. In addition, the presence of a sublabral foramen and a non-cordlike MGHL had a higher prevalence of type II SLAP lesions. Other studies have also demonstrated that the Buford complex is highly predisposed toward superior labral lesions.[74,80] Each of these studies postulates a mechanism for the increased association with pathological conditions; however, there is no consensus.

Regardless, these variations are important because they need to be distinguished from true SLAP lesions, and repair of these anatomic variations can have adverse consequences. For instance, in the original description of the Buford

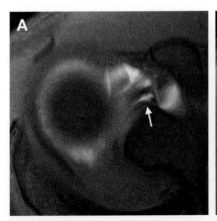
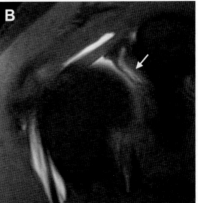

Fig. 3. A 27-year-old pitcher with superior labral tear. Axial (*A*) and coronal (*B*) T1 FS MR arthrogram images demonstrate irregular margins of the space interposed between the labrum and glenoid anterosuperiorly (*arrows*). Findings are consistent with arthroscopically confirmed SLAP IIA lesion.

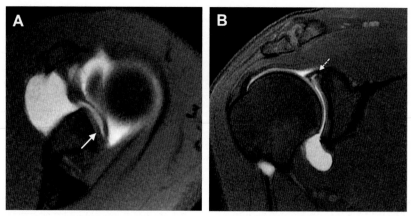

Fig. 4. Superior labral tear extending from 10 o'clock to 2 o'clock. (*A*) Axial T1 FS MR arthrogram image demonstrates uneven width of space anterosuperiorly versus posterosuperiorly (*arrow*), consistent with SLAP IIC lesion. (*B*) Tear is confirmed on coronal T1 FS image (*dashed arrow*).

lesion, when the cordlike MGHL was unknowingly shortened by attachment to the glenoid rim, the patient was left with constrained external rotation.[53]

SLAP LESIONS
Pathogenesis

The most common mechanisms for SLAP include direct compression loads, forceful traction loads to the arm, and repetitive overhead motion.[13] Impaction loading in cadavers has shown that SLAP tears are more frequent with forward falls (shoulder flexion) than with backwards falls (shoulder extension).[81] In another biomechanical study, traction on the biceps tendon reproducibly created a SLAP II lesion, with inferior glenohumeral subluxation facilitating the tear.[82]

With regard to the overhead athlete, several anatomic and biomechanical factors predispose this group to SLAP tears. As already described, some consider that repetitive contact and internal impingement of the labrum with the undersurface of the cuff in the abducted externally rotated position can cause abnormalities.[19] Although the exact mechanism remains to be elucidated, subsequent controlled laboratory studies have shown that SLAP II lesions were seen more frequently in this late cocking phase of throwing.[83,84] Another study found increased mechanical strain at the posterosuperior labrum in the late cocking phase, which was thought to be due to the anatomic orientation of the long head of the biceps tendon in this position.[85] Injury during the late cocking phase of throwing is not universally accepted, however. In the first published series on superior labral injury in the overhead athlete, Andrews and colleagues[11] postulated a deceleration mechanism for labral injuries as the biceps contract to slow down the rapidly extending elbow in follow-through. In

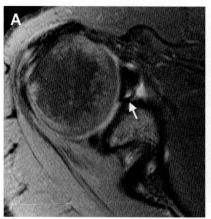
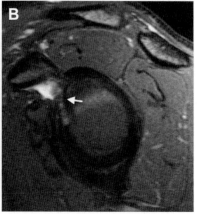

Fig. 5. A 19-year-old pitcher. (*A, B*) Axial T1 FS MR arthrogram images demonstrate labral tearing anterosuperiorly with associated small perilabral ganglion cysts (*arrows*), consistent with SLAP IIA lesion.

a laboratory study examining the stages of throwing during simulated biceps loading, Yeh and colleagues[86] found that the greatest stress at the superior labrum/biceps tendon interface occurred during the deceleration stage.

In an elegant series on the throwing shoulder, Burkart and colleagues[22,23,87] proposed a biomechanical cascade beginning with an acquired tight posteroinferior capsule, leading to a posterosuperior shift in the glenohumeral rotation point, which results in increased clearance of the greater tuberosity over the glenoid during the lack cocking phase. This process causes increased shear forces at the biceps anchor/posterosuperior labral attachment and failure from their attachments via the peel-back mechanism.[12]

As discussed in the section on Labral Variants, it is unclear how labral variants such as the sublabral foramen or the Buford complex predispose to labral tearing. In addition, from the functional point of view, injury may propagate along the PAFS. At the anterior and anterosuperior labrum, the connecting band as described by Huber and Putz[43] consists of fibers connecting the labrum with the superior and inferior glenohumeral ligaments. At the anterosuperior labrum, fibers of the elastic sheetlike structure, which is subject to constant tensile stress, connect with the rotator interval.[26] At the posterosuperior labrum, fibers of the long head of the biceps tendon intermingle with labrum fibers and form a major component of the labrum.[26,35,43,54] However, individual variants of the PAFS and mechanisms for direction of propagation beyond the 4 types of SLAP originally described have not been well described in the literature.

Superior Labral Tears and SLAP Classification

In 1983, Pappas and colleagues[88] presented one of the earliest descriptions of superior labral injury. They proposed the concept that a damaged labrum could cause functional glenohumeral instability and described findings on arthrography. Two years later, Andrews and colleagues[11] reported the first series of superior labral injury in the overhead athlete in 73 baseball pitchers, and described the classic mechanism of labral tearing caused by forces transmitted through the long head of the biceps tendon. In 1990, the term SLAP lesion was introduced to the literature by Snyder and colleagues[13] who described 4 subtypes, occurring with 2 distinct mechanisms of injury: compression force from a fall onto an outstretched arm and traction force caused by a sudden pull on the arm or during overhead sports motion. In type I, the superior labrum is frayed but the peripheral labral edge remains attached to the glenoid (**Fig. 6**). In type II, the superior labrum and attached biceps tendon are stripped from the glenoid (see **Fig. 4**). In type III, a bucket-handle tear of the superior labrum is present. At least half of the time, SLAP III lesions show the characteristic Cheerio sign, which is a rounded core of soft tissue surrounded by a rim of contrast material (**Fig. 7**).[89,90] In type IV, a bucket-handle tear is present with additional extension into the biceps tendon (**Fig. 8**).

Since 1991, several additional types of SLAP lesions have been described (**Table 1**). In 1998, Morgan and colleagues[91] described 3 subtypes of SLAP II, type IIA being primarily anterior (see **Figs. 3** and **5**), type IIB being primarily posterior, and type IIC representing combined anterior and posterior tears (see **Fig. 4**). These investigators noted that type IIB and IIC lesions were more frequently observed than SLAP IIA lesions in throwing athletes. Maffet and colleagues[92] described 3 additional types of SLAP after observing other patterns of biceps tendon-superior labrum injury: type V, described as an anterior-inferior Bankart lesion, continues superiorly to include separation of the biceps anchor (**Fig. 9**); type VI, an unstable flap tear of the superior labrum in addition to biceps tendon separation; and type VII, a superior labrum biceps tendon separation that extends anteriorly beneath the MGHL. In 2004, Nord and colleagues[93] described type VIII, an extended SLAP lesion along the posterior glenoid labrum (**Fig. 10**); type IX, a circumferential labral tear (**Fig. 11**); and

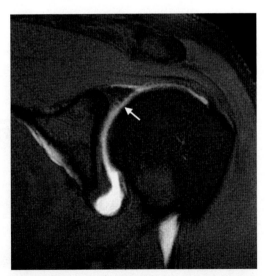

Fig. 6. Coronal T1 FS MR arthrogram image demonstrates irregular morphology of the superior labrum (*arrow*), consistent with fraying and SLAP I lesion.

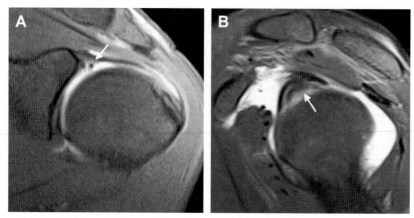

Fig. 7. Coronal (*A*) and sagittal (*B*) T1 FS MR arthrogram images demonstrate a bucket-handle tear of the superior labrum (*arrows*) characterized by high signal intensity contrast surrounding a core of hypointense labrum, an appearance designated the Cheerio sign, consistent with SLAP III lesion.

type X, a SLAP lesion associated with a reverse Bankart lesion (**Fig. 12**). Another type X lesion exists in the literature, which was described in 2000 as a SLAP lesion that extends into the rotator

interval in the form of a lesion of the SGHL, coracohumeral ligament, capsule, or synovium.[40]

The original classification by Snyder and colleagues remains the most widely recognized.[94]

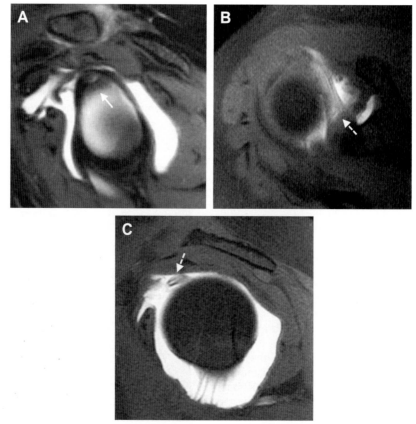

Fig. 8. (*A*) Sagittal T1 FS MR arthrogram image demonstrates a displaced bucket-handle tear of the superior labrum (*arrow*). Axial (*B*) and additional sagittal (*C*) T1 FS MR arthrogram images demonstrate extension into the proximal portion of the long head of the biceps tendon (*dashed arrows*), consistent with SLAP IV lesion.

Type	Clock Position if Designated in Literature	Quoted Description in Literature (Initial Description if Available)
Table 1 **SLAP Classification**		
Snyder et al[13,a]		
I	10–2[41]	"The superior labrum had marked fraying with a degenerative appearance, but the peripheral labral edge remained firmly attached to the glenoid"
II	10–2[41]	"Fraying and degenerative changes were similar to those of Type I. In addition, the superior labrum and attached biceps tendon were stripped off the underlying glenoid"
III	10–2[41]	"A bucket handle tear was noted in the superior labrum"
IV	10–2[41]	"Bucket-handle tears of the superior labrum similar to those of Type III were noted, but in addition, the tear extended into the biceps tendon. The biceps tendon had an attached partial tear, which tended to displace with the labral flap into the joint"
Morgan et al[91]		
IIA	—	Snyder SLAP II that is "primarily anterior"
IIB	—	Snyder SLAP II that is "primarily posterior"
IIC	—	Snyder SLAP II that is "combined anterior and posterior"
Maffet et al[92]		
V	—	"Anterior-inferior Bankart lesion continues superiorly to include separation of the biceps tendon"
VI	—	"Unstable flap tear of the [superior] labrum is present in addition to biceps tendon separation"
VII	—	"Superior labrum-biceps tendon separation extends anteriorly beneath the middle glenohumeral ligament"
Powell et al[131,b]		
VIII	6–2	"SLAP extension along the posterior glenoid labrum as far as 6 o'clock"
IX	Entire	"Pan-labral SLAP injury extending the entire circumference of the glenoid"
X	—	"Superior labral tear associated with posterior-inferior labral tear (reverse Bankart lesion)"
Beltran et al[40,c]		
X	10–2+	"Extension of the superior labral abnormalities into the rotator interval. This extension may be in the form of a lesion of the superior glenohumeral ligament, a lesion of the coracohumeral ligament, a lesion of the interval capsule and synovium, or some combination of these"

[a] Initially presented at the Annual Meeting on Arthroscopic Surgery of the Shoulder, San Diego, CA, May 1989.
[b] Initially presented at the Annual Meeting of the Arthroscopy Association of North America, Orlando, FL, April 2004.
[c] Initially presented at the Annual Meeting of the Radiological Society of North America, Chicago, IL, December 2000.

Regarding frequency of SLAP lesions, in Snyder and colleagues' original article[13] the most common was type II (41%) followed by type III (33%), type IV (15%), and type I (11%). In accord with these data, Handelberg and colleagues[95] retrospectively reviewed 530 arthroscopies and discovered 32 SLAP lesions, 53% of which were type II. Kim and colleagues[96] prospectively reviewed 544 shoulder arthroscopy procedures and found 139 SLAP lesions, the most common being type I (74%) followed by type II (21%), type IV (6%), and type III (0.7%).

The tremendous variability between reports is due not only to selection bias and varying patient populations but also to observer variability. Snyder and colleagues[13] described the superior labrum in

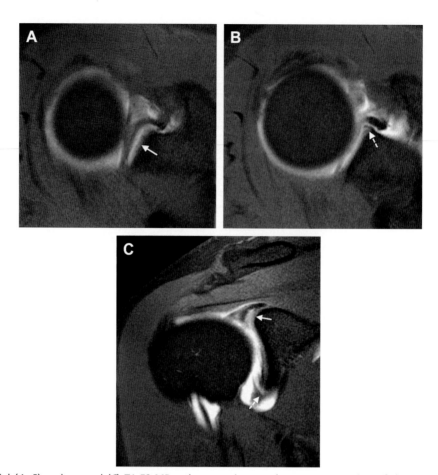

Fig. 9. Axial (*A, B*) and coronal (*C*) T1 FS MR arthrogram images demonstrate tearing of the superior labrum (*arrows*), which extends anteroinferiorly (*dashed arrows*), consistent with SLAP V lesion.

type I as "marked fraying with a degenerative appearance." However, Kohn[97] found an abundance of labral fibrillation and fissuring (76%) in his study of 106 cadaveric shoulders. In the clinical portion of his study, 46 of 72 (64%) shoulders demonstrated a damaged labrum arthroscopically. Forty-five of these 46 damaged labra were left untreated and the remaining abnormalities corrected. Surprisingly, none of the patients had symptoms that could be related to this structure, leading to the conclusion that labral lesions were of little clinical relevance.

Handelberg and colleagues[95] acknowledged Kohn's findings and carefully interpreted labral lesions in an older population. It may not be surprising that in their study a relatively low incidence of type I lesions was found (9.5%). On the other hand, Kim and colleagues[96] discovered that the most common type in their series was type I and this was significantly associated with age.

The topic of variability of diagnosis among experienced arthroscopists was studied by Gobezie and colleagues[98] who, after viewing video vignettes of arthroscopies, found considerable intraobserver and interobserver variability among those deemed experts regarding both SLAP classification and treatment. As arthroscopy is considered the gold standard on which many studies base their sensitivity, specificity, and predictive values, it is clear that any reported values must be carefully scrutinized.

Diagnosis of Microinstability and SLAP Lesion

Diagnosis of microinstability is clinical,[10] diagnosis of SLAP lesions is suspected clinically and arthroscopy and imaging are used for confirmation.[4,14,99] There are numerous findings on physical examination to suggest SLAP lesions; however, there is no definitive clinical sign or symptom that is diagnostic.[4,100] A large part of the difficulty of diagnosis using history and physical examination lies in the high likelihood of concurrent abnormality in the shoulder.[13] In one

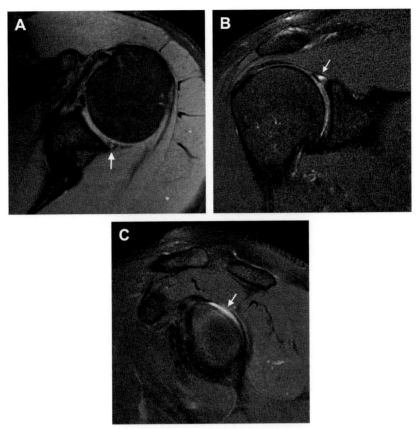

Fig. 10. Axial proton-density FS (*A*), coronal T2-weighted (T2) FS (*B*), and sagittal T2 FS (*C*) MR images demonstrate tearing of the superior labrum extending along the posterior labrum (*arrows*), consistent with SLAP VIII lesion.

prospective review, 88% of SLAP lesions were associated with other intra-articular lesions.[96]

Imaging

Numerous studies have demonstrated a moderate to high degree of accuracy of radiologists in detecting labral abnormalities. Kim and colleagues[67] reported sensitivity, specificity, and accuracy of direct computed tomographic arthrography to be 94% to 97%, 73% to 77%, and 86%, respectively. However, in the study by Kim and colleagues, SLAP type I was not included in the analysis because they considered this to be a degenerative process and often not clinically important. Sensitivity, specificity, and accuracy of unenhanced MR imaging have been reported to be between 66% and 98%, 71% and 90%, and 77% and 96%, respectively.[101–103] Sensitivity, specificity, and accuracy of indirect MR arthrography have been reported to be between 84% and 91%, 58% and 85%, and 78% and 89%, respectively.[102,103] Sensitivity, specificity, and accuracy of direct MR arthrography have been reported to

be between 82% and 100%, 69% and 98%, and 74% and 94%, respectively.[104–107]

Although multiple studies have demonstrated imaging to be accurate in the diagnosis of labral tears, there has been somewhat less impressive accuracy in defining the particular type of SLAP, regardless of modality.[67] Given the amount of variability in practice and experience among arthroscopists,[98] this may not be surprising, even with the more recent 20-power magnification arthroscopes with a resolution that current imaging cannot match.

Different patient positioning has also been advocated to increase detection and improve characterization of superior labral abnormality in conjunction with MR arthrography. Improved detection of SLAP lesions is possible with the arm adducted and in external rotation,[108] in an abducted and externally rotated position (ABER),[109,110] and with arm traction.[111] Furthermore, imaging of the arm in an abducted externally rotated view (ABER) has been shown to demonstrate greater than 3 mm of posterior glenohumeral translation in unstable SLAP lesions.[112]

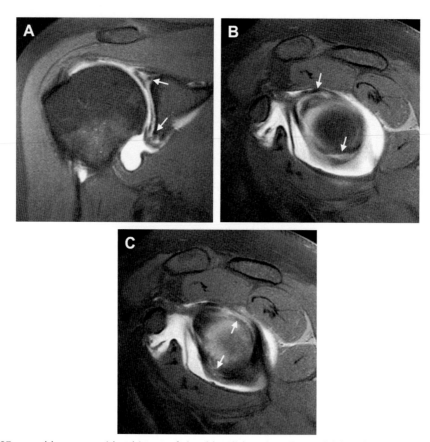

Fig. 11. A 37-year-old woman with a history of shoulder dislocation. Coronal (*A*) and sagittal (*B, C*) T1 FS MR arthrogram images demonstrate circumferential labral tearing (*arrows*), consistent with SLAP IX lesion.

However, this is one isolated report in the literature; a previous report indicated that the humeral head can demonstrate a few degrees of posterior translation in the ABER position in normal individuals.[113] Borrero and colleagues[114] demonstrated that the ABER position was helpful in the detection of posterosuperior labral peel-back on MR arthrography, which can indicate the presence of superior labral instability. In this study, the MR sign of labral peel-back (defined as a posterosuperior labrum medial and caudal to a line tangential to the glenoid rim) allowed identification of a labral abnormality not seen in standard planes in the neutral position in several cases.

Magnetic Resonance Imaging of SLAP

Most of the studies in the literature describing MR imaging accuracy used a 1.5-T magnet. Since the introduction of higher field strengths, several studies have demonstrated that 3-T magnets are also accurate.[115] However, to the best of the authors' knowledge, no head-to-head comparisons of 1.5-T and 3-T magnets have been performed. Regarding 3-T magnets, a single

three-dimensional isotropic dataset (see **Fig. 2**) can also be performed, with shorter imaging times than 3-plane two-dimensional sequences, and similar results between these 2 modes have been found with the use of indirect MR arthrography.[116]

Several studies have advocated for the use of direct intra-articular contrast, at both 1.5 T[117,118] and 3 T.[119,120] Nondisplaced labral tears may coapt, simulating an intact labrum. Intra-articular contrast allows controlled distention of the glenohumeral joint, which can aid in the detection of these nondisplaced labral tears.[119,120] However, there exist factors beyond image quality when considering direct MR arthrography. Patient's reluctance to undergo an invasive procedure, risk, time, cost, and labor must also be considered.[121] Some have advocated that young athletes (<40 years old) are a subgroup of patients for whom direct MR arthrography yields considerably more diagnostic information.[118,121] Joint distention with saline has been shown to provide equivalent diagnostic information to gadolinium in one report.[122]

Indirect MR arthrography involves intravenous administration of contrast medium followed by

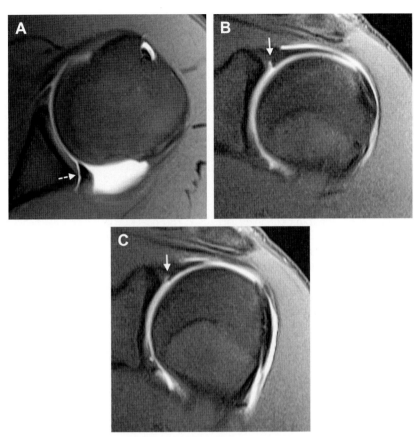

Fig. 12. A 20-year-old pitcher with shoulder pain. Axial (*A*) and coronal (*B*, *C*) T1 FS MR arthrogram images demonstrate superior labral tearing (*arrows*) with posterior extension (*dashed arrow*), consistent with SLAP X lesion as described by Powell and colleagues[131] in 2004.

10 to 15 minutes of joint movement. Some reports have indicated this technique to be more sensitive and specific than noncontrast MR imaging.[103,123] However, one report on unexercised shoulders indicated that indirect MR imaging had decreased specificity for superior labral tearing compared with noncontrast MR imaging.[102]

Treatment

Treatment of microinstability and clinically suspected SLAP is often initially conservative, consisting of nonsteroidal antiinflammatory medications, stretching exercises, and muscle strengthening.[124] However, surgery is often required and is considered after failure of nonsurgical treatment lasting longer than 3 months.[94] Surgical therapy depends on the type of tear, age and activity of the patient, stability of the superior labrum as determined arthroscopically, and integrity of the biceps anchor.[125] Clinically favorable results have been shown with surgically repaired unstable isolated SLAP lesions,[126] and those concomitantly repaired

with coexisting shoulder abnormalities.[125] Paralabral ganglion cysts associated with SLAP lesions can also usually be treated arthroscopically.[94] Detailed treatment of individual types of SLAP lesions is variable,[125,127,128] even among experienced shoulder arthroscopic specialists,[98,129] and is beyond the scope of this article.

Treatment of anatomic variants has been discouraged in the literature, even in the setting of an arthroscopically mobile superior glenoid labrum.[55] As described earlier, repair of anatomic variants can have adverse consequences, particularly with deficits in range of motion. However, there is debate in the literature about how to treat SLAP lesions in the setting of an anatomic variant. More recently, a novel surgical technique has been proposed in those with SLAP lesions and Buford complexes, whereby a standard SLAP repair is used in conjunction with transection of the cordlike MGHL, with the proximal remnant affixed to the anterosuperior glenoid and the distal remnant left free.[130] Nearly all 21 patients treated with this technique showed improvement after surgery without evidence of instability or decreased range of motion.

SUMMARY

Labral abnormalities and SLAP lesions are an important cause of shoulder pain and the clinical entity of microinstability. Knowledge of the anatomic variants and an understanding of the anatomy can help in distinguishing SLAP lesions from variant normal anatomy. However, even with improved understanding of the patho-biomechanics of SLAP tears, there remain unanswered questions related to their development, extension, and effects on the biomechanics of the shoulder.

Although 13 types of SLAP lesion exist, the radiologist should keep in mind that classification is designed to stratify patients with the goal of optimizing treatment options and prognosis. A complete description of the variants and extent of labral abnormality as well as associated shoulder pathology is mandatory in helping the arthroscopist to manage the patient and maximize clinical outcome.

REFERENCES

1. Wilk KE, Reinold MM, Andrews JR. The athlete's shoulder. 2nd edition. Philadelphia: Churchill Livingstone/Elsevier; 2009.

2. McGinty JB, Burkhart SS. Operative arthroscopy. 3rd edition. Philadelphia: Lippincott Williams & Wilkins; 2003.

3. Nottage WM. Microinstability. Presented at the American Academy of Orthopaedic Surgeons AANA Specialty Day. San Francisco, March 2001.

4. Ruotolo C, Nottage WM, Flatow EL, et al. Controversial topics in shoulder arthroscopy. Arthroscopy 2002;18(2 Suppl 1):65–75.

5. Silliman JF, Hawkins RJ. Classification and physical diagnosis of instability of the shoulder. Clin Orthop Relat Res 1993;(291):7–19.

6. Burkhart SS, Morgan CD, Kibler WB. Shoulder injuries in overhead athletes. The "dead arm" revisited. Clin Sports Med 2000;19(1):125–58.

7. Woertler K, Waldt S. MR imaging in sports-related glenohumeral instability. Eur Radiol 2006;16(12): 2622–36.

8. Townley CO. The capsular mechanism in recurrent dislocation of the shoulder. J Bone Joint Surg Am 1950;32A(2):370–80.

9. Savoie FH 3rd, Papendik L, Field LD, et al. Straight anterior instability: lesions of the middle glenohumeral ligament. Arthroscopy 2001;17(3):229–35.

10. Castagna A, Nordenson U, Garofalo R, et al. Minor shoulder instability. Arthroscopy 2007;23(2):211–5.

11. Andrews JR, Carson WG Jr, McLeod WD. Glenoid labrum tears related to the long head of the biceps. Am J Sports Med 1985;13(5):337–41.

12. Burkhart SS, Morgan CD. The peel-back mechanism: its role in producing and extending posterior type II SLAP lesions and its effect on SLAP repair rehabilitation. Arthroscopy 1998; 14(6):637–40.

13. Snyder SJ, Karzel RP, Del Pizzo W, et al. SLAP lesions of the shoulder. Arthroscopy 1990;6(4): 274–9.

14. Savoie FH 3rd, Field LD, Atchinson S. Anterior superior instability with rotator cuff tearing: SLAC lesion. Orthop Clin North Am 2001;32(3):457–61, ix.

15. Steinbeck J, Liljenqvist U, Jerosch J. The anatomy of the glenohumeral ligament complex and its contribution to anterior shoulder stability. J Shoulder Elbow Surg 1998;7(2):122–6.

16. Chung CB, Steinbach LS. MRI of the upper extremity: shoulder, elbow, wrist and hand. Philadelphia: Wolters Kluwer Health/Lippincott Williams & Wilkins; 2010.

17. Jobe FW, Tibone JE, Jobe CM. The shoulder in sports. In: Rockwood CA, Matson FA, editors. The shoulder. Philadelphia: WB Saunders; 1990. p. 963–7.

18. Walch G, Liotard JP, Boileau P, et al. Postero-superior glenoid impingement. Another shoulder impingement. Rev Chir Orthop Reparatrice Appar Mot 1991;77(8):571–4 [in French].

19. Walch G, Boileau C, Noel E. Impingement of the deep surface of the supraspinatus tendon on the posterior superior glenoid rim: an arthroscopic study. J Shoulder Elbow Surg 1992;1:238–45.

20. Jobe CM. Posterior superior glenoid impingement: expanded spectrum. Arthroscopy 1995;11(5): 530–6.

21. Jobe FW, Giangarra CE, Kvitne RS, et al. Anterior capsulolabral reconstruction of the shoulder in athletes in overhand sports. Am J Sports Med 1991;19(5):428–34.

22. Burkhart SS, Morgan CD, Kibler WB. The disabled throwing shoulder: spectrum of pathology Part I: pathoanatomy and biomechanics. Arthroscopy 2003;19(4):404–20.

23. Burkhart SS, Morgan CD, Kibler WB. The disabled throwing shoulder: spectrum of pathology Part III: The SICK scapula, scapular dyskinesis, the kinetic chain, and rehabilitation. Arthroscopy 2003;19(6): 641–61.

24. Bowen MK, Warren RF. Ligamentous control of shoulder stability based on selective cutting and static translation experiments. Clin Sports Med 1991;10(4):757–82.

25. Speer KP. Anatomy and pathomechanics of shoulder instability. Clin Sports Med 1995;14(4): 751–60.

26. Arai R, Kobayashi M, Toda Y, et al. Fiber components of the shoulder superior labrum. Surg Radiol Anat 2012;34(1):49–56.

27. Gaskill TR, Braun S, Millett PJ. The rotator interval: pathology and management. Arthroscopy 2011; 27(4):556–67.

28. Nobuhara K, Ikeda H. Rotator interval lesion. Clin Orthop Relat Res 1987;(223):44–50.

29. Field LD, Savoie FH 3rd. Arthroscopic suture repair of superior labral detachment lesions of the shoulder. Am J Sports Med 1993;21(6):783–90 [discussion: 790].

30. Harryman DT 2nd, Sidles JA, Clark JM, et al. Translation of the humeral head on the glenoid with passive glenohumeral motion. J Bone Joint Surg Am 1990;72(9):1334–43.

31. Harryman DT 2nd, Sidles JA, Harris SL, et al. The role of the rotator interval capsule in passive motion and stability of the shoulder. J Bone Joint Surg Am 1992;74(1):53–66.

32. Field LD, Warren RF, O'Brien SJ, et al. Isolated closure of rotator interval defects for shoulder instability. Am J Sports Med 1995;23(5):557–63.

33. Hara H, Ito N, Iwasaki K. Strength of the glenoid labrum and adjacent shoulder capsule. J Shoulder Elbow Surg 1996;5(4):263–8.

34. Howell SM, Galinat BJ. The glenoid-labral socket. A constrained articular surface. Clin Orthop Relat Res 1989;(243):122–5.

35. Nishida K, Hashizume H, Toda K, et al. Histologic and scanning electron microscopic study of the glenoid labrum. J Shoulder Elbow Surg 1996;5(2 Pt 1): 132–8.

36. Gray H, Williams PL, Bannister LH. Gray's anatomy: the anatomical basis of medicine and surgery. 38th edition. New York: Churchill Livingstone; 1995.

37. Levine WN, Flatow EL. The pathophysiology of shoulder instability. Am J Sports Med 2000;28(6): 910–7.

38. Hertz H, Weinstabl R, Grundschober F, et al. Macroscopic and microscopic anatomy of the shoulder joint and the limbus glenoidalis. Acta Anat (Basel) 1986;125(2):96–100 [in German].

39. Habermeyer P, Schuller U, Wiedemann E. The intra-articular pressure of the shoulder: an experimental study on the role of the glenoid labrum in stabilizing the joint. Arthroscopy 1992;8(2):166–72.

40. Resnick D, Kang HS, Pretterklieber ML. Internal derangements of joints. 2nd edition. Philadelphia: Saunders/Elsevier; 2007.

41. Tibone JE, Savoie FH, Shaffer B. Shoulder arthroscopy. New York: Springer-Verlag; 2003.

42. Vangsness CT Jr, Jorgenson SS, Watson T, et al. The origin of the long head of the biceps from the scapula and glenoid labrum. An anatomical study of 100 shoulders. J Bone Joint Surg Br 1994; 76(6):951–4.

43. Huber WP, Putz RV. Periarticular fiber system of the shoulder joint. Arthroscopy 1997;13(6):680–91.

44. Pal GP, Bhatt RH, Patel VS. Relationship between the tendon of the long head of biceps brachii and the glenoidal labrum in humans. Anat Rec 1991; 229(2):278–80.

45. MacDonald PB. Congenital anomaly of the biceps tendon and anatomy within the shoulder joint. Arthroscopy 1998;14(7):741–2.

46. Hyman JL, Warren RF. Extra-articular origin of biceps brachii. Arthroscopy 2001;17(7):E29.

47. Mariani PP, Bellelli A, Botticella C. Arthroscopic absence of the long head of the biceps tendon. Arthroscopy 1997;13(4):499–501.

48. Moseley HF, Overgaard B. The anterior capsular mechanism in recurrent anterior dislocation of the shoulder. J Bone Joint Surg Br 1962;44: 913–27.

49. Park YH, Lee JY, Moon SH, et al. MR arthrography of the labral capsular ligamentous complex in the shoulder: imaging variations and pitfalls. AJR Am J Roentgenol 2000;175(3):667–72.

50. Chandnani VP, Gagliardi JA, Murnane TG, et al. Glenohumeral ligaments and shoulder capsular mechanism: evaluation with MR arthrography. Radiology 1995;196(1):27–32.

51. Beltran J, Bencardino J, Padron M, et al. The middle glenohumeral ligament: normal anatomy, variants and pathology. Skeletal Radiol 2002; 31(5):253–62.

52. Kask K, Poldoja E, Lont T, et al. Anatomy of the superior glenohumeral ligament. J Shoulder Elbow Surg 2010;19(6):908–16.

53. Williams MM, Snyder SJ, Buford D Jr. The Buford complex–the "cord-like" middle glenohumeral ligament and absent anterosuperior labrum complex: a normal anatomic capsulolabral variant. Arthroscopy 1994;10(3):241–7.

54. Cooper DE, Arnoczky SP, O'Brien SJ, et al. Anatomy, histology, and vascularity of the glenoid labrum. An anatomical study. J Bone Joint Surg Am 1992;74(1):46–52.

55. Davidson PA, Rivenburgh DW. Mobile superior glenoid labrum: a normal variant or pathologic condition? Am J Sports Med 2004;32(4):962–6.

56. Neumann CH, Petersen SA, Jahnke AH. MR imaging of the labral-capsular complex: normal variations. AJR Am J Roentgenol 1991;157(5): 1015–21.

57. Sasaki T, Yodono H, Prado GL, et al. Increased signal intensity in the normal glenoid labrum in MR imaging: diagnostic pitfalls caused by the magic-angle effect. Magn Reson Med Sci 2002; 1(3):149–56.

58. Li T, Mirowitz SA. Manifestation of magic angle phenomenon: comparative study on effects of varying echo time and tendon orientation among

various MR sequences. Magn Reson Imaging 2003;21(7):741–4.

59. Hayes CW, Parellada JA. The magic angle effect in musculoskeletal MR imaging. Top Magn Reson Imaging 1996;8(1):51–6.

60. Bydder M, Rahal A, Fullerton GD, et al. The magic angle effect: a source of artifact, determinant of image contrast, and technique for imaging. J Magn Reson Imaging 2007;25(2):290–300.

61. McCauley TR, Pope CF, Jokl P. Normal and abnormal glenoid labrum: assessment with multi-planar gradient-echo MR imaging. Radiology 1992;183(1):35–7.

62. Waldt S, Metz S, Burkart A, et al. Variants of the superior labrum and labro-bicipital complex: a comparative study of shoulder specimens using MR arthrography, multi-slice CT arthrography and anatomical dissection. Eur Radiol 2006;16(2):451–8.

63. Smith DK, Chopp TM, Aufdemorte TB, et al. Sublabral recess of the superior glenoid labrum: study of cadavers with conventional nonenhanced MR imaging, MR arthrography, anatomic dissection, and limited histologic examination. Radiology 1996;201(1):251–6.

64. Harzmann HC, Burkart A, Wortler K, et al. Normal anatomical variants of the superior labrum biceps tendon anchor complex. Anatomical and magnetic resonance findings. Orthopade 2003;32(7):586–94 [in German].

65. Jin W, Ryu KN, Kwon SH, et al. MR arthrography in the differential diagnosis of type II superior labral anteroposterior lesion and sublabral recess. AJR Am J Roentgenol 2006;187(4):887–93.

66. Holzapfel K, Waldt S, Bruegel M, et al. Inter- and intraobserver variability of MR arthrography in the detection and classification of superior labral anterior posterior (SLAP) lesions: evaluation in 78 cases with arthroscopic correlation. Eur Radiol 2010; 20(3):666–73.

67. Kim YJ, Choi JA, Oh JH, et al. Superior labral anteroposterior tears: accuracy and interobserver reliability of multidetector CT arthrography for diagnosis. Radiology 2011;260(1):207–15.

68. Tuite MJ, Rutkowski A, Enright T, et al. Width of high signal and extension posterior to biceps tendon as signs of superior labrum anterior to posterior tears on MRI and MR arthrography. AJR Am J Roentgenol 2005;185(6):1422–8.

69. Jin W, Ryu KN, Park YK, et al. Cystic lesions in the posterosuperior portion of the humeral head on MR arthrography: correlations with gross and histologic findings in cadavers. AJR Am J Roentgenol 2005;184(4):1211–5.

70. Tuite MJ, Cirillo RL, De Smet AA, et al. Superior labrum anterior-posterior (SLAP) tears: evaluation of three MR signs on T2-weighted images. Radiology 2000;215(3):841–5.

71. Tirman PF, Feller JF, Janzen DL, et al. Association of glenoid labral cysts with labral tears and glenohumeral instability: radiologic findings and clinical significance. Radiology 1994;190(3):653–8.

72. Detrisac DA, Johnson LL. Arthroscopic shoulder anatomy: pathologic and surgical implications. Thorofare (NJ): Slack; 1986.

73. De Maeseneer M, Van Roy F, Lenchik L, et al. CT and MR arthrography of the normal and pathologic anterosuperior labrum and labral-bicipital complex. Radiographics 2000;20(Spec No):S67–81.

74. Ilahi OA, Labbe MR, Cosculluela P. Variants of the anterosuperior glenoid labrum and associated pathology. Arthroscopy 2002;18(8):882–6.

75. Shortt CP, Morrison WB, Shah SH, et al. Association of glenoid morphology and anterosuperior labral variation. J Comput Assist Tomogr 2009;33(4): 584–6.

76. Lapner PL, Lapner MA, Uhthoff HK. The anatomy of the superior labrum and biceps origin in the fetal shoulder. Clin Anat 2010;23(7):821–8.

77. Fealy S, Rodeo SA, Dicarlo EF, et al. The developmental anatomy of the neonatal glenohumeral joint. J Shoulder Elbow Surg 2000;9(3):217–22.

78. Tena-Arregui J, Barrio-Asensio C, Puerta-Fonolla J, et al. Arthroscopic study of the shoulder joint in fetuses. Arthroscopy 2005;21(9):1114–9.

79. Rao AG, Kim TK, Chronopoulos E, et al. Anatomical variants in the anterosuperior aspect of the glenoid labrum: a statistical analysis of seventy-three cases. J Bone Joint Surg Am 2003;85-A(4):653–9.

80. Bents RT, Skeete KD. The correlation of the Buford complex and SLAP lesions. J Shoulder Elbow Surg 2005;14(6):565–9.

81. Clavert P, Bonnomet F, Kempf JF, et al. Contribution to the study of the pathogenesis of type II superior labrum anterior-posterior lesions: a cadaveric model of a fall on the outstretched hand. J Shoulder Elbow Surg 2004;13(1):45–50.

82. Bey MJ, Elders GJ, Huston LJ, et al. The mechanism of creation of superior labrum, anterior, and posterior lesions in a dynamic biomechanical model of the shoulder: the role of inferior subluxation. J Shoulder Elbow Surg 1998;7(4):397–401.

83. Kuhn JE, Lindholm SR, Huston LJ, et al. Failure of the biceps superior labral complex: a cadaveric biomechanical investigation comparing the late cocking and early deceleration positions of throwing. Arthroscopy 2003;19(4):373–9.

84. Shepard MF, Dugas JR, Zeng N, et al. Differences in the ultimate strength of the biceps anchor and the generation of type II superior labral anterior posterior lesions in a cadaveric model. Am J Sports Med 2004;32(5):1197–201.

85. Pradhan RL, Itoi E, Hatakeyama Y, et al. Superior labral strain during the throwing motion. A cadaveric study. Am J Sports Med 2001;29(4):488–92.

86. Yeh ML, Lintner D, Luo ZP. Stress distribution in the superior labrum during throwing motion. Am J Sports Med 2005;33(3):395–401.

87. Burkhart SS, Morgan CD, Kibler WB. The disabled throwing shoulder: spectrum of pathology. Part II: evaluation and treatment of SLAP lesions in throwers. Arthroscopy 2003;19(5):531–9.

88. Pappas AM, Goss TP, Kleinman PK. Symptomatic shoulder instability due to lesions of the glenoid labrum. Am J Sports Med 1983;11(5):279–88.

89. Hunter JC, Blatz DJ, Escobedo EM. SLAP lesions of the glenoid labrum: CT arthrographic and arthroscopic correlation. Radiology 1992;184(2): 513–8.

90. Monu JU, Pope TL Jr, Chabon SJ, et al. MR diagnosis of superior labral anterior posterior (SLAP) injuries of the glenoid labrum: value of routine imaging without intraarticular injection of contrast material. AJR Am J Roentgenol 1994;163(6): 1425–9.

91. Morgan CD, Burkhart SS, Palmeri M, et al. Type II SLAP lesions: three subtypes and their relationships to superior instability and rotator cuff tears. Arthroscopy 1998;14(6):553–65.

92. Maffet MW, Gartsman GM, Moseley B. Superior labrum-biceps tendon complex lesions of the shoulder. Am J Sports Med 1995;23(1):93–8.

93. Nord KD, Brady PC, Yazdani RS, et al. The anatomy and function of the low posterolateral portal in addressing posterior labral pathology. Arthroscopy 2007;23(9):999–1005.

94. Keener JD, Brophy RH. Superior labral tears of the shoulder: pathogenesis, evaluation, and treatment. J Am Acad Orthop Surg 2009;17(10):627–37.

95. Handelberg F, Willems S, Shahabpour M, et al. SLAP lesions: a retrospective multicenter study. Arthroscopy 1998;14(8):856–62.

96. Kim TK, Queale WS, Cosgarea AJ, et al. Clinical features of the different types of SLAP lesions: an analysis of one hundred and thirty-nine cases. J Bone Joint Surg Am 2003;85-A(1):66–71.

97. Kohn D. The clinical relevance of glenoid labrum lesions. Arthroscopy 1987;3(4):223–30.

98. Gobezie R, Zurakowski D, Lavery K, et al. Analysis of interobserver and intraobserver variability in the diagnosis and treatment of SLAP tears using the Snyder classification. Am J Sports Med 2008; 36(7):1373–9.

99. Francavilla G, Sutera R, Iovane A, et al. Role of MR arthrography in shoulder micro-instability: personal experience. Medicina Dello Sport 2010;63(4): 547–56.

100. Stetson WB, Snyder SJ. Clinical presentation and follow-up of isolated SLAP lesions of the shoulder (SS-04). Arthroscopy 2011;27(5 Suppl 1):e30–1.

101. Connell DA, Potter HG, Wickiewicz TL, et al. Non-contrast magnetic resonance imaging of superior labral lesions. 102 cases confirmed at arthroscopic surgery. Am J Sports Med 1999;27(2):208–13.

102. Dinauer PA, Flemming DJ, Murphy KP, et al. Diagnosis of superior labral lesions: comparison of non-contrast MRI with indirect MR arthrography in unexercised shoulders. Skeletal Radiol 2007; 36(3):195–202.

103. Herold T, Hente R, Zorger N, et al. Indirect MR-arthrography of the shoulder-value in the detection of SLAP-lesions. Rofo 2003;175(11):1508–14 [in German].

104. Applegate GR, Hewitt M, Snyder SJ, et al. Chronic labral tears: value of magnetic resonance arthrography in evaluating the glenoid labrum and labral-bicipital complex. Arthroscopy 2004;20(9):959–63.

105. Bencardino JT, Beltran J, Rosenberg ZS, et al. Superior labrum anterior-posterior lesions: diagnosis with MR arthrography of the shoulder. Radiology 2000;214(1):267–71.

106. Waldt S, Burkart A, Lange P, et al. Diagnostic performance of MR arthrography in the assessment of superior labral anteroposterior lesions of the shoulder. AJR Am J Roentgenol 2004;182(5): 1271–8.

107. Jee WH, McCauley TR, Katz LD, et al. Superior labral anterior posterior (SLAP) lesions of the glenoid labrum: reliability and accuracy of MR arthrography for diagnosis. Radiology 2001;218(1):127–32.

108. Jung JY, Ha DH, Lee SM, et al. Displaceability of SLAP lesion on shoulder MR arthrography with external rotation position. Skeletal Radiol 2011; 40(8):1047–55.

109. Choi JA, Suh SI, Kim BH, et al. Comparison between conventional MR arthrography and abduction and external rotation MR arthrography in revealing tears of the antero-inferior glenoid labrum. Korean J Radiol 2001;2(4):216–21.

110. Cvitanic O, Tirman PF, Feller JF, et al. Using abduction and external rotation of the shoulder to increase the sensitivity of MR arthrography in revealing tears of the anterior glenoid labrum. AJR Am J Roentgenol 1997;169(3):837–44.

111. Chan KK, Muldoon KA, Yeh L, et al. Superior labral anteroposterior lesions: MR arthrography with arm traction. AJR Am J Roentgenol 1999;173(4): 1117–22.

112. Chhadia AM, Goldberg BA, Hutchinson MR. Abnormal translation in SLAP lesions on magnetic resonance imaging abducted externally rotated view. Arthroscopy 2010;26(1):19–25.

113. Howell SM, Galinat BJ, Renzi AJ, et al. Normal and abnormal mechanics of the glenohumeral joint in the horizontal plane. J Bone Joint Surg Am 1988; 70(2):227–32.

114. Borrero CG, Casagranda BU, Towers JD, et al. Magnetic resonance appearance of posterosuperior labral peel back during humeral abduction

and external rotation. Skeletal Radiol 2010;39(1): 19–26.

115. Magee TH, Williams D. Sensitivity and specificity in detection of labral tears with 3.0-T MRI of the shoulder. AJR Am J Roentgenol 2006;187(6): 1448–52.

116. Oh DK, Yoon YC, Kwon JW, et al. Comparison of indirect isotropic MR arthrography and conventional MR arthrography of labral lesions and rotator cuff tears: a prospective study. AJR Am J Roentgenol 2009;192(2):473–9.

117. Flannigan B, Kursunoglu-Brahme S, Snyder S, et al. MR arthrography of the shoulder: comparison with conventional MR imaging. AJR Am J Roentgenol 1990;155(4):829–32.

118. Magee T, Williams D, Mani N. Shoulder MR arthrography: which patient group benefits most? AJR Am J Roentgenol 2004;183(4):969–74.

119. Major NM, Browne J, Domzalski T, et al. Evaluation of the glenoid labrum with 3-T MRI: is intraarticular contrast necessary? AJR Am J Roentgenol 2011; 196(5):1139–44.

120. Magee T. 3-T MRI of the shoulder: is MR arthrography necessary? AJR Am J Roentgenol 2009; 192(1):86–92.

121. Jbara M, Chen Q, Marten P, et al. Shoulder MR arthrography: how, why, when. Radiol Clin North Am 2005;43(4):683–92, viii.

122. Helms CA, McGonegle SJ, Vinson EN, et al. Magnetic resonance arthrography of the shoulder: accuracy of gadolinium versus saline for rotator cuff and labral pathology. Skeletal Radiol 2011; 40(2):197–203.

123. Sommer T, Vahlensieck M, Wallny T, et al. Indirect MR arthrography in the diagnosis of lesions of the labrum glenoidale. Rofo 1997;167(1):46–51 [in German].

124. Bedi A, Allen AA. Superior labral lesions anterior to posterior-evaluation and arthroscopic management. Clin Sports Med 2008;27(4):607–30.

125. Gregush RV, Snyder SJ. Superior labral repair. Sports Med Arthrosc 2007;15(4):222–9.

126. Rhee YG, Lee DH, Lim CT. Unstable isolated SLAP lesion: clinical presentation and outcome of arthroscopic fixation. Arthroscopy 2005;21(9):1099.

127. Higgins LD, Warner JJ. Superior labral lesions: anatomy, pathology, and treatment. Clin Orthop Relat Res 2001;(390):73–82.

128. Nam EK, Snyder SJ. The diagnosis and treatment of superior labrum, anterior and posterior (SLAP) lesions. Am J Sports Med 2003;31(5):798–810.

129. Wolf BR, Britton CL, Vasconcellos DA, et al. Agreement in the classification and treatment of the superior labrum. Am J Sports Med 2011;39(12): 2588–94.

130. Crockett HC, Wingert NC, Wright JM, et al. Repair of SLAP lesions associated with a Buford complex: a novel surgical technique. Arthroscopy 2011; 27(3):314–21.

131. Powell SE, Nord KD, Ryu RK. The diagnosis, classification, and treatment of SLAP lesions. Oper Tech Sports Med 2004;12:99–110.

Magnetic Resonance Imaging in Glenohumeral Instability

Peter J. MacMahon, MD*, William E. Palmer, MD

KEYWORDS

- Shoulder • Glenohumeral instability • MR Imaging
- MR arthrography • Labrum • Glenohumeral ligaments
- Bankart

The glenohumeral joint is one of the least anatomically constrained in the body,[1] conferring an advantage in mobility but causing a propensity for instability.[2,3] In patients with unstable shoulders, symptoms such as apprehension, looseness, slipping, or "going out" usually correlate with objective signs on physical examination.[4–6] These clinical features may warrant imaging studies for lesion characterization, preoperative planning, and prognosis, and the detection of secondary degenerative change.[4–6]

Historically, glenohumeral instability has been classified by both directionality (anterior, posterior, or multidirectional) and origin (traumatic or atraumatic).[4] Trauma typically causes unidirectional instability and results from single inciting events (eg, fall on an out-stretched hand) or repeated high-load activities (eg, weight-lifting).[4] After trauma, orthopedists can usually determine the predominant direction of instability based on history, symptoms, and signs,[5] whereas atraumatic instability is more difficult to characterize. Causes include connective tissue disorders or repeated low-load activities (eg, swimming) that lead to generalized ligamentous laxity and multidirectional instability (MDI), often affecting both shoulders equally.[7] Although trauma-related instability can be obvious clinically, shoulder hypermobility caused by atraumatic instability has proved difficult to distinguish from hypermobility caused by benign capsular laxity. The differentiation is important because true instability eventually leads to debilitation and progressive joint degeneration. Regardless of whether it is causing instability, capsular laxity remains a difficult imaging diagnosis.

This article first reviews the anatomic structures most important in glenohumeral stability and the most common instability patterns. Subsequently, the focus shifts to MR imaging findings in unstable shoulders.

FUNCTIONAL STABILITY

The normal shoulder maintains stable alignment because of osseous congruity, labrocapsular integrity, and synergistic muscle balance.[6] The osseous geometry of the glenohumeral joint contributes less to functional stability than in other joints, because the glenoid surface area is small and shallow compared with the humeral articular surface.[8] Glenoid hypoplasia further reduces glenoid surface area and predisposes toward instability.[6] For example, patients with an acquired or developmental deficiency of the posteroinferior glenoid rim have increased risk of posterior shoulder instability.[9]

The glenoid labrum encircles the glenoid, enhancing both depth and surface area of the glenoid cavity, and consequently improving congruity of the two articular surfaces (**Fig. 1**).[10] The glenoid labrum is commonly described as a fibrocartilaginous structure; however, histologic examinations have shown that the labrum consists of parallel collagen fibers and dense fibrous connective

Department of Musculoskeletal Imaging and Intervention, Massachusetts General Hospital, Harvard Medical School, 55 Fruit Street, YAW 6030, Boston, MA 02114, USA
* Corresponding author.
E-mail address: petermacmahon@yahoo.com

Magn Reson Imaging Clin N Am 20 (2012) 295–312
doi:10.1016/j.mric.2012.01.003

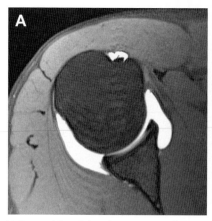
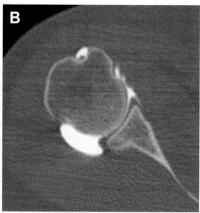

Fig. 1. Normal labrum. (A) Axial T1 fat-suppressed MR arthrogram showing normal anterior and posterior labrum outlined by contrast. The low-signal-intensity labrum lies on hyaline articular cartilage that is of intermediate signal intensity on T1-weighted and T2-weighted MR images. (B) Normal axial CT arthrogram in a different patient showing the normal labrum and glenoid rim.

tissue without chondrocytes, an appearance that corresponds to the morphologic structure of a tendon.[11,12] The labrum functions as a "chock block" to resist translational forces during movement and, most importantly, acts as a point of attachment for the joint capsule, glenohumeral ligaments (GHLs), and biceps tendon.[3,13,14] As a capsular attachment site, the labrum helps to create a suction seal. Negative intraarticular pressure boosts shoulder stability unless the seal is lost because of rotator cuff tear or labral tear.[1,6] Compared with the anteroinferior labrocapsular complex, the anterosuperior labrocapsular complex is less important in shoulder stabilization.[15] Superior labral lesions occur in patients with clinically stable shoulders and are often debrided without shoulder destabilization.[14,16,17] Developmental variations of the anterosuperior labrum,

due to a sublabral foramen or Buford complex (Fig. 2), are not associated with shoulder instability.[3]

The glenohumeral joint capsule has ligamentous thickenings (Fig. 3) that are consistently shown on MR arthrography.[18] The most important ligaments serve important biomechanical roles through limiting excessive translation and rotation of the humeral head.[19] Numerous in vivo and in vitro studies have investigated the complex anatomic configurations and biomechanical contributions of these structures.[20–28] The coracohumeral ligaments (CHLs), superior GHLs, and middle GHLs are less important than the inferior GHL. If the inferior GHL is attached to a labrum that is torn from the glenoid rim, it becomes incompetent and the shoulder becomes unstable.

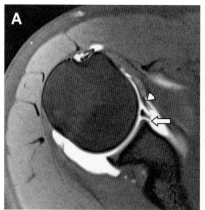
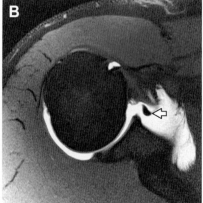

Fig. 2. Labral pseudotears. Axial T1 fat-suppressed MR arthrograms in two different patients. (A) Contrast undercuts the anterosuperior labrum to form a sublabral foramen (arrow). A normal flattened middle GHL is noted anteriorly (arrow head). (B) The anterior labrum is absent with a thickened cord-like middle GHL (arrow) anteriorly consistent with a Buford complex. When isolated, these normal variants are not associated with instability and should not be confused with labral tears.

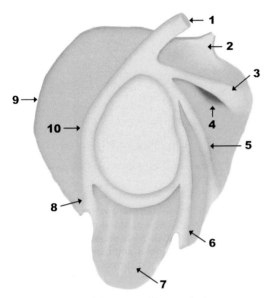

Fig. 3. Diagram of the normal intraarticular structures of the glenohumeral joint. 1. Long head of biceps tendon. 2. Coracohumeral ligamentous component of capsule. 3. Superior GHL blending with joint capsule. 4. Foramen of Weitbrecht (outpouching of the capsule between superior GHL and middle GHL forming entrance of the subscapularis bursa). 5. Middle GHL. 6. Anterior band of the GHL. 7. Axillary pouch. 8. Posterior band of the GHL. 9. Posterior joint capsule. 10. Posterior glenoid labrum.

On MR images, the CHL extends laterally from the dorsal base of the coracoid.[21,29] The superior GHL courses parallel to the coracoid process from its labral attachment site and merges with the CHL in the rotator interval, reinforcing the

biceps tendon sling (pulley).[30,31] The CHL also branches posteriorly to envelope the supraspinatus and infraspinatus tendons, forming the semicircular humeral ligament (rotator cable).[29,32] The middle GHL arises from the anterosuperior glenolabral rim with the superior GHL and courses caudally, merging with the subscapularis tendon near the lesser tuberosity (**Fig. 4**). The labrum, middle GHL, and inferior GHL share strong developmental relationships. Based on cadaver studies, the middle GHL is absent in approximately 30% of patients.[33] When present, it ranges in thickness from wafer-thin to cord-like. The cord-like middle GHL can be associated with absent anterosuperior labrum (Buford complex) (see **Fig. 2**). When the middle GHL is small or absent, there is often compensatory enlargement and superior takeoff of the inferior GHL.[34] Although the CHL, superior GHL, and middle GHL make limited stabilizing contributions, many authors associate laxity of these structures with microinstability and MDI.[35,36] Therefore, some surgeons tighten the rotator interval (capsulorrhaphy) in patients with MDI.[37]

Compared with other capsuloligamentous structures, the inferior GHL contributes most to passive glenohumeral stabilization. The inferior GHL includes an anterior band (aIGHL) (see **Fig. 4**), posterior band, and intervening axillary pouch.[38,39] The aIGHL resists anteroinferior translation of the humeral head and becomes taut when the shoulder is abducted and externally rotated (ABER position) (**Fig. 5**).[40,41] In most patients, the aIGHL arises from the labroglenoid rim inferior to the 3 o'clock position, though it may arise more

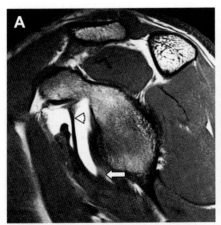
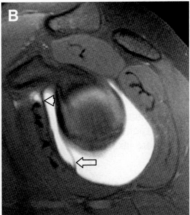

Fig. 4. Normal middle GHL and inferior GHL. (*A*) Sagittal oblique T1 fat-suppressed MR arthrogram showing the normal middle GHL (*arrowhead*), which in this patient extends inferiorly from the superior GHL to merge with the posterior surface of the subscapularis. The anterior band of the inferior GHL (aIGHL) (*arrow*) in this patient is a relatively thick structure. (*B*) Sagittal oblique T1 fat-suppressed arthrogram in a different patient showing a normal middle GHL (*arrowhead*) and normal aIGHL (*arrow*). These structures are thinner than in the previous patient but are still within normal limits.

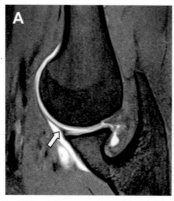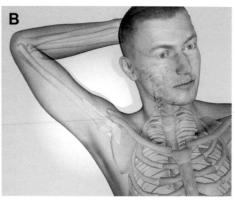

Fig. 5. Normal aIGHL. (*A*) ABER positioned T1 fat-suppressed arthrogram image showing a normal anterior inferior GHL glenoid attachment (*arrow*). The aIGHL resists anteroinferior translation of the humeral head and is under greatest tension when in the ABER position. (*B*) Illustration of the ABER position and imaging plane. The patient places the hand behind the head, which externally rotates the humerus and markedly abducts the shoulder. The imaging plane (*light green shaded region*) is parallel to the humeral diaphysis. The ABER position has a potential role in increasing sensitivity to subtle injuries at the aIGHL insertion.

superiorly. The aIGHL usually attaches to the labrum and glenoid rim,[41,42] forming a sleeve of continuous tissue between the labrum, capsule, and periosteum.[43] Lesions involving this periosteal sleeve are often associated with instability. The posterior band of the inferior GHL more commonly arises directly from the posteroinferior glenoid rather than the labrum. The humeral attachment of the inferior GHL complex is either (1) collar-like, in which the anterior and posterior bands of the inferior GHL fan out and create a ring-like insertion slightly caudal to the articular edge of the humeral head, or (2) V-shaped, in which the anterior and posterior bands of the inferior GHL come together and create a point-like insertion.[44]

The dynamic stabilizers of the shoulder include the rotator cuff, deltoid, periscapular muscles and the biceps tendon (long head).[2] During normal shoulder movements, these structures maintain a delicate contractile balance to center and compress the humeral head into the labroglenoid socket and counter the translational forces inherent in shoulder motion.[6,45,46] This "compression concavity" mechanism is most important in the middle ranges of motion when the capsuloligamentous structures are lax.[6]

INSTABILITY PATTERNS: CLINICAL PERSPECTIVE
Anterior Instability

The glenohumeral joint dislocates more commonly than any other, occurring in 11.2 per 100,000 persons per year. Most dislocations (90%) are directed anteriorly.[47,48] The mechanism can involve falling on an outstretched arm or colliding with players during contact sports, such as American football or rugby.[49] At the time of injury, the shoulder is often forced anteriorly in abduction, external rotation, and extension. A patient may not realize that the shoulder has dislocated and spontaneously relocated. First-time dislocations can be difficult to diagnose unless confirmed through reduction maneuvers or radiographs. In a recent study of young athletes, first-time trauma-related shoulder injuries were clinically categorized as subluxations in 85% of cases and as dislocations in only 15% of cases.[50] Although structural damage is commonly associated with dislocations,[51] the authors also reported a high rate of labral, capsular, and osseous lesions in their patients with anterior subluxations.

After traumatic shoulder dislocation (treated nonoperatively), the likelihood of repeat dislocation depends on patient age and the date of initial injury. Patients younger than 20 years have a higher risk of recurrent dislocation (>90% when subluxation events are included) than those older than 40 years (<10%).[52–55] The likelihood of recurrent dislocation also depends on behavior modification. If an athlete returns to a collision sport, such as football and hockey, or a contact sport, such as lacrosse and basketball, the incidence of recurrent dislocation approaches 100% at the same level of competition.[56] Older individuals are much more willing to modify behavior to avoid repeated dislocations, chronic anterior instability, and progressive functional disability.

Posterior Instability

Posterior instability is much less common than anterior instability. An incidence of 2% to 4% is generally accepted, but a higher incidence (11.6%) was reported more recently when recurrent posterior subluxation was taken into account.[57,58] Traumatic posterior dislocation typically occurs after a blow to the upper arm when the humerus is flexed, adducted, and internally rotated (opposite to anterior dislocation). Bilateral posterior dislocation can occur after an epileptic seizure or high-voltage electric shock from the strong contraction of internal rotators.

MDI

MDI represents a complex condition without consistent diagnostic and treatment criteria.[4,59,60] In 1980, Neer and Foster[61] reported that patients treated surgically for MDI presented with predominantly inferior signs and symptoms. More recently, authors have recommended that the diagnosis of MDI requires symptoms and signs of instability in an inferior direction and at least one other direction (anterior or posterior).[62] MDI often develops in the absence of trauma (atraumatic instability), involves both shoulders, and indicates joint hypermobility from generalized capsular laxity. Acquired causes may reflect repetitive overstretching activities (eg, swimming, gymnastics),[7,61] proprioceptive imbalances,[63] connective tissue disorders, or multifactorial conditions.[64–68] Some authors argue that all shoulder instabilities show some degree of excessive multidirectional translation and, therefore, propose that the multidirectional descriptor should be dropped so that instabilities are described based only on the predominant direction of abnormal motion.[4,69]

IMAGING TECHNIQUES

At the authors' institution, referring physicians request the imaging modality. In patients with suspected shoulder instability, the cross-sectional modality could be CT, CT arthrography, MR imaging, or MR arthrography.[34,35,70–78] It is extremely rare for a radiologist to change the request. Some orthopedists depend on nonarthrographic studies, but others strongly prefer arthrographic techniques unless recent acute trauma has occurred, in which case joint effusion, edema, and hemorrhage are usually present.[79] MR arthrography is more commonly requested in younger individuals with clinical evidence of shoulder instability. Although certain referrers exclusively select MR, others are balanced in their choice of MR versus CT, depending on the suspicion of glenoid rim fracture and the likelihood of performing Latarjet reconstruction of the glenoid rim.

In the assessment of the labrocapsular complex, MR arthrography has shown sensitivities of 86% to 91% and specificities of 86% to 98%,[70,80–82] whereas conventional MR imaging has shown sensitivities and specificities ranging from 44% to 100% and 66% to 95%, respectively.[72,83] MR arthrography can add confidence in the diagnosis of labral tear compared with conventional MR imaging, even at 3T.[81,84] A potential advantage of MR arthrography is ABER positioning (see **Fig. 4**).[85] If the position can be tolerated, it may improve the detection of subtle anteroinferior labral tears, while also revealing tendon delamination involving the rotator cuff.[85,86] Studies comparing CT arthrography and MR arthrography have shown similar performance in unstable shoulders (see **Fig. 1**).[3,79,87,88] CT is preferable to MR imaging when evaluating for small fracture fragments of the glenoid rim and assessing bone stock in patients with recurrent dislocation.[35,89,90]

INSTABILITY PATTERNS: MR IMAGING
Traumatic Anterior Instability

Increased experience in arthroscopy and cross-sectional imaging has led to refinements in the nomenclature used to describe lesions of the inferior labrocapsular complex. Many of these variants are important for the radiologist to understand, depending on the level of specialization among orthopedic referrers. Others are irrelevant. The most important lesions are Bankart, Perthes, anterior labral-ligamentous periosteal sleeve avulsion (ALPSA), and humeral avulsion of glenohumeral ligament (HAGL) (**Fig. 6**). Although Bankart and Bankart variant lesions have been correctly classified with 77% sensitivity, 91% specificity, and 84% accuracy on MR arthrograms, it is not possible to categorize all labral-ligamentous injuries.[91] In the same MR arthrographic study, 22% of all anteroinferior labral lesions were non-classifiable. This situation was most common in patients with histories of chronic instability and advanced secondary changes, such as capsular scarring, synovitis, and joint degeneration.

Bankart lesion

During glenohumeral dislocation or subluxation, the anteroinferior labrum can be avulsed by the inferior GHL or crushed and torn by the humeral head. Although this injury pattern was originally described by Broca and Hartmann[92] in 1890, and later by Perthes[93] in 1906, it is recognized today as the Bankart lesion because Bankart first emphasized it as the most important cause of recurrent shoulder dislocation.[94,95] At arthroscopy and imaging, the classic Bankart lesion indicates focal detachment of the anteroinferior labral-ligamentous complex

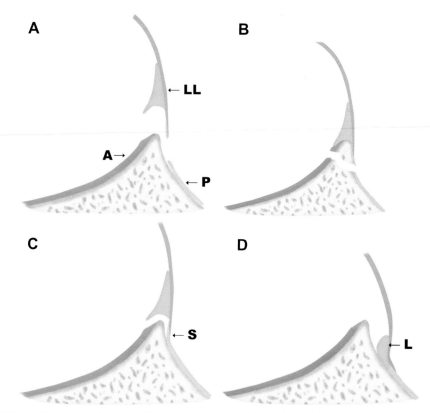

Fig. 6. Diagrammatic representation of the commonest instability-related injuries in the anterior shoulder. (*A*) Classic Bankart lesion. The anteroinferior capsulolabral ligamentous complex is completely detached from the glenoid rim with rupture of the capsule-periosteal sleeve. (*B*) The bony Bankart lesion. The instability injury has avulsed the glenoid rim at the capsulolabral attachment and ruptured the capsule-periosteal sleeve. (*C*) Perthes lesion. The instability event has resulted in a tear of the labroligamentous complex at the glenoid rim; however, the capsule-periosteal sleeve remains intact. (*D*) ALPSA. The labroligamentous complex has detached from the glenoid rim, displaced medially (from progressive stripping of the periosteal sleeve), and scarred onto the scapular neck. A, articular cartilage; L, displaced and deformed labrum; LL, labroligamentous complex; P, periosteum; S, capsule periosteal sleeve.

from the glenoid rim (**Fig. 7**).[74,96] The Bankart lesion typically occurs between the 3 and 6 o'clock positions, and represents the most common labral abnormality in patients with first-time traumatic dislocations.[97,98] On MR images, the labrum shows focal detachment from the glenoid rim but remains continuous with the aIGHL (see **Fig. 7**).[76,91] On arthrographic MR images, the Bankart lesion is readily classified based on the presence of sublabral contrast. Because of displacement from the glenoid rim, the lesion shows little tendency to heal and, therefore, often requires an anterior stabilization procedure (Bankart repair).[94,97,98]

Perthes lesion

The Perthes lesion, a potentially less-debilitating variant of the Bankart lesion, is characterized by tear of the anteroinferior labrum from its osteochondral attachment but not from its periosteal sleeve.[76,99] The Perthes lesion is important for

radiologists to consider because it can be difficult to identify at arthroscopy without prior knowledge.[100] It is easily overlooked on both MR and arthrographic MR images when the torn labral fragment remains closely apposed to the glenoid rim in its normal anatomic position. Despite labrocapsular insufficiency and clinical signs of instability, scarring can prevent contrast from entering the tear (**Fig. 8**).[91,100] ABER positioning may improve the detection of Perthes lesions because traction on the aIGHL transmits tension to the labrum, displacing it from the glenoid rim (see **Fig. 8**).[91,100–102] The ABER position may also help to distinguish a nondisplaced Bankart lesion from a Perthes lesion by more clearly showing the integrity of the periosteal sleeve.

ALPSA lesion

Bankart and Perthes lesions can reflect acute or remote injuries, but the ALPSA lesion indicates

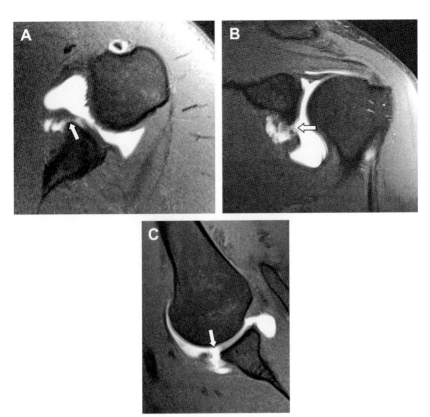

Fig. 7. Classic Bankart lesion sustained after traumatic anterior shoulder dislocation. (*A*) Axial T1 fat-suppressed MR arthrogram showing separation of the anteroinferior labroligamentous complex from the glenoid rim (*arrow*), including disruption of the periosteal sleeve. (*B*) Coronal oblique T1 fat-suppressed MR arthrogram of same patient showing the Bankart lesion (*arrow*). The anteroinferior labral tear extends superiorly to involve the biceps anchor. (*C*) ABER-positioned T1 fat-suppressed arthrogram in same patient showing the classic Bankart lesion (*arrow*) with displacement of the labroligamentous complex from the glenoid rim.

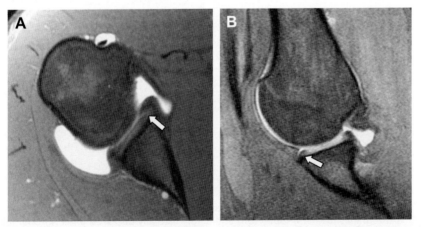

Fig. 8. Perthes lesion in a patient with history of anterior dislocation. (*A*) This axial T1 fat-suppressed MR arthrogram shows very subtle undercutting of the anteroinferior labrum with intraarticular contrast (*arrow*). (*B*) The ABER-positioned T1 fat-suppressed arthrogram image more clearly shows the Perthes lesion (*arrow*) by creating tension in the aIGHL.

chronic instability. In contrast to the classic Bankart lesion, this Bankart variant rarely occurs after a single dislocation, leading some authors to suggest that the ALPSA lesion reflects an advanced stage of the Perthes lesion.[103,104] The ALPSA lesion is characterized by medial displacement of the torn anteroinferior labral-ligamentous complex, which scars onto the scapular neck and becomes synovialized with its attached periosteum.[74] Axial and coronal images both can show the thickened labral-ligamentous complex on the scapular neck (**Fig. 9**). On arthrographic MR images, the aIGHL is outlined by contrast and followed to the abnormal periosteal sleeve. Periosteal mineralization is often missed on MR images but is obvious on CT images. Over time, the periosteal sleeve is stripped along the neck of the glenoid from repeated dislocation or subluxation, resulting in a severely deficient anteroinferior glenoid rim. The deformed resynovialized labral tissue on the scapular neck may be subtle in chronic untreated cases (**Fig. 10**).[74] Compared with Perthes lesions, ALPSA lesions are more frequently associated with instability, Hill-Sachs fractures, cartilage defects, synovitis, and joint degeneration.[103,105] ALPSA lesions have a worse prognosis because of poor capsular tissue quality that increases the technical difficulty of the surgical repair. After an anterior stabilization procedure, failed repair and recurrent instability occur nearly twice as often in ALPSA lesions compared with Bankart lesions.[104]

HAGL lesion

During dislocation, extreme tension is transmitted across the length of the aIGHL. Ligamentous

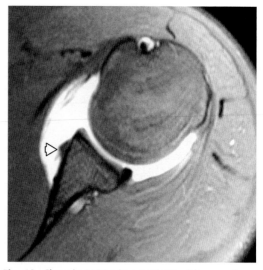

Fig. 10. Chronic ALPSA in a patient with several-year history of multiple prior anterior shoulder dislocations. Axial T1 fat-suppressed MR arthrogram. In this patient, the torn and displaced anteroinferior labrum (*arrow head*) is more subtle because it has become flattened and resynovialized along the scapular neck. Note the absence of the labrum at the anteroinferior glenoid rim compared with the posterior glenoid.

failure usually occurs at the labral attachment site, but when it occurs at the humeral attachment site it is called a *HAGL lesion*.[44,106] HAGL lesions usually occur in men involved in contact sports, such as rugby, American football, and ice hockey.[107,108] Despite symptoms and signs of anterior instability, this injury is difficult to identify at both arthroscopy and open shoulder surgery

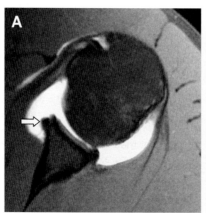

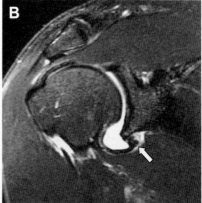

Fig. 9. ALPSA lesion in a patient with history of recurrent anterior shoulder dislocations. (A) Axial T1 fat-suppressed MR arthrogram showing a subtly torn and mildly medially displaced anteroinferior labrum (*arrow*). The periosteal sleeve seems intact, consistent with an ALPSA lesion. (B) Coronal oblique T2 fat-suppressed MR arthrogram in the same patient, again showing the torn anteroinferior glenoid labrum, nodular in shape and medially displaced (*arrow*). The coronal image can sometimes show the medially displaced labral tissue to better advantage compared with axial images.

unless there is elevated suspicion and targeted examination.[44,107] In the acute setting, the HAGL lesion is obvious on MR images because extra-articular edema and hemorrhage localize to the humeral neck and frequently outline the stump of the detached aIGHL. In the chronic setting, unfortunately, once edema has resolved and scarring has occurred, imaging findings are extremely limited. The ligament remains incompetent, but its torn stump cannot be distinguished from re-modeled scar. Rarely, a pseudo-pouch fills with fluid and extends distally along the humeral neck into the quadrilateral space near the axillary nerve and inferior circumflex neurovascular bundle. On arthrographic and arthrographic MR images, this pseudo-pouch becomes distended by contrast, outlining the aIGHL stump, which has a character-istic "J" configuration (**Fig. 11**).[35] In approximately 20% of HAGL lesions, a small bony fragment is avulsed from the humerus (bony HAGL or BHAGL).[109] Rarely, the HAGL and Bankart lesions occur together, resulting in a "floating" aIGHL.[110]

Bony Bankart lesion

During anterior glenohumeral dislocation, the humeral head impacts the glenoid rim and can

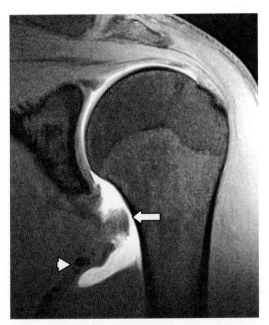

Fig. 11. HAGL lesion in patient who sustained trau-matic shoulder injury while playing contact sports. Coronal oblique T2 fat-suppressed MR arthrogram showing severe disruption of the humeral attachment of the aIGHL with extravasation of contrast along the humeral neck (*arrow*) and loss of the normal U-shaped inferior capsule. The contrast extends toward the quadrilateral space containing the axillary nerve and inferior circumflex neurovascular bundle (*arrowhead*).

shear off an osseous fragment. When the inferior labrocapsular complex is attached to the fracture fragment, it is commonly called a *bony Bankart lesion* (although Bankart never described these osseous defects).[94,95] Although CT reveals even tiny osseous fragments (**Fig. 12**), MR can only show larger fractures and contour defects. Corti-cally based fragments are particularly difficult to identify but are best seen on sagittal MR images (see **Fig. 12**).[34,35] The size of the glenoid defect influences treatment. Most studies conclude that a defect measuring more than 20% to 30% of total glenoid surface area precludes arthroscopic repair, and represents an indication for fragment fixation or bone grafting (eg, Latarjet procedure).[2,108,111] Although patients with minimal glenoid bone loss successfully undergo arthroscopic Bankart repair,[3] soft tissue stabilization procedures typically fail if a fracture fragment is not addressed, particularly in contact athletes.[108,112]

Hill-Sachs fracture

Hill-Sachs fracture also results from impaction by the humeral head against the glenoid rim, causing a depressed fracture in 47% to 80% of new dislo-cations, and nearly 100% of repeated dislocations (**Fig. 13**).[113–115] Located at the posterosuperolat-eral margin of the humeral head, they are named for Hill and Sachs,[116] who described the radio-graphic appearance in 1940. In the weeks following acute injury, MR shows bone marrow edema that dissipates distally, even when the degree of depression is minimal at CT.[34] In a study from 1992, MR imaging was 97% sensitive, 91% specific, and 94% accurate in showing Hill-Sachs lesions, and was superior to arthros-copy.[117] An indentation at the anatomic neck of the humerus can be confused with a small Hill-Sachs lesion.[118] This normal groove usually lies at least 20 mm distal to the top of the humeral head, whereas the Hill-Sachs lesion is usually located in the most cranial 18 mm of the humeral head. Larger Hill-Sachs defects can cause locking and mechanical symptoms from glenoid capture during shoulder motion.[108] Although these "engaging" defects must be corrected to prevent persistent mechanical symptoms after a stabiliza-tion procedure,[108,115] no widely accepted methods exist to quantify the Hill-Sachs lesion and assess its probability of engagement.[119,120]

Posterior instability

Different MR imaging criteria apply in the diagnosis of posterior glenohumeral instability compared with anterior instability. Although anterior insta-bility is likely if the labrum is torn at the aIGHL attachment site, posterior unidirectional instability

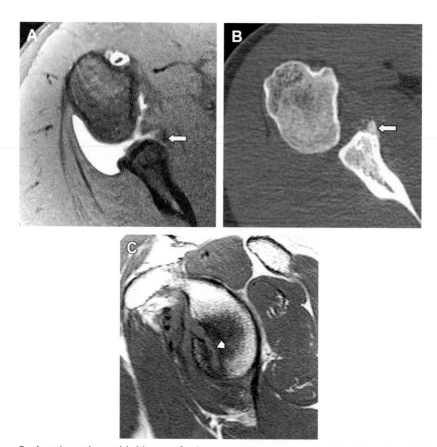

Fig. 12. Bony Bankart in patient with history of prior traumatic anterior shoulder dislocation. (*A*) Axial T1 fat-suppressed MR arthrogram showing contrast undercutting low signal tissue at the anteroinferior glenoid rim (*arrow*). The abrupt contour change of the glenoid rim in this region is most consistent with a bony Bankart lesion. (*B*) Axial CT of the same patient more clearly shows the fracture of the anteroinferior glenoid rim (*arrow*). (*B, C*) Sagittal oblique T1-weighted MR in a different patient showing a large fracture (*arrow head*) of the anteroinferior glenoid. This patient will likely require osseous reconstruction to resolve instability symptoms.

cannot be predicted based on the presence of labral tear alone. The posterior band of the inferior GHL is variable in size and often not visualized. Nondisplaced posterior labral tears may be associated with pain but not instability. Abnormalities of the periosteum, glenoid rim, and humeral head increase the probability of posterior instability.[121]

At arthroscopy, two findings that are most frequently associated with unidirectional posterior instability include detachment of the posteroinferior labrum and, in most cases, coexistent stretching and stripping of the joint capsule and periosteum along the glenoid neck (analogous to the anterior Perthes or ALPSA lesions).[122,123] The longer the detached labral segment (>15 mm in craniocaudal length), the closer the association with instability and the greater the need for a posterior stabilization procedure.[124] As nondisplaced posterior labral tears do not predispose to instability they may only require arthroscopic debridement.

On MR images, these arthroscopic findings correlate with posterior labral displacement from the glenoid rim. Although the torn labral fragment becomes detached from the glenoid, it remains attached to the periosteal sleeve and, therefore, simulates a Perthes lesion (**Fig. 14**). Longer segments of displaced labrum correspond to greater degrees of periosteal stripping along the glenoid neck. The periosteum can become thickened, but the posterior joint capsule remains paper-thin and attaches to the base of labrum at the junction with periosteum. The posterior labro-capsular periosteal sleeve avulsion (POLPSA) lesion is similar to a nondisplaced ALPSA lesion and represents avulsion of an intact posterior labrum with capsule–periosteal sleeve stripping (**Fig. 15**).[125,126] The posterior labrum rarely avulses completely from both the glenoid rim and the periosteal sleeve (so-called reverse Bankart lesion) (**Fig. 16**).[127,128]

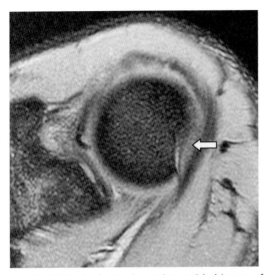

Fig. 13. Hill-Sachs lesion in patient with history of prior anterior shoulder dislocation. Axial gradient-echo T2* nonarthrographic MR showing a large Hill-Sachs deformity of the posterolateral humeral head (*arrow*) without associated marrow edema.

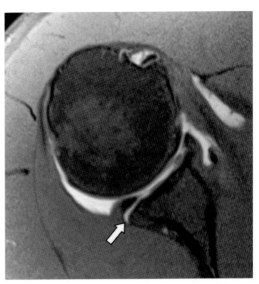

Fig. 15. Posterior labrocapsular periosteal sleeve avulsion (POLPSA) lesion. Axial T1 fat-suppressed MR arthrogram showing detachment of an otherwise intact posterior labrum with stripping/avulsion of the posterior scapular periosteum (*arrow*), which remains attached to the posterior glenoid. This structure creates a redundant recess that communicates with the joint.

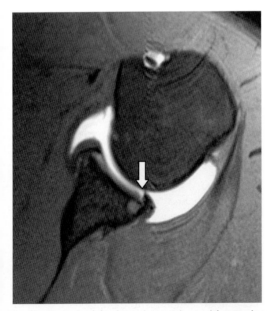

Fig. 14. Posterior labral tear in a patient with ongoing shoulder discomfort. Axial T1 fat-suppressed MR arthrogram showing minimally displaced tear (*arrow*) of the posterior labrum at the chondrolabral junction. No substantial periosteal stripping is present and the periosteal sleeve remains intact. Subchondral cyst formation is seen in the adjacent glenoid. The shoulder cannot be determined to be unstable based on these imaging findings, although the lesion may be painful.

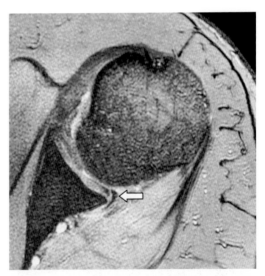

Fig. 16. Posterior labral tear in a patient with recent history of traumatic posterior shoulder dislocation. Axial gradient-echo T2* nonarthrographic MR showing surgically confirmed complete detachment of the posterior labrum (*arrow*) from the glenoid rim consistent with a posterior Bankart lesion. Acute changes in the posterior soft tissues are also present, probably related to recent posterior dislocation.

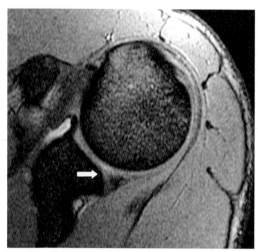

Fig. 17. Posterior glenoid dysplasia. Axial gradient-echo T2* nonarthrographic MR showing sharp posterior truncation of the inferior glenoid rim with a delta-shaped defect (*arrow*) replaced by hypertrophied labrum and articular cartilage.

MR images show glenoid shape and orientation. Posterior glenoid dysplasia, or hypoplasia, may predispose shoulders to labral tear and instability.[129,130] In an arthrographic MR study, moderate to severe dysplastic configurations were identified in 14% of patients (40% including milder cases).[130] The dysplastic glenoid rim shows bony deficiency

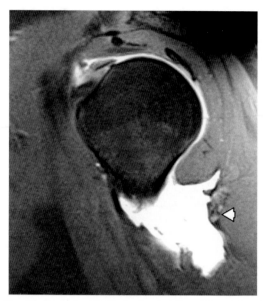

Fig. 19. Posterior HAGL. Sagittal oblique T1-weighted MR arthrogram showing extravasation of contrast into the posterior soft tissues of the shoulder secondary to a tear at the humeral attachment of the posterior inferior GHL (a posterior HAGL). The arrowhead shows the neurovascular bundle containing axillary nerve and posterior humeral circumflex artery.

with compensatory thickening of both overlying articular cartilage and labrum (**Fig. 17**).[2,9,129–133] The retroverted glenoid, in contrast, shows abnormal orientation without deficiency of the glenoid rim or compensatory changes in articular cartilage.

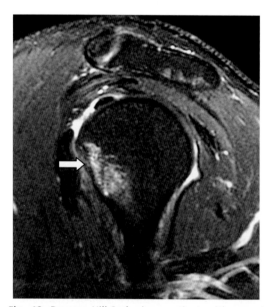

Fig. 18. Reverse Hill-Sachs in a patient with recent history of traumatic posterior shoulder instability event. Sagittal oblique T2-weighted fat-suppressed MR showing pronounced marrow edema and flattening of the anterior humeral head (*arrow*) consistent with a reverse Hill-Sachs injury.

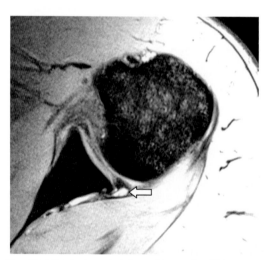

Fig. 20. Kim lesion. Axial gradient-echo T2* nonarthrographic MR showing a flattened posteroinferior labrum, with grossly intact chondrolabral junction and a deep paralabral cyst (*arrow*) consistent with a Kim lesion in this patient with MDI and posterior predominant symptoms.

Several imaging findings are only seen after traumatic posterior shoulder dislocation. Reverse Hill-Sachs fracture (McLaughlin fracture) results from impaction of the anteromedial humeral head against the posterior glenoid rim (**Fig. 18**).[57,128,134,135] Larger humeral defects, similar to Hill-Sachs fractures, can engage the glenoid rim during internal rotation.[123] Some authors distinguish between a posterior HAGL and reverse HAGL, though both are difficult to confirm on MR images.[136] The posterior HAGL is analogous to the anterior HAGL and results from forced posterior subluxation or dislocation of the abducted shoulder (**Fig. 19**).[137] The reverse HAGL represents an avulsion of the posterior joint capsule from the humerus superior to the posterior band of the inferior GHL.[136] Bony avulsion at the humeral attachment site of the posterior band of inferior GHL has been termed the posterior BHAGL lesion. A nondisplaced posterior labral tear with intact and

nonavulsed periosteal sleeve (Kim lesion) is an important imaging finding (**Fig. 20**).[138] This lesion may be concealed at arthroscopy but should be taken into account because anterior capsular tightening may cause the tear to extend along the periosteum, thereby exacerbating posterior instability.

MDI (Atraumatic)

The clinical diagnosis of MDI depends on symptoms and signs indicating instability in an inferior direction and at least one other direction (anterior or posterior).[62] Findings at arthroscopy and imaging reflect the dominant direction of instability. In a study of athletes with MDI, the most common arthroscopic finding was increased capsular volume based on redundant axillary recess.[62] Anterior Bankart lesions were identified in 53%, and posterior labral lesions were seen in

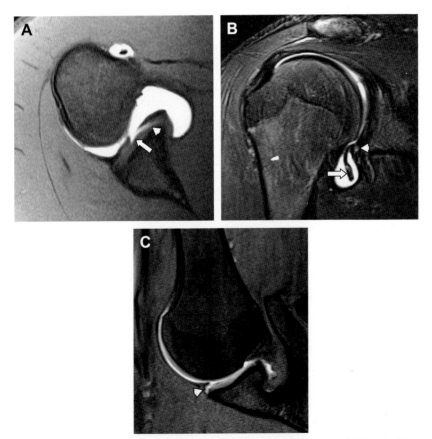

Fig. 21. Perthes lesion with articular cartilage fragment. This patient is a professional baseball pitcher who had a first-time anterior dislocation during a high-velocity (98 mph) pitch. (*A*) Axial T1 fat-suppressed MR arthrogram showing articular cartilage defect (*arrow*) in the inferior glenoid with extension of contrast deep to the anteroinferior labrum (*arrow head*). (*B*) Coronal oblique T2 fat-suppressed MR arthrogram in same patient showing the large partially detached articular cartilage and labral fragment (*arrow*) in the axillary recess. The arrowhead denotes the Perthes lesion of the labrum. (*C*) ABER T1 fat-suppressed MR arthrogram confirming the presence of a Perthes-type tear (*arrow head*) of the anteroinferior labrum.

the remainder. On MR images, including MR arthrography, no criteria allow the definite diagnosis of increased capsular volume.[139] MR imaging may be most valuable in excluding or showing intraarticular lesions that should also be addressed at capsulorrhaphy.[74]

ASSOCIATED FINDINGS IN GLENOHUMERAL INSTABILITY

In chronic glenohumeral instability, abnormal load distribution may damage articular cartilage. On MR images, focal cartilage defects can involve the anterior or posterior glenoid fossa, depending on the direction of instability. Lesions include fissuring and delamination, with or without cartilage fragment displacement, detachment, and intraarticular loose bodies (**Fig. 21**). Glenoid lesions are more common than humeral defects.[140] The glenolabral articular disruption (GLAD) lesion indicates focal cartilage disruption at the anteroinferior glenoid fossa, adjacent to the inferior labral-ligamentous complex. Although the appearance can be identical to cartilage defects seen in unstable shoulders, the GLAD lesion was reported in a small subset of patients who did not have instability symptoms.[141,142] Rotator cuff tears may be present, especially in patients older than 40 years.[3]

SUMMARY

Glenohumeral instability is a common cause of shoulder disability. Imaging findings often correlate closely with clinical symptoms and signs. MR and MR arthrography can accurately show the extent of soft tissue and osseous injury in unstable shoulders. This information provides prognostic information and enables the surgeon to plan conservative treatment or operative intervention.

REFERENCES

1. Veeger HE, van der Helm FC. Shoulder function: the perfect compromise between mobility and stability. J Biomech 2007;40(10):2119–29.
2. Bushnell BD, Creighton RA, Herring MM. Bony instability of the shoulder. Arthroscopy 2008; 24(9):1061–73.
3. Omoumi P, Teixeira P, Lecouvet F, et al. Glenohumeral joint instability. J Magn Reson Imaging 2011; 33(1):2–16.
4. Kuhn JE. A new classification system for shoulder instability. Br J Sports Med 2010;44(5):341–6.
5. Cadet ER. Evaluation of glenohumeral instability. Orthop Clin North Am 2010;41(3):287–95.
6. Doukas WC, Speer KP. Anatomy, pathophysiology, and biomechanics of shoulder instability. Orthop Clin North Am 2001;32(3):381–91, vii.
7. Bell JE. Arthroscopic management of multidirectional instability. Orthop Clin North Am 2010;41(3): 357–65.
8. Lugo R, Kung P, Ma CB. Shoulder biomechanics. Eur J Radiol 2008;68(1):16–24.
9. Weishaupt D, Zanetti M, Nyffeler RW, et al. Posterior glenoid rim deficiency in recurrent (atraumatic) posterior shoulder instability. Skeletal Radiol 2000; 29(4):204–10.
10. Howell SM, Galinat BJ. The glenoid-labral socket. A constrained articular surface. Clin Orthop Relat Res 1989;(243):122–5.
11. Moseley HF, Overgaard B. The anterior capsular mechanism in recurrent anterior dislocation of the shoulder. J Bone Joint Surg 1962;44(4):913–27.
12. Huber WP, Putz RV. Periarticular fiber system of the shoulder joint. Arthroscopy 1997;13(6):680–91.
13. Harryman DT, Sidles JA, Harris SL, et al. The effect of articular conformity and the size of the humeral head component on laxity and motion after glenohumeral arthroplasty. A study in cadavera. J Bone Joint Surg Am 1995;77(4):555–63.
14. Pouliart N, Gagey O. The effect of isolated labrum resection on shoulder stability. Knee Surg Sports Traumatol Arthrosc 2006;14(3):301–8.
15. Cooper DE, Arnoczky SP, O'Brien SJ, et al. Anatomy, histology, and vascularity of the glenoid labrum. An anatomical study. J Bone Joint Surg Am 1992;74(1):46–52.
16. Altchek DW, Warren RF, Wickiewicz TL, et al. Arthroscopic labral debridement. A three-year follow-up study. Am J Sports Med 1992;20(6): 702–6.
17. Andrews JR, Kupferman SP, Dillman CJ. Labral tears in throwing and racquet sports. Clin Sports Med 1991;10(4):901–11.
18. Palmer WE, Caslowitz PL, Chew FS. MR arthrography of the shoulder: normal intraarticular structures and common abnormalities. AJR Am J Roentgenol 1995;164(1):141–6.
19. Boardman ND, Debski RE, Warner JJ, et al. Tensile properties of the superior glenohumeral and coracohumeral ligaments. J Shoulder Elbow Surg 1996;5(4):249–54.
20. Kask K, Poldoja E, Lont T, et al. Anatomy of the superior glenohumeral ligament. J Shoulder Elbow Surg 2010;19(6):908–16.
21. Gaskill TR, Braun S, Millett PJ. The rotator interval: pathology and management. Arthroscopy 2011; 27(4):556–67.
22. Itoi E, Berglund LJ, Grabowski JJ, et al. Superior-inferior stability of the shoulder: role of the coracohumeral ligament and the rotator interval capsule. Mayo Clin Proc 1998;73(6):508–15.

23. Nobuhara K, Ikeda H. Rotator interval lesion. Clin Orthop Relat Res 1987;(223):44–50.

24. Harryman DT II, Sidles JA, Harris SL, et al. The role of the rotator interval capsule in passive motion and stability of the shoulder. J Bone Joint Surg Am 1992;74(1):53–66.

25. Cueff F, Ropars M, Chagneau F, et al. Interest of complementary inferior glenohumeral ligament fixation in capsulo-labral repair for shoulder instability: a biomechanical study. Orthop Traumatol Surg Res 2010;96(Suppl 8):S94–8.

26. Ticker JB, Flatow EL, Pawluk RJ, et al. The inferior glenohumeral ligament: a correlative investigation. J Shoulder Elbow Surg 2006;15(6):665–74.

27. Kuhn JE, Huston LJ, Soslowsky LJ, et al. External rotation of the glenohumeral joint: ligament restraints and muscle effects in the neutral and abducted positions. J Shoulder Elbow Surg 2005; 14(1 Suppl S):39S–48S.

28. Malicky DM, Kuhn JE, Frisancho JC, et al. Neer Award 2001: nonrecoverable strain fields of the anteroinferior glenohumeral capsule under subluxation. J Shoulder Elbow Surg 2002;11(6):529–40.

29. Yang HF, Tang KL, Chen W, et al. An anatomic and histologic study of the coracohumeral ligament. J Shoulder Elbow Surg 2009;18(2):305–10.

30. Arai R, Mochizuki T, Yamaguchi K, et al. Functional anatomy of the superior glenohumeral and coracohumeral ligaments and the subscapularis tendon in view of stabilization of the long head of the biceps tendon. J Shoulder Elbow Surg 2009;19(1):58–64.

31. Nakata W, Katou S, Fujita A, et al. Biceps pulley: normal anatomy and associated lesions at MR arthrography. Radiographics 2011;31(3):791–810.

32. Clark JM, Harryman DT II. Tendons, ligaments, and capsule of the rotator cuff. Gross and microscopic anatomy. J Bone Joint Surg Am 1992;74(5):713–25.

33. Wall MS, O'Brien SJ. Arthroscopic evaluation of the unstable shoulder. Clin Sports Med 1995;14(4): 817–39.

34. Steinbach LS. MRI of shoulder instability. Eur J Radiol 2008;68(1):57–71.

35. Bergin D. Imaging shoulder instability in the athlete. Magn Reson Imaging Clin N Am 2009; 17(4):595–615, v.

36. Ferrari DA. Capsular ligaments of the shoulder. Anatomical and functional study of the anterior superior capsule. Am J Sports Med 1990;18(1):20–4.

37. Moon YL, Singh H, Yang H, et al. Arthroscopic rotator interval closure by purse string suture for symptomatic inferior shoulder instability. Orthopedics 2011;34(4):269–72.

38. Bencardino JT, Beltran J. MR imaging of the glenohumeral ligaments. Radiol Clin North Am 2006; 44(4):489–502, vii.

39. Ide J, Maeda S, Takagi K. Normal variations of the glenohumeral ligament complex: an anatomic study for arthroscopic Bankart repair. Arthroscopy 2004;20(2):164–8.

40. Turkel SJ, Panio MW, Marshall JL, et al. Stabilizing mechanisms preventing anterior dislocation of the glenohumeral joint. J Bone Joint Surg Am 1981; 63(8):1208–17.

41. Eberly VC, McMahon PJ, Lee TQ. Variation in the glenoid origin of the anteroinferior glenohumeral capsulolabrum. Clin Orthop Relat Res 2002;(400): 26–31.

42. Ramirez Ruiz FA, Baranski Kaniak BC, Haghighi P, et al. High origin of the anterior band of the inferior glenohumeral ligament: MR arthrography with anatomic and histologic correlation in cadavers. Skeletal Radiol 2011. [Epub ahead of print].

43. Dwek JR. The periosteum: what is it, where is it, and what mimics it in its absence? Skeletal Radiol 2010;39(4):319–23.

44. Bui-Mansfield LT, Taylor DC, Uhorchak JM, et al. Humeral avulsions of the glenohumeral ligament: imaging features and a review of the literature. AJR Am J Roentgenol 2002;179(3):649–55.

45. Matsen FA III, Harryman DT II, Sidles JA. Mechanics of glenohumeral instability. Clin Sports Med 1991;10(4):783–8.

46. Halder AM, Kuhl SG, Zobitz ME, et al. Effects of the glenoid labrum and glenohumeral abduction on stability of the shoulder joint through concavity-compression: an in vitro study. J Bone Joint Surg Am 2001;83(7):1062–9.

47. Simonet WT, Melton LJ II, Cofield RH, et al. Incidence of anterior shoulder dislocation in Olmsted County, Minnesota. Clin Orthop Relat Res 1984;(186):186–91.

48. Goss TP. Anterior glenohumeral instability. Orthopedics 1988;11(1):87–95.

49. Longo UG, Huijsmans PE, Maffulli N, et al. Video analysis of the mechanisms of shoulder dislocation in four elite rugby players. J Orthop Sci 2011;16(4): 389–97.

50. Owens BD, Duffey ML, Nelson BJ, et al. The incidence and characteristics of shoulder instability at the United States Military Academy. Am J Sports Med 2007;35(7):1168–73.

51. Owens BD, Nelson BJ, Duffey ML, et al. Pathoanatomy of first-time, traumatic, anterior glenohumeral subluxation events. J Bone Joint Surg Am 2010; 92(7):1605–11.

52. McLaughlin HL, Cavallaro WU. Primary anterior dislocation of the shoulder. Am J Surg 1950; 80(6):615–21; passim.

53. Rowe CR. Acute and recurrent anterior dislocations of the shoulder. Orthop Clin North Am 1980;11(2): 253–70.

54. Neviaser RJ, Neviaser TJ. Recurrent instability of the shoulder after age 40. J Shoulder Elbow Surg 1995;4(6):416–8.

55. Simonet WT, Cofield RH. Prognosis in anterior shoulder dislocation. Am J Sports Med 1984; 12(1):19–24.

56. Romeo AA, Cohen BS, Carreira DS. Traumatic anterior shoulder instability. Orthop Clin North Am 2001;32(3):399–409.

57. McLaughlin HL. Posterior dislocation of the shoulder. J Bone Joint Surg Am 1952;24-A-3:584–90.

58. Wolf EM, Eakin CL. Arthroscopic capsular plication for posterior shoulder instability. Arthroscopy 1998; 14(2):153–63.

59. Richards RR. The diagnostic definition of multidirectional instability of the shoulder: searching for direction. J Bone Joint Surg Am 2003;85(11): 2145–6.

60. Joseph TA, Williams JS Jr, Brems JJ. Laser capsulorrhaphy for multidirectional instability of the shoulder. An outcomes study and proposed classification system. Am J Sports Med 2003;31(1): 26–35.

61. Neer CS II, Foster CR. Inferior capsular shift for involuntary inferior and multidirectional instability of the shoulder. A preliminary report. J Bone Joint Surg Am 1980;62(6):897–908.

62. Baker CL III, Mascarenhas R, Kline AJ, et al. Arthroscopic treatment of multidirectional shoulder instability in athletes: a retrospective analysis of 2- to 5-year clinical outcomes. Am J Sports Med 2009;37(9):1712–20.

63. Hewitt M, Getelman MH, Snyder SJ. Arthroscopic management of multidirectional instability: pancapsular plication. Orthop Clin North Am 2003;34(4): 549–57.

64. Bigliani LU, Kurzweil PR, Schwartzbach CC, et al. Inferior capsular shift procedure for anterior-inferior shoulder instability in athletes. Am J Sports Med 1994;22(5):578–84.

65. Lebar RD, Alexander AH. Multidirectional shoulder instability. Clinical results of inferior capsular shift in an active-duty population. Am J Sports Med 1992; 20(2):193–8.

66. Treacy SH, Savoie FH III, Field LD. Arthroscopic treatment of multidirectional instability. J Shoulder Elbow Surg 1999;8(4):345–50.

67. Pollock RG, Owens JM, Flatow EL, et al. Operative results of the inferior capsular shift procedure for multidirectional instability of the shoulder. J Bone Joint Surg Am 2000;82(7):919–28.

68. Gartsman GM, Roddey TS, Hammerman SM. Arthroscopic treatment of multidirectional glenohumeral instability: 2- to 5-year follow-up. Arthroscopy 2001;17(3):236–43.

69. Kuhn JE, Helmer TT, Dunn WR, et al. Development and reliability testing of the frequency, etiology, direction, and severity (FEDS) system for classifying glenohumeral instability. J Shoulder Elbow Surg 2011;20(4):548–56.

70. Palmer WE, Brown JH, Rosenthal DI. Labral-ligamentous complex of the shoulder: evaluation with MR arthrography. Radiology 1994;190(3):645–51.

71. Hayes ML, Collins MS, Morgan JA, et al. Efficacy of diagnostic magnetic resonance imaging for articular cartilage lesions of the glenohumeral joint in patients with instability. Skeletal Radiol 2010; 39(12):1199–204.

72. Magee T, Williams D, Mani N. Shoulder MR arthrography: which patient group benefits most? AJR Am J Roentgenol 2004;183(4):969–74.

73. Van der Woude HJ, Vanhoenacker FM. MR arthrography in glenohumeral instability. JBR-BTR 2007; 90(5):377–83.

74. Woertler K, Waldt S. MR imaging in sports-related glenohumeral instability. Eur Radiol 2006;16(12): 2622–36.

75. Roger B, Skaf A, Hooper AW, et al. Imaging findings in the dominant shoulder of throwing athletes: comparison of radiography, arthrography, CT arthrography, and MR arthrography with arthroscopic correlation. AJR Am J Roentgenol 1999;172(5): 1371–80.

76. Beltran J, Rosenberg ZS, Chandnani VP, et al. Glenohumeral instability: evaluation with MR arthrography. Radiographics 1997;17(3):657–73.

77. Elentuck D, Palmer WE. Direct magnetic resonance arthrography. Eur Radiol 2004;14(11):1956–67.

78. Shankman S, Bencardino J, Beltran J. Glenohumeral instability: evaluation using MR arthrography of the shoulder. Skeletal Radiol 1999;28(7):365–82.

79. Farber JM, Buckwalter KA. Sports-related injuries of the shoulder: instability. Radiol Clin North Am 2002;40(2):235–49.

80. Tirman PF, Stauffer AE, Crues JV III, et al. Saline magnetic resonance arthrography in the evaluation of glenohumeral instability. Arthroscopy 1993;9(5): 550–9.

81. Major NM, Browne J, Domzalski T, et al. Evaluation of the glenoid labrum with 3-T MRI: is intraarticular contrast necessary? AJR Am J Roentgenol 2011; 196(5):1139–44.

82. Dietrich TJ, Zanetti M, Saupe N, et al. Articular cartilage and labral lesions of the glenohumeral joint: diagnostic performance of 3D water-excitation true FISP MR arthrography. Skeletal Radiol 2009;39(5):473–80.

83. Tuite MJ, De Smet AA, Norris MA, et al. MR diagnosis of labral tears of the shoulder: value of T2*-weighted gradient-recalled echo images made in external rotation. AJR Am J Roentgenol 1995; 164(4):941–4.

84. Magee T. 3-T MRI of the shoulder: is MR arthrography necessary? AJR Am J Roentgenol 2009; 192(1):86–92.

85. Saleem AM, Lee JK, Novak LM. Usefulness of the abduction and external rotation views in shoulder

MR arthrography. AJR Am J Roentgenol 2008; 191(4):1024–30.

86. Tirman PF, Bost FW, Steinbach LS, et al. MR arthrographic depiction of tears of the rotator cuff: benefit of abduction and external rotation of the arm. Radiology 1994;192(3):851–6.

87. Waldt S, Metz S, Burkart A, et al. Variants of the superior labrum and labro-bicipital complex: a comparative study of shoulder specimens using MR arthrography, multi-slice CT arthrography and anatomical dissection. Eur Radiol 2006;16(2):451–8.

88. Oh JH, Kim JY, Choi JA, et al. Effectiveness of multidetector computed tomography arthrography for the diagnosis of shoulder pathology: comparison with magnetic resonance imaging with arthroscopic correlation. J Shoulder Elbow Surg 2009; 19(1):14–20.

89. Huijsmans PE, de Witte PB, de Villiers RV, et al. Recurrent anterior shoulder instability: accuracy of estimations of glenoid bone loss with computed tomography is insufficient for therapeutic decision-making. Skeletal Radiol 2011;40(10):1329–34.

90. Stevens KJ, Preston BJ, Wallace WA, et al. CT imaging and three-dimensional reconstructions of shoulders with anterior glenohumeral instability. Clin Anat 1999;12(5):326–36.

91. Waldt S, Burkart A, Imhoff AB, et al. Anterior shoulder instability: accuracy of MR arthrography in the classification of anteroinferior labroligamentous injuries. Radiology 2005;237(2):578–83.

92. Broca A, Hartmann H. Contribution a l'etude des luxations de l'epaule (luxations dites incompletes, decollements periostiques, luxations directes et luxations indirectes). Bulletins de la Société Anatomique de Paris 1890;65:312–36 [in French].

93. Perthes G. Operationen bei habitueller Schulterluxation. Deutsche Zeitschr f Chir 1906;85:199–207 [in German].

94. Bankart AS. Recurrent or habitual dislocation of the shoulder-joint. Br Med J 1923;2(3285):1132–3.

95. Bankart AS. The pathology and treatment of recurrent dislocation of the shoulder joint. Br J Surg 1938;26:23–9.

96. Neviaser TJ. The anterior labroligamentous periosteal sleeve avulsion lesion: a cause of anterior instability of the shoulder. Arthroscopy 1993;9(1):17–21.

97. Taylor DC, Arciero RA. Pathologic changes associated with shoulder dislocations. Arthroscopic and physical examination findings in first-time, traumatic anterior dislocations. Am J Sports Med 1997;25(3):306–11.

98. Norlin R. Intraarticular pathology in acute, first-time anterior shoulder dislocation: an arthroscopic study. Arthroscopy 1993;9(5):546–9.

99. Perthes G. Zur therapie der habituellen schulterluxation. Münchener medizinische Wochenschrif 1905; 16 [in German].

100. Wischer TK, Bredella MA, Genant HK, et al. Perthes lesion (a variant of the Bankart lesion): MR imaging and MR arthrographic findings with surgical correlation. AJR Am J Roentgenol 2002; 178(1):233–7.

101. Schreinemachers SA, van der Hulst VP, Jaap Willems W, et al. Is a single direct MR arthrography series in ABER position as accurate in detecting anteroinferior labroligamentous lesions as conventional MR arthrography? Skeletal Radiol 2009; 38(7):675–83.

102. Cvitanic O, Tirman PF, Feller JF, et al. Using abduction and external rotation of the shoulder to increase the sensitivity of MR arthrography in revealing tears of the anterior glenoid labrum. AJR Am J Roentgenol 1997;169(3):837–44.

103. Lee BG, Cho NS, Rhee YG. Anterior labroligamentous periosteal sleeve avulsion lesion in arthroscopic capsulolabral repair for anterior shoulder instability. Knee Surg Sports Traumatol Arthrosc 2011;19(9):1563–9.

104. Ozbaydar M, Elhassan B, Diller D, et al. Results of arthroscopic capsulolabral repair: Bankart lesion versus anterior labroligamentous periosteal sleeve avulsion lesion. Arthroscopy 2008;24(11):1277–83.

105. Habermeyer P, Gleyze P, Rickert M. Evolution of lesions of the labrum-ligament complex in posttraumatic anterior shoulder instability: a prospective study. J Shoulder Elbow Surg 1999;8(1):66–74.

106. Wolf EM, Cheng JC, Dickson K. Humeral avulsion of glenohumeral ligaments as a cause of anterior shoulder instability. Arthroscopy 1995;11(5):600–7.

107. Bokor DJ, Conboy VB, Olson C. Anterior instability of the glenohumeral joint with humeral avulsion of the glenohumeral ligament. A review of 41 cases. J Bone Joint Surg Br 1999;81(1):93–6.

108. Burkhart SS, De Beer JF. Traumatic glenohumeral bone defects and their relationship to failure of arthroscopic Bankart repairs: significance of the inverted-pear glenoid and the humeral engaging Hill-Sachs lesion. Arthroscopy 2000;16(7):677–94.

109. Oberlander MA, Morgan BE, Visotsky JL. The BHAGL lesion: a new variant of anterior shoulder instability. Arthroscopy 1996;12(5):627–33.

110. Warner JJ, Beim GM. Combined Bankart and HAGL lesion associated with anterior shoulder instability. Arthroscopy 1997;13(6):749–52.

111. Bigliani LU, Newton PM, Steinmann SP, et al. Glenoid rim lesions associated with recurrent anterior dislocation of the shoulder. Am J Sports Med 1998;26(1):41–5.

112. Itoi E, Lee SB, Berglund LJ, et al. The effect of a glenoid defect on anteroinferior stability of the shoulder after Bankart repair: a cadaveric study. J Bone Joint Surg Am 2000;82(1):35–46.

113. Chen AL, Hunt SA, Hawkins RJ, et al. Management of bone loss associated with recurrent anterior

glenohumeral instability. Am J Sports Med 2005; 33(6):912–25.

114. Calandra JJ, Baker CL, Uribe J. The incidence of Hill-Sachs lesions in initial anterior shoulder dislocations. Arthroscopy 1989;5(4):254–7.

115. Lynch JR, Clinton JM, Dewing CB, et al. Treatment of osseous defects associated with anterior shoulder instability. J Shoulder Elbow Surg 2009;18(2): 317–28.

116. Hill HA, Sachs MD. The groove defect of the humeral head. A frequently unrecognized complication of dislocations of the shoulder joint. Radiology 1940;35:690–700.

117. Workman TL, Burkhard TK, Resnick D, et al. Hill-Sachs lesion: comparison of detection with MR imaging, radiography, and arthroscopy. Radiology 1992;185(3):847–52.

118. Richards RD, Sartoris DJ, Pathria MN, et al. Hill-Sachs lesion and normal humeral groove: MR imaging features allowing their differentiation. Radiology 1994;190(3):665–8.

119. Yamamoto N, Itoi E, Abe H, et al. Effect of an anterior glenoid defect on anterior shoulder stability: a cadaveric study. Am J Sports Med 2009;37(5): 949–54.

120. Rowe CR, Zarins B, Ciullo JV. Recurrent anterior dislocation of the shoulder after surgical repair. Apparent causes of failure and treatment. J Bone Joint Surg Am 1984;66(2):159–68.

121. Shah N, Tung GA. Imaging signs of posterior glenohumeral instability. AJR Am J Roentgenol 2009; 192(3):730–5.

122. Kim SH, Ha KI, Park JH, et al. Arthroscopic posterior labral repair and capsular shift for traumatic unidirectional recurrent posterior subluxation of the shoulder. J Bone Joint Surg Am 2003;85(8):1479–87.

123. Savoie FH III, Holt MS, Field LD, et al. Arthroscopic management of posterior instability: evolution of technique and results. Arthroscopy 2008;24(4): 389–96.

124. Tung GA, Hou DD. MR arthrography of the posterior labrocapsular complex: relationship with glenohumeral joint alignment and clinical posterior instability. AJR Am J Roentgenol 2003;180(2):369–75.

125. Simons P, Joekes E, Nelissen RG, et al. Posterior labrocapsular periosteal sleeve avulsion complicating locked posterior shoulder dislocation. Skeletal Radiol 1998;27(10):588–90.

126. Yu JS, Ashman CJ, Jones G. The POLPSA lesion: MR imaging findings with arthroscopic correlation in patients with posterior instability. Skeletal Radiol 2002;31(7):396–9.

127. el-Hardary MS, Kamar AD, Ibrahim MM, et al. Morphological variations of root canals of distal root of lower second molar. Alex Dent J 1976; 1(3):148–63.

128. Finnoff JT, Doucette S, Hicken G. Glenohumeral instability and dislocation. Phys Med Rehabil Clin N Am 2004;15(3):v–vi, 575–605.

129. Harish S, Nagar A, Moro J, et al. Imaging findings in posterior instability of the shoulder. Skeletal Radiol 2008;37(8):693–707.

130. Harper KW, Helms CA, Haystead CM, et al. Glenoid dysplasia: incidence and association with posterior labral tears as evaluated on MRI. AJR Am J Roentgenol 2005;184(3):984–8.

131. Smith SP, Bunker TD. Primary glenoid dysplasia. A review of 12 patients. J Bone Joint Surg Br 2001; 83(6):868–72.

132. Trout TE, Resnick D. Glenoid hypoplasia and its relationship to instability. Skeletal Radiol 1996; 25(1):37–40.

133. Wirth MA, Lyons FR, Rockwood CA Jr. Hypoplasia of the glenoid. A review of sixteen patients. J Bone Joint Surg Am 1993;75(8):1175–84.

134. Antoniou J, Harryman DT II. Posterior instability. Orthop Clin North Am 2001;32(3):463–73, ix.

135. Petersen SA. Posterior shoulder instability. Orthop Clin North Am 2000;31(2):263–74.

136. Bokor DJ, Fritsch BA. Posterior shoulder instability secondary to reverse humeral avulsion of the glenohumeral ligament. J Shoulder Elbow Surg 2010; 19(6):853–8.

137. Chung CB, Sorenson S, Dwek JR, et al. Humeral avulsion of the posterior band of the inferior glenohumeral ligament: MR arthrography and clinical correlation in 17 patients. AJR Am J Roentgenol 2004;183(2):355–9.

138. Kim SH, Ha KI, Yoo JC, et al. Kim's lesion: an incomplete and concealed avulsion of the posteroinferior labrum in posterior or multidirectional posteroinferior instability of the shoulder. Arthroscopy 2004;20(7):712–20.

139. Meister K. Injuries to the shoulder in the throwing athlete. Part one: biomechanics/pathophysiology/ classification of injury. Am J Sports Med 2000; 28(2):265–75.

140. Carroll KW, Helms CA, Speer KP. Focal articular cartilage lesions of the superior humeral head: MR imaging findings in seven patients. AJR Am J Roentgenol 2001;176(2):393–7.

141. Sanders TG, Tirman PF, Linares R, et al. The glenolabral articular disruption lesion: MR arthrography with arthroscopic correlation. AJR Am J Roentgenol 1999;172(1):171–5.

142. Neviaser TJ. The GLAD lesion: another cause of anterior shoulder pain. Arthroscopy 1993;9(1): 22–3.

Postoperative Shoulder Magnetic Resonance Imaging

Laura W. Bancroft, MD[a],*, Christopher Wasyliw, MD[b],
Christopher Pettis, MD[b], Timothy Farley, MD[b]

KEYWORDS

- Postoperative • Shoulder • Rotator cuff tear • Labral tear
- Magnetic resonance imaging • Complications

Magnetic resonance imaging (MRI) and MR arthrography have proven invaluable for the management of the postoperative shoulder, particularly in relation to the rotator cuff and labrum. MRI has proven to be an accurate imaging technique for the differentiation of expected findings versus complications in the postoperative setting. The transition from metallic hardware to bioabsorbable suture anchors used in orthopedic surgery has rendered less metallic susceptibility artifact over the years, allowing a more accurate interpretation of MR images. This article gives a pictorial review of various expected postoperative findings in the shoulder and complications related to repair of the rotator cuff and labrum.

TECHNICAL CONSIDERATIONS

The preferred imaging methods for evaluating the postoperative shoulder include MR arthrography, conventional MRI, and sonography (depending on the expertise of the interpreting radiologist).[1] When bioabsorbable anchors and other nonmetallic devices have been used, shoulder MR arthrography or conventional MRI are acquired in a similar fashion as in the preoperative patient, as outlined in the American College of Radiology-Society of Skeletal Radiology (ACR-SSR) Practice Guideline for the Performance and interpretation of Magnetic Resonance Imaging (MRI) of the Shoulder.[2] Metallic

suture anchors and shoulder arthroplasties do not pose an MRI safety risk for patients, but techniques should be implemented to decrease metallic artifact.[3,4] These include increasing the bandwidth, increasing the of echo train, using a small field of view, increasing the matrix, using fast STIR (short tau inversion recovery) sequences as opposed to fat suppressed sequences, and avoiding gradient echo imaging.[2]

Although this article is limited to the use of MRI for evaluating the postoperative shoulder, computed tomography (CT) arthrography is regarded as superior to MRI or MR arthrography in the evaluation of the rotator cuff in the setting of a previous shoulder arthroplasty.[1] However, CT arthrography is viewed as a second-line procedure for evaluating shoulders with suspected instability or labral disorders when MRI is not available or contraindicated.[1] Contraindications to MRI include the presence of non-MRI compatible intracranial aneurysm clips, pacemakers, implanted cardioverter defibrillators, intraorbital metal, and a variety of electronic and magnetically activated implants, devices, stents, and coils.[3,4]

EXPECTED POSTOPERATIVE FINDINGS
Rotator Cuff Repair

Arthroscopic repair of rotator cuff tears generally yields excellent pain relief and improvement in the ability to perform daily activities, despite structural

Dr Bancroft receives book royalties from Lippincott and is a speaker for the Institute for International Continuing Medical Education. The remaining authors have nothing to disclose.
a Department of Radiology, University of Central Florida School of Medicine, Florida State University School of Medicine, Florida Hospital, 601 East Rollins, Orlando, FL 32803, USA
b Department of Radiology, University of Central Florida School of Medicine, Florida Hospital, 601 East Rollins, Orlando, FL 32803, USA
* Corresponding author.
E-mail address: Laura.bancroft.md@flhosp.org

Magn Reson Imaging Clin N Am 20 (2012) 313–325
doi:10.1016/j.mric.2012.01.010

failure demonstrated on MRI.[5] Early repair of traumatic rotator cuff tears provides better results in terms of shoulder function, in comparison with delayed tendon repair.[6] The factors affecting tendon healing are patient age, the size and extent of the tear, and the presence of fatty degeneration of the rotator cuff muscle.[5] Although functional status tends to improve with time after 6 months, the structural status of repaired cuffs remains unchanged and can be well evaluated with MRI.[7] Repaired rotator cuff tendons will have a variable appearance on MRI, with temporal evolution on serial imaging.[8,9] Within 3 months of operating, tendons appear most disorganized compared with native tendons, and intermediate signal intensity within the surgical bed will correspond to granulation tissue.[8,9] With time, the development of fibrotic tissue will yield areas of low signal intensity on all sequences. Of note, only 10% of repaired tendons demonstrate normal signal intensity on MRI.[8,9]

Partial-Thickness Rotator Cuff Tendon Tear Repair

If partial-thickness rotator cuff tears are treated surgically, they may be debrided, repaired with a transtendon technique, or repaired after tear completion. When tears are bursal sided and there are morphologic changes in the coracoacromial arch, a subacromial decompression may also be performed.[10,11] Repair of high-grade articular sided tears may also be accompanied by anterior acromioplasty.[11] When tears are debrided, they typically have a defect that is longer than deep relative to the long axis of the tendon on MRI (**Fig. 1**). If the converse is true, then a recurrent tear is likely. In a study of 48 patients treated for high-grade partial-thickness rotator cuff tears, repair after conversion to a full-thickness tear showed less postoperative morbidity compared with those treated with transtendon technique; however, recurrent tears developed in 8% of those repaired tendons after tear completion.[12]

The transosseous equivalent repair technique is designed for small to medium U-shaped tears and for iatrogenically completed partial articular supraspinatus tendon avulsions of moderate to large size.[13] The use of selective knot placement allows the surgeon to convert a linear construct into a V configuration, which will optimize repair strength and allow earlier rehabilitation due to increased footprint contact dimensions and less repair gap.[13]

Full-Thickness Rotator Cuff Tendon Tear Repair

Direct suture repair

Rotator cuff tendon tears involving the myotendinous junction or critical zone may be treated with

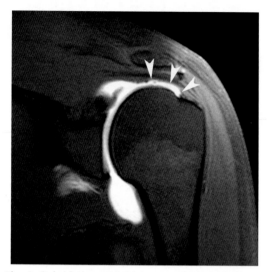

Fig. 1. Debrided partial thickness articular sided tear. Coronal image from magnetic resonance (MR) arthrogram shows a smooth defect that is longer than deep (*arrowheads*), consistent with prior debridement of partial-thickness articular sided supraspinatus tendon tear. No tendon retear was found at second look arthroscopy.

direct suture repair. There is often a slight difference in tendon caliber at the reattachment (**Fig. 2**), and, as with any repaired tendon, only 10% of repaired tendons will maintain the normal, native low signal intensity.

Single Row Technique

Most small full-thickness rotator cuff repairs are performed by using the tendon-to-bone repair technique, and various surgical tacks and suture material are available on the market. Assessment of the integrity of repaired rotator cuff tendon on postoperative MRI must address both the suture anchors and the tendon. Osteolysis around bioabsorbable suture anchors is an expected reaction (**Fig. 3**), and this is caused by mechanical forces or focal necrosis resulting from drilling. These osseous lucencies may double in size at 6 months, but should eventually stabilize and become replaced with bone at 2 years.[14]

Two-tendon tears of the rotator cuff can heal at a high rate with the use of transosseous-equivalent (TOE) suture bridge repair technique.[15] In a study by Sethi and colleagues, 83% of the repairs demonstrated intact rotator cuff repairs at a mean of 16 months postoperatively. Larger tears (3.5 vs 2.8 cm) were associated with failure ($P = .01$), as was more advanced fatty infiltration (Goutallier 1.3 vs 0.3, $P = .01$).[11] Furthermore, the modified transosseous equivalent procedure, otherwise known as surface holding repair with transosseous

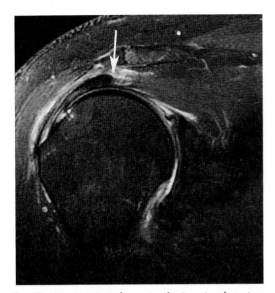

Fig. 2. Intact sutured supraspinatus tendon tear. Coronal oblique fast spin echo (FSE) T2-weighted fat-suppressed (FS) image shows a transition in caliber and signal intensity at the primarily repaired supraspinatus tendon (*arrow*), near the myotendinous junction. Only 10% of repaired rotator cuff tendons will demonstrate normal signal intensity. Note the partial thickness tearing of the distal supraspinatus tendon.

sutures, has also been used for massive rotator cuff tears involving at least 2 tendons, with a 92% continuous rotator cuff on postoperative MRI scans.[16]

Of note, asymptomatic patients may have signal changes suggestive of tendinopathy and have clinically silent partial and complete rotator cuff tears.[8] In addition, mild bone marrow edema-like signal changes may be present up to 5 years after surgery in asymptomatic patients who have undergone rotator cuff repair.[8] Patients can have marked improvement in symptoms without a watertight seal. Suspension bridge repair of massive rotator cuff tears can be effective, and complete coverage is not essential to convert debilitating tears into functional cuff tears.

Double-Row Technique

Double-row suture anchor repair is done in conjunction with creation of an implantation trough at the junction of the humeral head and greater tuberosity, which allows optimal apposition of tendon to bone (**Fig. 4**).[17–19] Intact tendons will have heterogeneous signal on postoperative MRI in the majority of cases (**Fig. 5**). Ma and colleagues[20] compared the MR arthrographic follow-up of 53 repaired rotator cuff tears that were performed with either single- or double-row technique. Although there was better shoulder strength demonstrated in patients who underwent double-row repair for larger size tears, there was no significant difference in postoperative structural integrity between the 2 groups at 6-month and 2-year follow-up with MR arthrography, regardless of tear size.[20] Koh and colleagues[21] did not find a statistically significant difference between the retear rates of arthroscopic single-row and double-row suture anchor repair in rotator cuff tears measuring between 2 and 4 cm. The short-term results of the clinical outcomes and structural integrity of TOE double-row rotator cuff repair (the suture–bridge technique) have results that compare favorably with those reported for other double-row suture anchor techniques employed in rotator cuff repairs.[22] The geometry of the TOE mattress suture configuration construct compresses the tendon, optimizing tendon-to-tuberosity contact dimensions in an attempt to restore the native footprint,

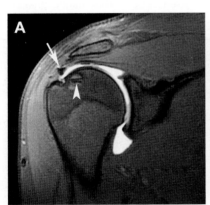
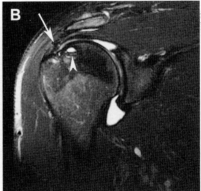

Fig. 3. Intact rotator cuff tendon repair with osteolysis about the suture anchor. (*A, B*) Coronal oblique magnetic resonance (MR) arthrogram (*A*) and FSE T2-weighted fat-suppressed (FS) image demonstrate susceptibility artifact from the suture (*arrows*) within the intact, repaired supraspinatus tendon. Notice the focal, well-demarcated increased T2-weighted signal intensity about the intact anchor (*arrowheads*) due to expected osteolysis from reaction to bioabsorbable material.

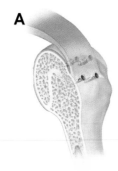
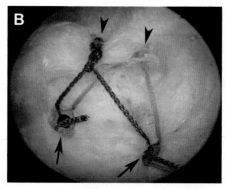

Fig. 4. Double-row technique for rotator cuff repair. (*A*) Schematic representation of double-row suture anchor repair, which is done in conjunction with creation of an implantation trough at the junction of the humeral head and greater tuberosity, to allow optimal apposition of tendon to bone. (*B*) Intraoperative photograph shows the overlapping, knotted sutures connecting the lateral (*arrowheads*) and medial (*arrows*) anchors, as viewed from above.

while providing strength sufficient to withstand immediate postoperative rehabilitation.[15]

Patch Grafting

Irreparable massive rotator cuff tears can be repaired using arthroscopic rotator cuff reconstruction with a variety of patch grafts, although there is limited postoperative imaging available to date in the literature. Patch grafts may be composed of allogenic freeze-dried tissues, artificial synthetic grafts, porcine small intestine submucosa, or autografts (such as the long head of the biceps).[23] Of note, all of the allografts have the potential to incite an aseptic inflammatory or foreign body reaction, which is evidenced by edema-like signal changes throughout the soft tissues and potentially the osseous structures on MRI.

Certain centers are now using polycarbonate polyurethane patches secured in a 6-point fixation construct to augment rotator cuff repairs.[24] In a study of 10 patients at 1 year follow-up, Encaalada-Diaz and colleages[24] found a 10% retear rate,on small and medium sized tears, and no visible subacromial adhesions on follow-up MRI using these nonresorbable scaffolds for permanent structural support. Since these constructs are so thin and are adherent to the repaired tendons, they are not well visualized on postoperative MRI. GraftJacket (Wright Medical Group, Incorporated, Arlington, TN, USA) is 1 type of bridging allograft that is composed of acellular human dermal matrix. This construct is implanted along the greater tuberosity and provides added support to the reattached tendons.[25]

Biceps Tenotomy/Tenodesis

Tenotomy or tenodesis of the long head of the biceps is performed if there are irreversible structural changes in the tendon, significant atrophy or hypertrophy, partial tearing greater than 25% of

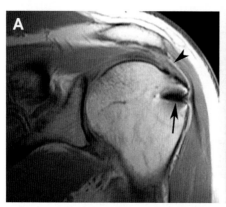
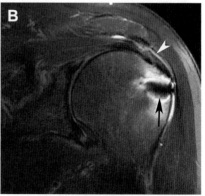

Fig. 5. Intact rotator cuff repair. (*A*, *B*) Coronal oblique FSE PD (*A*) and T2-weighted fat-suppressed (FS) (*B*) images show slight heterogeneity within the intact, repaired supraspinatus tendon (*arrowheads*). (*Arrows* = susceptibility artifact from suture anchor).

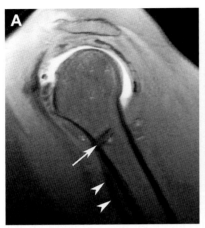
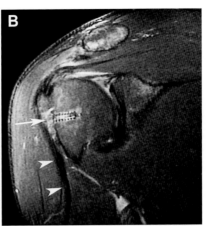

Fig. 6. Intact biceps tenodesis. (*A*) Sagittal FSE T2-weighted fat-suppressed (FS) image demonstrates an intact biceps tenodesis, with the long head of the biceps tendon (*arrowheads*) anchored to the proximal humeral shaft by a bioabsorbable suture anchor (*arrow*). (*B*) Coronal oblique FSE T2-weighted FS image in a different patient shows intermediate signal intensity in the proximal reattached biceps tendon (*arrow*), with slightly thickened, hypointense remaining tendon (*arrowheads*). Notice the type 2 superior labral anterior and posterior labral (SLAP) tear.

the width of the tendon, subluxation of tendon from the groove, or if there are certain disorders of the biceps origin.[26] Tenodesis remains the preferred treatment for younger patients with biceps dysfunction (**Fig. 6**).

Labral Tear Repair

Direct anatomic repair of labral tears usually occurs by suturing the anterior labrum and joint capsule, and the anterior band of the inferior band of the inferior glenohumeral ligament (IGHL) to the glenoid rim. With MRI or MR arthrography, there should be no separation of the labrocapsular complex and glenoid margin in intact labral repairs (**Figs. 7–9**).[27] Susceptibility artifact from metallic fixation should be minimized with MRI metal reduction techniques. Capsular thickening with an irregular nodular contour is an expected postoperative finding. Granulation tissue within the repaired labral tear may prevent joint fluid or injected contrast from outlining a persistent defect, resulting in false-negative MR examinations. Comparison with prior MRI studies is of utmost importance to evaluate for retear. The overall accuracy of MR arthrography for detecting labral tears after prior instability repair varies in the literature, but is generally greater than 90%.[28]

Paralabral cysts can develop through labral tears and extend along the spinoglenoid or suprascapular notches. These are known as spinoglenoid notch or suprascapular notch ganglia. Gains in

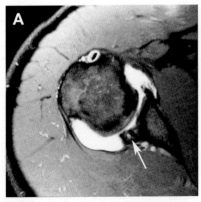
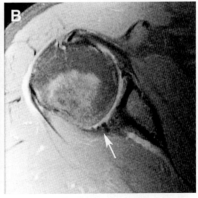

Fig. 7. Posterior labral repair. (*A*) Preoperative axial FSE T2-weighted fat-suppressed (FS) image shows joint fluid extending into the substance of the deformed, torn posterior labrum (*arrow*). (*B*) Postoperative axial image shows multifocal susceptibility artifact in the posterior labrum (*arrow*), caused by the suture used for primary repair.

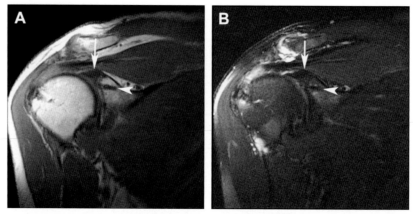

Fig. 8. Intact superior labral repair. (*A, B*) Coronal oblique FSE PD (*A*) and T2-weighted fat-suppressed (FS) (*B*) images show fairly uniform low signal throughout the repaired superior labrum (*arrows*), consistent with healed, repaired tear. Linear signal void in the superior glenoid corresponds to intact anchor (*arrowheads*). Notice the increased T2-weighted signal in the repaired distal supraspinatus tendon and humeral head suture anchor.

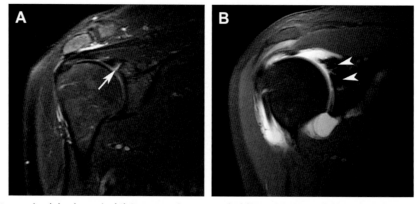

Fig. 9. Intact superior labral repair. (*A*) Preoperative coronal oblique FSE T2-weighted fat-suppressed (FS) image shows linear detachment of the superior labrum, evidenced by fluid (*arrow*) extending beneath the labrum. (*B*) Coronal image from postoperative magnetic resonance (MR) arthrogram shows susceptibility artifact from glenoid suture anchors (*arrowheads*). Fluid is no longer tracking beneath the labrum, consistent with healed repair.

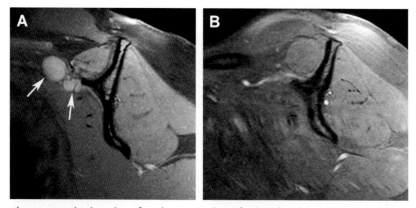

Fig. 10. Pre- and postoperative imaging after decompression of spinoglenoid notch ganglion and repair of superior labral anterior and posterior labral (SLAP) lesion. (*A*) Sagittal oblique FSE PD fat-suppressed (FS) image demonstrates a multiloculated spinoglenoid notch ganglion (*arrows*) that has extended medially from a SLAP tear. (*B*) Repeat sagittal oblique image was obtained after percutaneous cyst decompression and repair of the SLAP tear. Greater strength increase has been shown in patients who are treated with cyst decompression and SLAP repair, as opposed to SLAP repair alone.

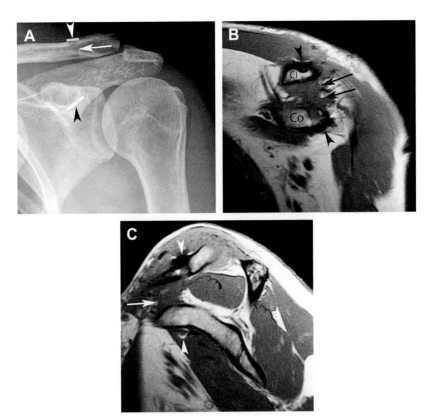

Fig. 11. Coracoclavicular cable fixation for grade 3 acromioclavicular (AC joint) separation. (*A*) Anteroposterior radiograph of the right shoulder obtained after coracoclavicular cable fixation demonstrates the intact fixation devices superior to the distal clavicle and inferior to the coracoids process (*arrowheads*). Notice the fixation cable tract through the distal clavicle (*arrow*) and nearly congruent AC joint. (*B, C*) Correlating coronal oblique (*B*) and sagittal oblique (*C*) images show susceptibility artifact (*arrowheads*) caused by the metallic fixation devices and intermediate signal intensity fibrosis (*arrows*) that blends imperceptibly with the cable device. Cl, clavicle; Co, coracoid.

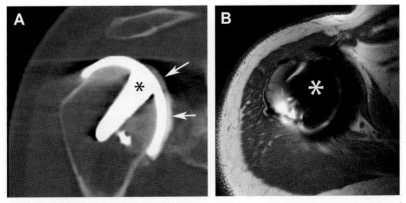

Fig. 12. Humeral head resurfacing performed for avascular necrosis. (*A*) Coronal reconstruction from computed tomography (CT) arthrogram delineates small capacity joint (*arrows*) after humeral head resurfacing (*asterisk*), consistent with clinical findings of adhesive capsulitis. (*B*) Despite techniques to minimize metallic artifact, susceptibility artifact from the implant (*asterisk*) obscured the adjacent glenoid and joint capsule.

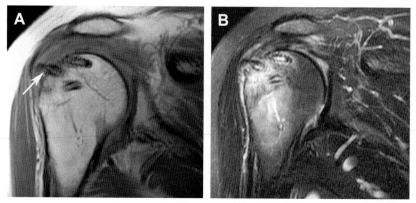

Fig. 13. Loosened and retracted rotator cuff suture anchor. (*A, B*) Coronal oblique FSE proton density (*A*) and T2-weighted fat-suppressed (FS) (*B*) images show that 1 of the bioabsorable suture anchors (*arrow*) has been partially pulled back into the substance of the supraspinatus tendon, consistent with loosening. Also note the marrow edema-like signal changes about the suture anchors, which can be seen in asymptomatic patients up to 5 years postoperatively.

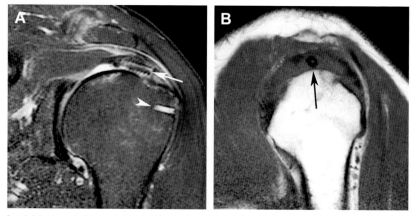

Fig. 14. Dislodged bioabsorbable rotator cuff suture anchor. (*A, B*) Coronal oblique FSE T2-weighted fat-suppressed (FS) (*A*) and sagittal T1-weighted (*B*) images demonstrate migration of the rotator cuff suture anchor (*arrows*) from its original placement in the greater tuberosity of the humerus (*arrowhead*) into the partial thickness, articular sided defect.

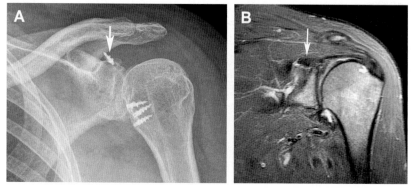

Fig. 15. Loose superior glenoid suture anchor. (*A*) Anteroposterior radiograph of the left shoulder delineates a loose, migrated glenoid suture anchor (*arrow*) as well as 3 intact medial humeral head anchors at site of prior capsulorraphy. (*B*) Coronal oblique FSE PD fat-suppressed (FS) image shows the susceptibility artifact from the suture anchor (*arrow*) extending into the inferior margin of the supraspinatus muscle.

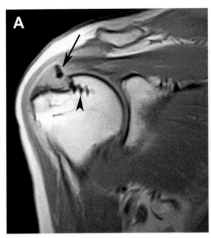
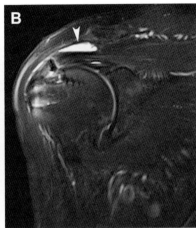

Fig. 16. Fragmented suture anchor and full-thickness retear after supraspinatus tendon reattachment. (*A*) Coronal oblique FSE proton density image shows a screw head fragment (*arrow*) migrated into a focal full-thickness supraspinatus defect. Notice the remaining screw (*arrowhead*) anchor medial to the lateral humeral head postsurgical trough. (*B*) Coronal oblique FSE T2-weighted fat-suppressed (FS) image shows focal fluid in the subacromial/subdeltoid bursa (*arrowhead*), due to communicating defect.

external rotation strength have been shown in patients who are treated with cyst decompression and superior labrum anterior and posterior (SLAP) repair, as opposed to SLAP repair alone (**Fig. 10**).[29]

Recurrent anterior shoulder dislocation typically results in combined Bankart and Hill-Sachs lesions, although concomitant SLAP lesions may also be present.[30] Arthroscopic Bankart repair after recurrent anterior shoulder dislocation may be performed in conjunction with the remplissage technique for treatment of instability with engaging Hill-Sachs lesions.[31] This technique transfers the posterior capsule and infraspinatus tendon into

the Hill-Sachs lesion to prevent engagement of the lesion on the glenoid rim. MRI will show corresponding findings of reattachment of the posterior structures into the defect, along with the metallic or bioabsorbable anchor embedded in the trough.[31]

Other Postoperative Conditions

MRI may be helpful to assess the integrity of soft tissue reconstructions, such as reconstructed coracoclavicular ligaments after grade 3 or higher acromioclavicular (AC) joint separation (**Fig. 11**). MRI allows for direct visualization of the cable

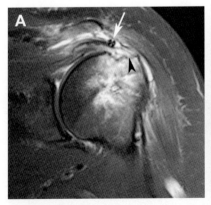
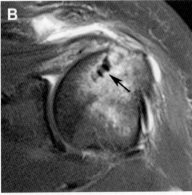

Fig. 17. Bioabsorbable screw fragment in the subacromial/subdeltoid bursa. (*A*) Coronal oblique FSE T2-weighted fat-suppressed (FS) image depicts a screw head fragment (*arrow*) from prior supraspinatus tendon repair. Notice the high signal within the distal supraspinatus tendon (*arrowhead*), consistent with high-grade tear. Notice the diffuse marrow edema-like signal changes throughout the lateral and central femoral head and neck, which are expected postsurgical findings. (*B*) Coronal oblique image obtained more anteriorly shows the bioabsorable screw base (*arrow*) remaining.

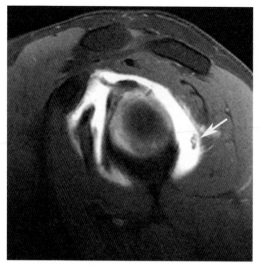

Fig. 18. Loose anchor in the posterior glenohumeral joint. Sagittal oblique image from magnetic resonance (MR) arthrogram outlines the loose anchor (*arrow*) in the posterior glenohumeral joint, which had been perceived as a moving joint mouse by the patient.

components and anatomic alignment of the AC joint, confirming that the construct is intact.

MRI is mainly used preoperative planning for shoulder arthroplasty to detect any rotator cuff tears.[32] MRI after shoulder arthroplasty can result in various degrees of susceptibility artifact,

depending on the type of metallic construct (**Fig. 12**). MRI may be a helpful adjunct to radiographs and CT in select cases to determine the extent of particle disease in the adjacent bones and soft tissues.

COMPLICATIONS

Complications in the postoperative shoulder may include failure of the repair, hematoma or seroma, adhesive capsulitis, septic arthritis or osteomyelitis, as well as regional complex pain syndrome.[33] Of interest, patients with structural failure or rerupture may still have significant improvement in pain and function. When rerupture does occur, the retear is usually smaller than the original tear. Furthermore, subtle changes in the rotator cuff signal intensity may not be as relevant after surgery.[34]

Recurrent Tears

Most recurrent tendon tears occur in the first 3 months after surgical repair.[35] Rotator cuff failure has a myriad of causes, including suture-bone or suture-anchor pullout (**Figs. 13–15**), suture breakage, knot slippage, tendon pullout, poor quality tendon or bone, muscle atrophy, inadequate initial repair, and improper physical therapy.[36,37] The bioabsorbable anchors may fragment before they are resorbed, and may act like intra-articular loose bodies (**Figs. 16–18**) and causes synovitis (**Fig. 19**). Occasionally, a retracted full-thickness

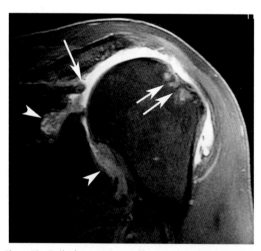

Fig. 19. Failed rotator cuff repair and synovitis. Coronal oblique FSE T2-weighted fat-suppressed (FS) image shows retraction of the tendionous remnant (*single arrow*) to the level of the glenohumeral joint. Heterogeneous signal intensity in the lateral humeral head (*double arrows*) is due to postsurgical change from resorbed bioabsorbable suture anchors and trough. Notice the extensive synovitis (*arrowheads*) through the joint space.

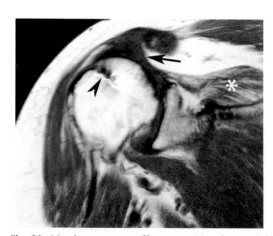

Fig. 20. Massive rotator cuff retear with subacromial fibrosis. Coronal oblique FSE PD image after prior rotator cuff repair shows marked fatty infiltration and moderate atrophy of the supraspinatus muscle (*asterisk*). The retracted supraspinatus tendon is retracted medially, and isointense soft tissue (*arrow*) extends to the undersurface of the acromion. This was found to be extensive scar tissue at second look arthroscopy. (*Arrowhead* = rotator cuff suture anchor).

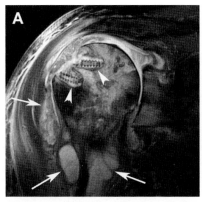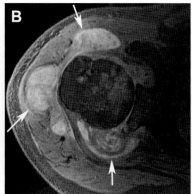

Fig. 21. Septic arthritis after failed rotator cuff repair. Coronal oblique (*A*) and axial (*B*) FSE T2-weighted fat-suppressed (FS) images show extensive complex fluid (*arrows*) within and around the shoulder joint, which proved to be pyarthrosis at surgical debridement. Notice the edema-like signal changes throughout the humeral head, osteolysis (*arrowheads*) around the suture anchors on coronal image, and retracted and torn supraspinatus tendon.

rotator cuff tear may adhere to the subacromial soft tissues via scar tissue (**Fig. 20**), giving a somewhat confusing MRI appearance.

Complications of labral repair include migration of either the bioabsorbable tacks or the suture anchors, loosened and/or protruding anchors that can contact the articular cartilage, resulting in early cartilage degeneration and synovitis induced by bioabsorbable tacks.[32]

Muscle Atrophy

The likelihood of recurrent tear is much greater if the repaired tendons have associated muscle fatty degeneration and atrophy (see **Fig. 20**). Muscle atrophy and fatty involution of the rotator cuff may occur after tendon rupture as well as after surgical procedures, including arthroscopic or open shoulder stabilization.[38,39] After repair of isolated subscapularis tendon tears, atrophy of the upper subscapularis muscle is present in 25% of patients in the postoperative course.[40] MRI allows a reliable and reproducible semiquantitative assessment of both muscular atrophy and fatty involution, best evaluated on T1-weighted sagittal oblique images.[38]

Other Complications

The work-up of suspected postoperative infection of the shoulder ultimately requires an arthrocentesis. However, MRI can be helpful in the evaluation of infected patients by detecting the presence of a joint effusion or any loculated soft tissue abscesses (**Fig. 21**).[41]

Deltoid dehiscence is 1 of the complications after open rotator cuff repair (**Fig. 22**), and it occurs in about 8% of cases at about 3 months after

surgery.[42,43] Small detachments are usually merely cosmetic defects; however, defects larger than 3 cm usually require reattachment onto the acromion for restoration of function.[42]

Heterotopic ossification (HO) is uncommon after open surgery of the shoulder, and it is rarely reported after arthroscopic repair.[44] Developing heterotopic ossification can result in hyperintensity throughout the involved soft tissues, whereas

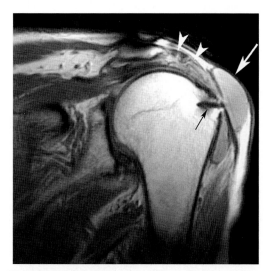

Fig. 22. Deltoid dehiscence after mini-open rotator cuff repair. Coronal oblique FSE proton density weighted image shows dehiscence of the central portion of the deltoid tendon (*arrowheads*) and focal lateral shoulder fluid collection (*white arrow*) after mini-open rotator cuff repair. Also, notice the marked thinning and retear of the supraspinatus tendon with intact rotator cuff suture anchor (*black arrow*).

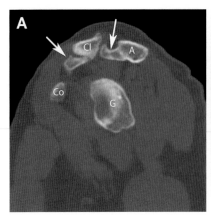
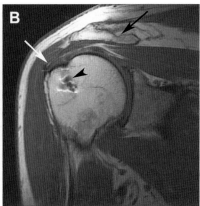

Fig. 23. Heterotopic ossification after rotator cuff repair. (*A*) Sagittal oblique computed tomography (CT) reconstruction of the right shoulder demonstrates well-organized heterotopic ossification (*arrows*) contiguous with the distal acromion (*A*) and clavicle (Cl). Co, coracoid; G, glenoid. (*B*) Corresponding coronal oblique T1-weighted image shows well-organized heterotopic ossification about the shoulder (*arrows*), which is isointense to marrow. (*Arrowhead* = rotator cuff suture anchor).

mature HO will parallel bone marrow on all MRI sequences (**Fig. 23**).

SUMMARY

In conclusion, MRI is an excellent technique to address complications after shoulder surgery, and it allows for evaluation for rotator cuff and labral retears, hardware integrity, infection, synovitis, deltoid dehiscence, and heterotopic ossification. With the advent of more widespread usage of bioabsorable suture anchors, MRI interpretation is proving to be an accurate imaging modality in the work-up of the complicated postoperative shoulder.

REFERENCES

1. Wise JN, Daffner RH, Weissman BN, et al. ACR appropriateness criteria on acute shoulder pain. J Am Coll Radiol 2011;8(9):602–9.
2. American College of Radiology (ACR), Society of Skeletal Radiology (SSR). ACR-SSR practice guideline for the performance and interpretation of magnetic resonance imaging (MRI) of the shoulder. Reston (VA): American College of Radiology (ACR); 2010. p. 11.
3. Kanal E, Barkovich AJ, Bell C, et al. ACR guidance document for safe MR practices: 2007. AJR Am J Roentgenol 2007;188:1–27.
4. Available at: www.MRIsafety.com. Accessed January 6, 2012.
5. Cho NS, Rhee YH. The factors affecting the clinical outcome and integrity of arthroscopically repaired rotator cuff tears of the shoulder. Clin Orthop Surg 2009;1:96–104.
6. Hantes ME, Karidakis GK, Vlychou M, et al. A comparison of early versus delayed repair of traumatic rotator cuff tears. Knee Surg Sports Traumatol Arthrosc 2011;19:1766–70.
7. Koh KH, Laddha MS, Lim TK, et al. Serial structural and functional assessments of rotator cuff repairs: do they differ at 6 and 19 months postoperatively? J Shoulder Elbow Surg 2011. [Epub ahead of print].
8. Spielmann AL, Forster BB, Kokan P, et al. Shoulder after rotator cuff repair: MR imaging findings in asymptomatic individuals—initial experience. Radiology 1999;213:705–8.
9. Crim J, Burks R, Manaster BJ, et al. Temporal evolution of MRI findings after arthroscopic rotator cuff repair. AJR Am J Roentgenol 2010;195:1361–6.
10. Koh KH, Shon MS, Lim TK, et al. Clinical and magnetic resonance imaging results of arthroscopic full-layer repair of bursal-side partial-thickness rotator cuff tears. Am J Sports Med 2011;39:1660–7.
11. Jacobson JA, Miller B, Bedi A, et al. Imaging of the postoperative shoulder. Semin Musculoskelet Radiol 2011;15:320–39.
12. Shin SJ. A comparison of 2 repair techniques for partial-thickness articular sided rotator cuff tears. Arthroscopy 2012;28(1):25–33.
13. Lewicky YM. "V"ictory transosseous equivalent suture configuration for arthroscopic rotator cuff tear repairs of iatrogenically completed PASTA lesions and full-thickness "U"-shaped tears. Orthopedics 2009;32:pii.
14. Glueck D, Wilson TC, Johnson DL. Extensive osteolysis after rotator cuff repair with a bioabsorbable suture abchor: a case report. Am J Sports Med 2005;33:742–4.
15. Sethi PM, Noonan BC, Cunningham J, et al. Repair results of 2-tendon rotator cuff tears utilizing the

transosseous equivalent technique. J Shoulder Elbow Surg 2010;19:1210–7.

16. Yamaguchi H, Suenanga N, Oizumi N, et al. Open repair for massive rotator cuff tear with a modified transosseous-equivalent procedure: preliminary results at short-term follow-up. J Orthop Sci 2011; 16:398–404.

17. Huijsmans PE, Pritchard MP, Berghs BM, et al. Arthroscopic rotator cuff repair with double-row fixation. J Bone Joint Surg Am 2007;89:1248–57.

18. Cho NS, Yi JW, Lee BG, et al. Retear patterns after arthroscopic rotator cuff repair: single-row versus suture bridge technique. Am J Sports Med 2010; 28:644–71.

19. El-Azab H, Buchmann S, Beitzel K, et al. Clinical and structural evaluation of arthroscopic double-row suture-bridge rotator cuff repair: early results of a novel technique. Knee Surg Sports Traumatol Arthrosc 2010;18:1720–7.

20. Ma HL, Chiang ER, Wu HT, et al. Clinical outcoming and imaging of arthroscopic single-row and double-row rotator cuff repair: a prospective randomized trial. Arthroscopy 2012;28(1):16–24.

21. Koh KH, Kang KC, Lim TK, et al. Prospective randomized clinical trial of single-versus double-row suture anchor repair in 2- and 4-cm rotator cuff tears: clinical and magnetic resonance imaging results. Arthroscopy 2011;27:453–62.

22. Touissant B, Schnaser W, Bosley J, et al. Early structural and functional outcomes for arthroscopic double-row transosseous-equivalent rotator cuff repair. Am J Sports Med 2011;39:1217–25.

23. Sano H, Mineta M, Kita A, et al. Tendon patch grafting using the long head of the biceps for irreparable massive rotator cuff tears. J Orthop Sci 2010;15:310–6.

24. Encalada-Diaz I, Cole BJ, Macgillivray JD, et al. Rotator cuff repair augmentation using a novel polycarbonate polyurethane patch: preliminary results at 12 months' follow-up. J Shoulder Elbow Surg 2011; 20:788–94.

25. Wong I, Burns J, Snyder S. Arthroscopic GraftJacket repair of rotator cuff tears. J Shoulder Elbow Surg 2010;19:104–9.

26. Ball C, Galatz LM, Yamaguchi K. Tenodesis or tenotomy of the biceps tendon: why and when to do it. Tech Shoulder Elbow Surg 2001;2:140–52.

27. Sugimoto H, Suzuki K, Mihara K, et al. MR arthrography of shoulder after suture-anchor Bankart repair. Radiology 2002;224:105–11.

28. Probyn LJ, White LM, Salonen DC, et al. Recurrent symptoms after shoulder instability repair: direct MR arthrographic assessment—correlation with second-look surgical evaluation. Radiology 2007;245:814–23.

29. Pillai G, Baynes JR, Gladstone J, et al. Greater strength increase with cyst decompression and SLAP repair than SLAP repair alone. Clin Orthop Relat Res 2011;469:1050–60.

30. Cho HL, Lee CK, Hwang TH, et al. Arthroscopic repair of combined Bankart and SLAP lesions: operative techniques and clinical results. Clin Orthop Surg 2010;2:39–46.

31. Zhu YM, Lu Y, Zhang J, et al. Arthroscopic Bankart repair combined with remplissage technique for the treatment of anterior shoulder instability with engaging Hill-Sachs lesion: a report of 49 cases with a minimum of 2-year follow-up. Am J Sports Med 2011;39:1640–7.

32. Buck FM, Jost B, Hodler J. Shoulder arthroplasty. Eur Radiol 2008;18:2937–48.

33. Major NM, Banks MC. MR imaging of complications of loose surgical tacks in the shoulder. AJR Am J Roentgenol 2003;180:377–80.

34. Mohtadi NG, Hollinshead RM, Sasyniuk TM, et al. A randomized clinical trial comparing open to arthroscopic acromioplasty with mini-open rotator cuff repair for full-thickness rotator cuff tears: disease-specific quality of life outcome at an average 2-year follow-up. Am J Sports Med 2008;36:1043–51.

35. Kluger R, Bock P, Mittlbock M, et al. Long-term survivorship of rotator cuff repairs using ultrasound and magnetic resonance imaging analysis. Am J Sports Med 2011;39:3071–81.

36. Magee TH, Shapiro M, Hewll G, et al. Complications of rotator cuff surgery in which bioabsorbable anchors are used. AJR Am J Roentgenol 2003; 181:1227–31.

37. Ruzek KA, Bancroft LW, Peterson JJ. Postoperative imaging of the shoulder. Radiol Clin North Am 2006;44:331–41.

38. Nikulka C, Goldmann A, Schroeder RJ. Magnetic resonance imaging analysis of the subscapularis muscle after arthroscopic and open shoulder stabilization. Clin Imaging 2010;34:269–76.

39. Goutallier D, Postel JM, Gleyze P, et al. Influence of cuff muscle fatty degeneration on anatomic and functional outcomes after simple suture of full-thickness tears. J Shoulder Elbow Surg 2003;12:550–4.

40. Bartl C, Salzmann GM, Seppel G, et al. Subscapularis function and structural integrity after arthroscopic repair of isolated subscapularis tears. Am J Sports Med 2011;39:1255–62.

41. Woertlwe K. Multimodality imaging of the postoperative shoulder. Eur Radiol 2007;17:3038–55.

42. Gumina D, Di Giorgio G, Perugia D, et al. Deltoid detachment consequent to open surgical repair of massice rotator cuff tears. Int Orthop 2008;32:81–4.

43. Mohana-Borges AV, Chung CB, Resnick D. MR imaging and MR arthrography of the postoperative shoulder: spectrum of normal and abnormal findings. Radiographics 2004;24:69–85.

44. Sanders BS, Wilcox RB 3rd, Higgins LD. Heterotopic ossification of the deltoid muscle after arthroscopic rotator cuff repair. Am J Orthop 2010;39: E67–71.

Magnetic Resonance Imaging of the Pediatric Shoulder

Nancy A. Chauvin, MD[a],*, Camilo Jaimes, MD[a],
Tal Laor, MD[b], Diego Jaramillo, MD, MPH[a]

KEYWORDS

- Shoulder MR imaging • Children • Shoulder development
- Brachial plexus palsy • Shoulder infection
- Shoulder inflammation

THE PEDIATRIC SHOULDER

Growth and development of the shoulder is complex. Appropriate interpretation of magnetic resonance (MR) images of the shoulder in children requires an understanding of normal skeletal maturation and how it results in different patterns of injury. The ability of MR imaging to depict cartilage, marrow, and soft tissues without using ionizing radiation makes it extremely useful in children. This article describes the MR appearance of normal developmental changes, common injuries, and unique conditions that affect the shoulder throughout childhood.

GENERAL DEVELOPMENTAL PRINCIPLES

The development of the shoulder starts during the fourth week of embryonic life. At this time, mesenchymal cells derived from somatic mesoderm condense and form the upper limb bud. These cells will eventually give origin to bone, cartilage, and other soft tissues of the upper extremity. By the eighth week of gestation, all structural components of the shoulder girdle are present.[1] Ossification of the diaphysis of the humerus starts between the seventh and ninth weeks of gestation, and is followed by the formation of the scapula and midportion of the clavicle.[2,3] Vascular invasion of the

humeral cartilaginous epiphysis, development of the marrow cavity, and somatic growth will continue to shape the shoulder throughout the remainder of fetal life.[4]

At birth, the proximal humeral epiphysis, acromion, coracoid, and lateral epiphysis of the clavicle are composed of hyaline cartilage, whereas the humeral diaphysis, midportion of the clavicle, and body of the scapula are ossified.[1] The primary physes of the clavicle and humerus are responsible for the longitudinal growth of these bones. The proximal physis of the humerus is responsible for approximately 80% of its overall elongation, whereas the lateral physis of the clavicle contributes little to the final length of the bone. Appositional growth of the diaphysis and metaphysis of the humerus and clavicle, and body of the scapula occurs by intramembranous ossification that originates from the periosteum and perichondrium.[5]

Throughout childhood, the cartilaginous epiphyses and apophyses of the shoulder develop secondary ossification centers.[6] These centers enlarge by endochondral ossification from a secondary physis.[7] The age at which each epiphysis or apophysis begins to ossify and grow varies between sites, which in turn results in the changing appearance of the shoulder at different stages of skeletal maturation. The subchondral marrow of a developing ossification center and its adjacent secondary

---

The authors have no financial disclosures.

[a] Department of Radiology, The Children's Hospital of Philadelphia, Perelman School of Medicine at the University of Pennsylvania, 34th Street and Civic Center Boulevard, Philadelphia, PA 19104, USA
[b] Musculoskeletal Imaging, Department of Radiology, Cincinnati Children's Hospital Medical Center, University of Cincinnati College of Medicine, 3333 Burnet Avenue, Cincinnati, OH 45229, USA
* Corresponding author.
E-mail address: chauvinn@email.chop.edu

physis is similar in architecture, composition, and MR imaging characteristics to the metaphysis and primary physis of long bones.[8] By the time skeletal maturity is reached, all epiphyseal cartilage has been replaced by mineralized bone, with the exception of articular cartilage.[6]

The growth of bones results in increased tension on the soft tissues of the shoulder girdle. The muscles, ligaments, tendons, and joint capsule, including the labroligamentous complex, grow in response to the traction exerted on them by the growing skeleton. The signal intensity (SI) on MR images of the subcutaneous tissues also changes during growth. In neonates and infants, there are prominent deposits of brown fat in the axillary, subscapular, and parascapular regions.[9] These normal deposits of brown fat show a slightly heterogeneous SI on T1-weighted images and may demonstrate patchy enhancement after the administration of intravenous contrast (**Fig. 1**), which can be a source of unnecessary concern.

TECHNIQUE

MR imaging of the pediatric shoulder is best performed with the patient in a supine position. Children younger than 7 years generally require sedation, whereas older patients are much more likely to tolerate the MR imaging examination without medication. The imaging protocol and the choice of appropriate coils depend on the size of the child and the clinical concern. In a young patient with a congenital or developmental abnormality, both shoulders should be imaged so that comparison can be made with the contralateral normal shoulder, as in the case of brachial plexus palsy. In these cases, a cardiac phased-array coil that covers both shoulder girdles is recommended. 3.0-T imaging is optimal. For a unilateral shoulder examination, infants and small children can be imaged using a small 4-channel multiflex coil. Older children (preteens) and adolescents are imaged using a small or large shoulder-array coil, respectively. A small field of view (FOV),

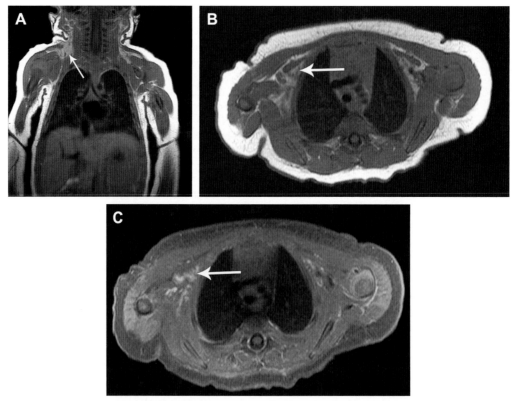

Fig. 1. Brown fat in a 1-month-old boy with a palpable right axillary mass. (*A*) Coronal and (*B*) axial T1-weighted MR images of the chest demonstrate intermediate SI in the subcutaneous tissues of the supraclavicular fossa, neck, and axilla (*arrows*). The absence of mass effect or infiltration of adjacent structures, as well as the location, are consistent with deposits of brown fat. (*C*) Axial fat-suppressed T1-weighted MR image following administration of intravenous gadolinium demonstrates patchy enhancement of these regions (*arrow*), secondary to the increased vascularity of brown adipose tissue.

such as 120 mm, is optimal for the very young patient. Older patients can be imaged adequately with a FOV ranging from 140 to 160 mm, depending on body size. When imaging a smaller child in a larger-diameter MR imaging system, it is useful to position the patient's body off midline thus bringing the shoulder closer to the center of the bore, to maximize the signal-to-noise ratio.[10]

SIGNAL CHARACTERISTICS OF THE IMMATURE SKELETON
Cartilage and Marrow

Transformation from red or hematopoietic to yellow or fatty marrow starts during the first year of life. Differences in marrow composition are depicted well on T1-weighted images, as red marrow is of intermediate to low SI and yellow marrow is of high SI. On fat-suppressed fluid-sensitive sequences, red marrow is of high SI and yellow marrow is of low SI. In the upper extremity, marrow transformation proceeds from distal to proximal (ie, from the fingers toward the shoulder). In an individual bone, this transformation begins in the epiphyses, continues in the diaphysis, and ends in the metaphyses. Marrow transformation in the epiphysis of the proximal humerus begins during the first year of life, soon after its radiographic appearance.[11,12] Residual foci of red marrow frequently can be seen in the metaphysis and epiphysis of the proximal humerus in older children and adolescents, even after skeletal maturity is reached.[13] In the proximal humeral metaphysis, these foci of residual red marrow tend to be vertically oriented and have sharp margins, whereas in the epiphysis they tend to have a curvilinear configuration along the humeral head (**Fig. 2**).[13] In the axial skeleton, marrow transformation occurs gradually and continuously throughout life. Marrow transformation in the clavicle starts between 6 and 10 years of age, and continues into the second and third decades of life.[11]

Hyaline cartilage of the epiphyses and apophyses is of intermediate SI on T1-weighted images and is of high SI on intermediate-weighted images (**Fig. 3**).[10] On fluid-sensitive sequences (short-tau inversion recovery [STIR] and T2-weighted images), the SI of epiphyseal cartilage is relatively low whereas that of the physis and articular cartilage remains high, thus providing contrast between the different forms of hyaline cartilage based on the relative content of free and bound water (**Fig. 4**).[8] The zone of provisional calcification can be appreciated as a thin band of very low SI on all pulse sequences, separating the physis from the metaphysis.[14] On gradient-echo (GRE) images, all forms of hyaline cartilage are of homogeneous intermediate or high SI, and the bone is of very low SI.[8,15]

As in the adult, the articular cartilage of the glenoid in children is of high SI, whereas the fibrocartilaginous labrum is of homogeneous low SI on all pulse sequences.

Anatomy

Humerus
The proximal humeral epiphysis is cartilaginous at birth, and with growth develops 3 separate ossification centers: the head, the greater tuberosity, and the lesser tuberosity.[1] The ossification center of the humeral head forms within the first months of life, but occasionally is present at birth in a full-term infant.[16,17] The ossification centers of the greater and lesser tuberosities develop between 9 and 12 months of age and 12 and 16 months of age, respectively.[18] Eventually the 3 ossification centers coalesce between 3 and 5 years of age, forming a single epiphyseal ossification center.[18] Initially the osseous contour of the proximal humeral epiphysis can be irregular, appearing bilobed or fragmented on coronal images and demonstrating a posterior notch on axial images. As the child grows, the ossification center develops a smoother contour, becomes more hemispheric, and abuts the primary proximal humeral physis (**Fig. 5**).[6]

In infants and younger children, the primary physis of the proximal humerus is smooth and gently arched.[15] With growth, it becomes increasingly undulated and multiplanar, and develops a characteristic tenting in the lateral aspect (**Fig. 6**). Closure of the proximal humeral physis occurs at approximately 14 to 16 years of age in girls and 15 to 17 years of age in boys.[1,19] Because of the substantial contribution of the proximal humeral physis to the final length of the bone, growth disturbances in this location can lead to marked deformity.[20]

Scapula
Coracoid In the neonatal period, the body of the scapula is ossified, but the coracoid and the acromion still are cartilaginous. During the first 3 months of life, a secondary ossification center develops in the coracoid.[17] With time, this spherical ossification center assumes a bipolar configuration with fronts of ossification advancing toward the body of the scapula and the distal end of the coracoid.[21] Around the age of 10 years, the proximal physis of the coracoid converges toward its base[21] and, because of its orientation, irregular contour, and proximity to the joint, may mimic an avulsion fracture or an injury to the glenoid labrum (**Fig. 7**).

Acromion Three distinct ossification centers merge to form the acromion: the pre-acromion, which is located more anteriorly; the meso-acromion, which

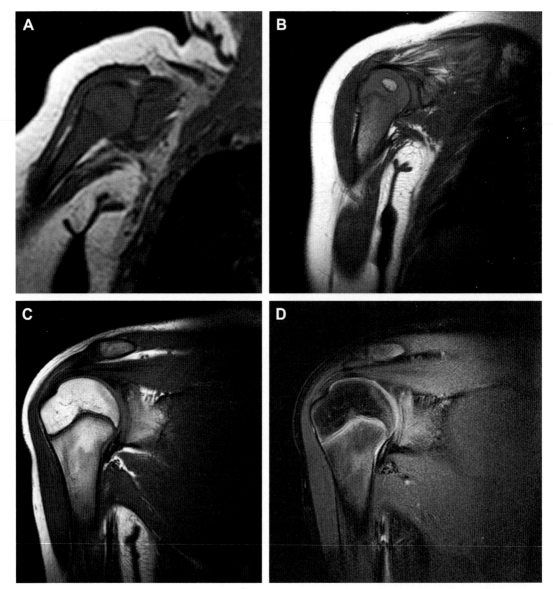

Fig. 2. Marrow transformation of the proximal humerus. (*A*) Coronal T1-weighted MR image of the shoulder in a 2-month-old boy shows hypointense red marrow in a recently formed secondary ossification center of the proximal humeral epiphysis. (*B*) Coronal T1-weighted MR image of the same boy, now 15 months old, shows high SI in the secondary ossification center of the humeral epiphysis, caused by the presence of yellow marrow. The metaphysis is still of relatively low SI because of persistent red marrow. (*C*) Coronal T1-weighted MR image in a different 11-year-old boy shows high SI in most of the epiphysis and the metaphysis of the humerus. Areas of low SI corresponding to persistent red marrow can be seen in the metaphysis and medial epiphysis of the humerus and in the glenoid. (*D*) Fat-suppressed intermediate-weighted MR image in the same boy shows high SI in these regions, caused by the high content of water in red marrow.

is located in the middle portion; and the meta-acromion, which is more posterior and forms the acromial angle (**Fig. 8**).[22–24] These ossification centers form during adolescence and fuse between 17 and 22 years of age.[21] At times, the variable pattern and rate of ossification in the acromion can simulate fractures in this location. Failure of the different ossification centers to fuse appropriately has been associated with the development of an os acromiale.[25]

Glenoid Early in life, the subchondral bone of the glenoid appears flattened or even convex on conventional radiography; however, on MR images the cartilaginous glenoid already demonstrates its

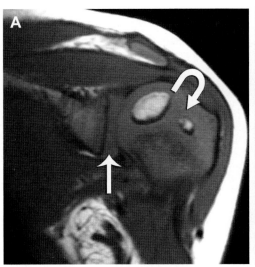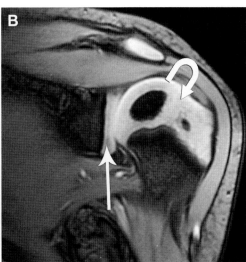

Fig. 3. Normal appearance of the cartilage in a 2-year-old girl. (*A*) Coronal T1-weighted MR image of the shoulder shows intermediate SI in the epiphyseal cartilage of the humeral head (*curved arrow*), the glenoid (*straight arrow*), and the tip of the acromion. The scapula, metaphysis of the humerus, and bony glenoid show intermediate SI caused by residual red marrow, and the ossification centers show high SI caused by the presence of yellow marrow. (*B*) Coronal gradient-echo (GRE) MR image shows very low SI in the bones caused by susceptibility arising from mineralized trabecula. By contrast, the cartilage is of very high SI (*arrows* point to the same structures as in *A*).

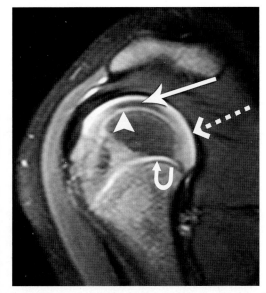

Fig. 4. Normal differentiation between regions of cartilage. Sagittal-oblique T2-weighted MR image of the shoulder in a 2-year-old boy shows a rim of high SI (*dotted arrow*) in the humeral epiphysis, which corresponds to articular cartilage. The primary physis (*curved arrow*) and the secondary physis (*arrowhead*) also demonstrate high SI. The epiphyseal hyaline cartilage (*straight arrow*) is of low and intermediate SI.

typical concave configuration and conforms to the shape of the humeral head. The bony glenoid develops from the fusion of 2 ossification centers. The first center appears at approximately 10 years of age in close proximity to the base of the coracoid, and the second one, which has a horseshoe configuration, appears at approximately 15 years of age.[1,21] These ossification centers fuse, undergo transformation to fatty marrow, and fuse with the subchondral bone plate. The articular surface of the glenoid remains cartilaginous and can be readily identified as a smooth rim of high SI on MR imaging fluid-sensitive sequences. Occasionally a focal well-marginated defect in the articular cartilage can be seen in the center of the glenoid fossa on MR images. This focal thinning, also known as the bare spot of the glenoid, is less commonly seen in children than in adults.[26]

During childhood, there is a change in the orientation of the glenoid relative to the angle of the scapula, termed the glenoid version. On MR imaging, the mean glenoid version in children younger than 2 years is −6°, or 6° of retroversion. Throughout childhood this value steadily increases, reaching adult standards of −1° by the end of the first decade of life. However, there is substantial variability in the normal values of glenoid version; approximately 68% of children have slightly retroverted glenoids, with the remaining 32% demonstrating mild anteversion.[27]

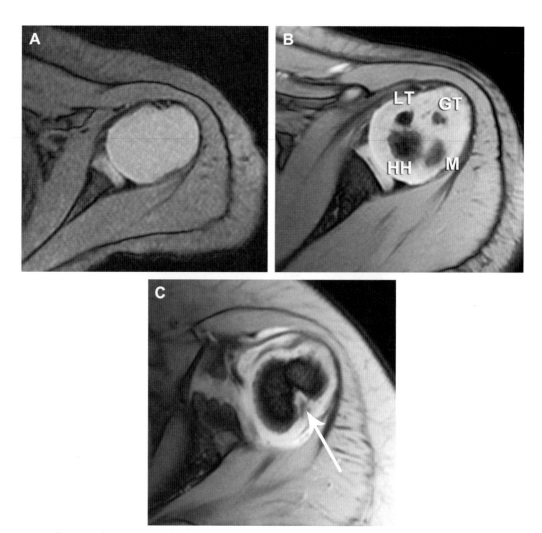

Fig. 5. Ossification of the proximal epiphysis of the humerus. (*A*) Axial GRE MR image in a 1-month-old girl shows an entirely cartilaginous epiphysis. (*B*) Axial GRE MR image in a 12-month-old boy depicts 4 low SI areas in the proximal humerus: the ossification centers in the head of the humerus (HH), lesser tuberosity (LT), greater tuberosity (GT), and the superior aspect of the humeral metaphysis (M). (*C*) Axial GRE MR image in a 4-year-old girl demonstrates a single ossification center in the proximal humeral epiphysis. This ossification center demonstrates a bilobed configuration and has a notch (*arrow*) in the posterolateral aspect.

CONGENITAL

Brachial Plexus Palsy

Neonatal brachial plexus palsy is caused by traction on the brachial plexus (C5-T1) during labor, which results in injury to 1 or more nerve levels. The prevalence of this complication has been reported as 1 to 1.5 per 1000 live births.[28] Predisposing factors for a brachial plexus injury include shoulder dystocia, instrumented delivery, breech delivery, and fetal macrosomia. Cesarean section has a significant protective effect. The diagnosis is made by observing arm weakness in a distribution consistent with a brachial plexus injury at birth.[29]

Shoulder dysfunction represents a major source of disability in infants with brachial plexus injuries. Most patients with brachial plexus birth palsy who begin to recover in the first 3 months of life can be expected to have improvement to nearly normal function. Although most infants recover, up to one-third have residual dysfunction.[30] The most common deficit involves weakness of the external rotators of the shoulder, namely the infraspinatus and teres minor muscles, which are innervated by nerves (supraspinatus and axillary nerves, respectively) that originate from the C5 to C6 nerve roots. This weakness leads to an internal rotation contracture of the shoulder. With long-standing internal rotation, significant periarticular

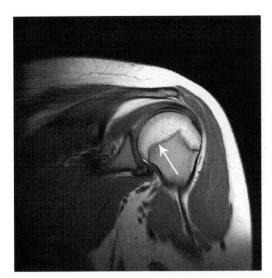

Fig. 6. Normal multiplanar course of the physis of the proximal humerus during adolescence. Coronal T1-weighted MR image of the shoulder in a 15-year-old girl with a history of shoulder instability shows normal beaked appearance of the proximal humeral physis. The band of low SI corresponding to the zone of provisional calcification (*arrow*) appears continuous, which confirms intact endochondral ossification.

capsuloligamentous tightness may develop. In turn, this can lead to a posteriorly directed force on the humeral head, causing a hypoplastic humeral head and posterior humeral head displacement.[31] On rare occasion only the C7, C8, and first thoracic nerve roots are affected, giving rise to paralysis of the lower arm.[32] If left untreated, brachial plexus palsy can lead ultimately to shoulder dislocation and even a fixed articular deformity of both the glenoid and humeral head, with overgrowth of the coracoid.[33]

Treatment options for neonatal brachial plexus palsy depend on the time of recognition and age at diagnosis, the degree of glenohumeral dysplasia, and the reducibility of the subluxation or dislocation if present. The goals of intervention include achieving full passive range of motion, maintenance of a stable glenohumeral articulation, and muscle re-balancing to facilitate glenoid remodeling.[33] Early treatments include physical therapy, abduction and external rotation splints and spica casts, and injections of botulinum toxin type A to prevent contracture and to maintain full passive range of motion. Early microneurosurgical reconstruction of the brachial plexus may improve functional outcomes in children younger than 2 years.[34] In the older child, capsular release, glenoid osteotomy, and extra-articular tendon transfers are used to restore active external rotation. Salvage options in the older child with advanced glenohumeral

dysplasia include a humeral external derotational osteotomy.[33]

Characterization of glenohumeral deformities with conventional radiographs is not possible, as the glenohumeral joint does not completely ossify until puberty. Ultrasonography has been shown to be an effective screening modality for depiction of posterior subluxation of the humeral head in infants, with optimal imaging performed at 3 and 6 months of age.[35] As the humeral head and glenoid are largely cartilaginous, MR imaging is the preferred method of evaluation in the young child (<5 years), whereas computed tomography scans generally are reserved for the older child.[30] The optimum protocol should include images of both shoulders to allow for comparison with the normal, unaffected shoulder. GRE sequences best demonstrate the hyaline cartilage of the humeral epiphysis and glenoid fossa, as well as the glenoid labrum in young infants.[36] High-resolution, 3-mm thick, axial and oblique coronal GRE images are obtained to assess the presence and the degree of incongruity of the glenohumeral joint, the shape of the humeral head, the degree of glenoid hypoplasia, and the glenoid version angle.[30] In children younger than 5 years, the cartilaginous normal glenoid shows increased SI on GRE sequences. The physis of the glenoid also will be of high SI and the labrum will be of low SI (similar to adults). The glenocapsular angle can be measured from the axial images to determine the degree of glenoid version. In the abnormal shoulder, there is thinning of the posterior aspect of the glenoid. With more severe dysplasia, the glenoid cavity often is poorly developed posteriorly, and the posterior labrum and humeral head are displaced posteriorly (**Fig. 9**). In addition, severely affected patients will show thinning of the superior aspect of the glenoid cartilage as well as atrophy of the muscles of the shoulder girdle.[30] The degree of rotator cuff muscle atrophy and fatty deposition, particularly the subscapularis muscle, directly correlates with development of secondary deformation of the glenohumeral joint.[37] Given its ability to assess the cartilaginous structures and soft tissues, MR imaging is an essential tool in the initial assessment, surveillance, presurgical planning, and postsurgical evaluation of skeletally immature children with a brachial plexus injury.

TRAUMA

Injury from trauma is influenced dramatically by the degree of skeletal maturation of the child and the offending activity. In children, most injuries occur at the chondro-osseous junctions of the physes and apophyses. These sites of transition are at greatest risk during adolescence, when the

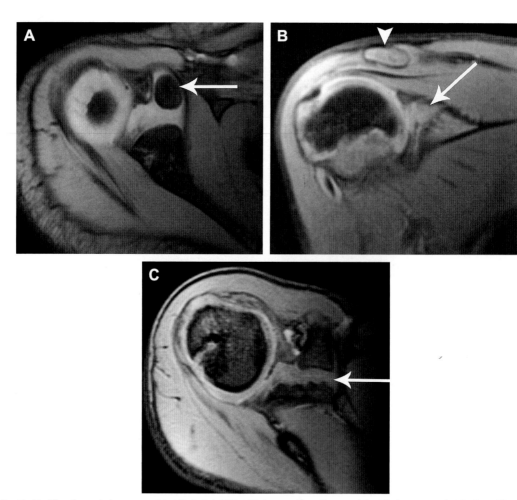

Fig. 7. Ossification of the coracoid. (*A*) Axial GRE MR image in a 2-year-old girl shows a spherical ossification center (*arrow*) in the coracoid. (*B*) Coronal intermediate-weighted MR image in a different 11-year-old girl with shoulder pain after a fall demonstrates irregular linear high SI (*arrow*) in close proximity to the superior anterior aspect of the glenoid and labrum. The cartilaginous tip of the acromion (*arrowhead*) also can be seen. (*C*) Axial GRE image at the corresponding level demonstrates that the high SI is continuous with the physis of the base of the coracoid (*arrow*).

teenage growth spurt makes the physes thicker and there is a rapid increase in muscle strength.[38] MR imaging demonstrates the extent of cartilaginous involvement and associated soft tissue injuries, and aids in early identification of complications such as physeal bridges.

The recent surge in participation in recreational and competitive sports has contributed to an increase in the incidence of sports-related injuries. Each year approximately 3% to 11% of schoolchildren sustain injuries related to sports.[39,40] Shoulder injuries are seen more commonly with throwing sports, martial arts, ice hockey, and tennis.[40]

Acute Injuries

Fractures of the shoulder are not uncommon in children, and often involve the clavicle. Clavicular fractures can be identified readily on conventional radiography and rarely require additional imaging. Less frequently, fractures of the proximal humerus and scapula result from acute trauma. Salter-Harris type I fractures or complete separation of the proximal humeral epiphysis occurs in neonates and infants in whom the physis is still relatively smooth.[38] These injuries have been described in association with obstetric, accidental, and nonaccidental trauma. Because of the great reparative capabilities of the immature skeleton and particularly the proximal humerus, these fractures can be treated conservatively and have an excellent prognosis.[41,42] Separations of the proximal humeral epiphysis are well depicted on MR imaging (Fig. 10) but also can be successfully documented with sonography, which is easier to perform and can be done portably.[43]

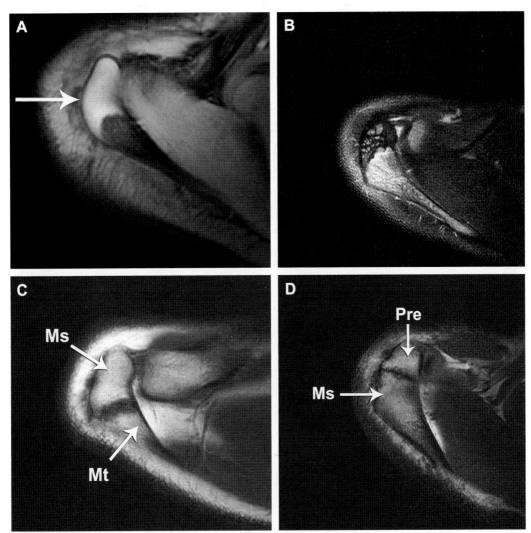

Fig. 8. Ossification patterns in the acromion. (*A*) Axial GRE MR image in a 2-year-old girl shows homogeneous high SI in the acromion (*arrow*), indicating that it is entirely cartilaginous. (*B*) Axial fat-suppressed T2-weighted MR image in a 15-year-old girl demonstrates multiple foci of ossification in the acromion. (*C*) Axial T1-weighted MR image in a 16-year-old boy shows a synchondrosis between the ossified meta-acromion (Mt) and meso-acromion (Ms). (*D*) Axial T1-weighted MR image in another15-year-old girl shows a synchondrosis between the ossified meso-acromion (Ms) and pre-acromion (Pre).

Approximately 3% of all physeal injuries occur in the proximal humerus.[44,45] In older children these fractures may be more severe than in the neonate, and usually are a Salter-Harris type II fracture, which includes a metaphyseal component. However, the overall prognosis of fractures in these locations is excellent, and surgical interventions are rarely warranted.[42]

In addition to fractures, trauma to the shoulder can result in dislocation of the humeral head. Dislocations are commonly seen in adolescents and young adults, with 40% of first episodes occurring before the third decade of life.[46] Skeletally immature children and those who resume sports activities soon after the injury have the highest recurrence rate.[47] First-time dislocation and recurrent episodes are associated with injuries to the glenoid labrum, best characterized by intra-articular contrast, and the rotator cuff muscles.[48]

Chronic Injuries

In little leaguer's shoulder, the chronic stress and traction associated with overhead throwing results in physeal widening and irregularity, which can be appreciated on conventional radiography.[49,50] On MR images, the physis is abnormally widened and of an irregular contour, and has increased SI

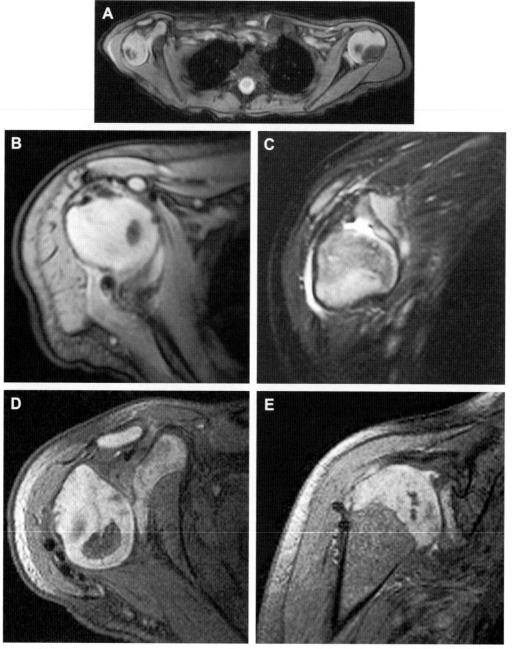

Fig. 9. Brachial plexus palsy in a 9-month-old boy. (A) Axial GRE image shows posterior dislocation of the right humeral head with flattening of the posterior aspect of the glenoid cartilage and overgrowth of the anterior glenoid cartilage. The left shoulder is normal. There is atrophy of the right shoulder muscles, particularly the deltoid and subscapularis muscles. (B) Axial GRE and (C) coronal oblique T2-weighted fat-suppressed images obtained postoperatively 2 months later for follow-up show mild inferior subluxation. There is flattening of the humeral head with thinning of the posterior and inferior glenoid cartilage. (D) Axial and (E) coronal GRE images at 2 years of age demonstrate continued posterior subluxation with a dysplastic glenoid fossa.

on fluid-sensitive sequences (Fig. 11).[51,52] Extension of unmineralized cartilage into the metaphysis also can be seen in severe cases.[53] Patients are typically tender to palpation directly over the proximal humeral physis. It is important to recognize that this chronic stress injury is not a form of physeal fracture, and has incorrectly been referred to as epiphysiolysis. Therapeutic rest usually

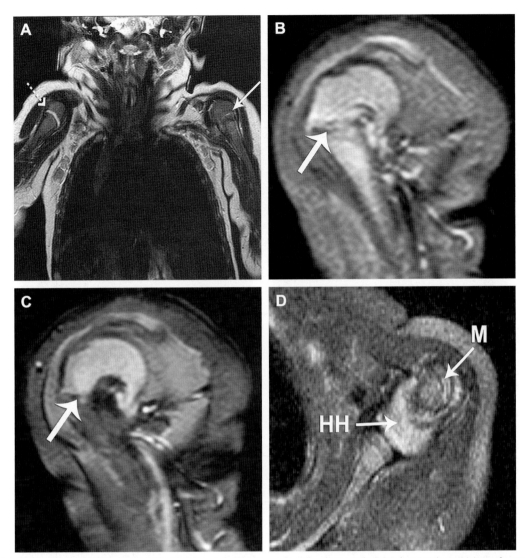

Fig. 10. Salter-Harris II fracture of the of the proximal humerus in a 7-month-old infant with suspicion of osteo-myelitis of the left shoulder. (*A*) Coronal T2-weighted MR image of the chest shows loss of the normal physeal SI in the proximal physis of the left humerus (*straight arrow*) compared with the normal right proximal humeral physis (*dashed arrow*). Sagittal (*B*) short-tau inversion recovery (STIR) and (*C*) GRE MR images show a fracture in the proximal metaphysis and physis of the left humerus with complete separation of epiphysis (*arrow*). (*D*) Axial fat-suppressed T2-weighted MR image demonstrates that the head of the humerus (HH) still articulates with the glenoid, despite the abnormal relationship with metadiaphysis (M) of the bone.

allows for healing without any permanent sequelae. However, if the inciting activity is not curtailed, growth disturbances and bony bridges may ensue.

INFECTION
Acute Osteomyelitis

Infections involving the bone and bone marrow can occur by 3 major pathways: hematogenous,

direct inoculation from trauma, and extension from adjacent soft tissue infection. In infants and children, acute osteomyelitis is most commonly acquired hematogenously. The most common organisms isolated are *Staphylococcus aureus*, with an increasing incidence of methicillin-resistant strains in recent years.[54,55] Other organisms include β-hemolytic *Streptococcus* and *Streptococcus pneumoniae*, *Escherichia coli*, and *Pseudomonas aeruginosa*.[56] In Europe, *Kingella*

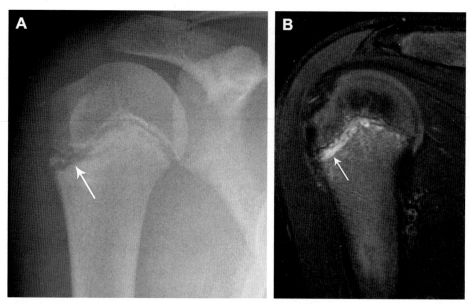

Fig. 11. Right shoulder pain in a 13-year-old male pitcher. (A) Conventional radiograph and (B) coronal oblique T2-weighted MR image of the right shoulder show widening (arrows) with increased SI primarily of the lateral aspect of the proximal humeral physis.

kingae has become one of the most frequent organisms in children younger than 4 years.[57–59]

Normal developmental changes in the growing skeleton influence the manifestations of osteomyelitis. In infants, diaphyseal vessels extend through the metaphysis and penetrate the cartilaginous physis to reach the epiphysis. As a result, blood flow through transphyseal blood vessels leads to an increased frequency of epiphyseal and joint infections in infants. By 18 months of age, however, the vascular connection through the physis is severed.[60] In children between the ages of 2 and 16 years, the physis becomes a partial barrier to the spread of infection; therefore, the metaphyses and metaphyseal equivalents are the most common location for acute hematogenous osteomyelitis. Once the physis is fused, the metaphyseal blood vessels terminate in the epiphysis and hematogenous infections are mainly localized to the epiphyseal portion of the humerus.

The clinical presentation of osteomyelitis varies according to age. Infection in the neonate and young infant is usually clinically silent, as they are unable to mount a significant inflammatory reaction. Diagnosis is often delayed at this age and multifocal osteomyelitis is frequent, occurring in 22% to 47% of cases.[60] The earliest manifestations of osteomyelitis of the shoulder are fever, pseudoparalysis of the arm, and pain with passive motion. MR imaging can delineate the full extent of disease by characterizing the marrow, cartilage, muscle, and subcutaneous tissues.[61] The sensitivity and specificity of MR imaging for the detection of osteomyelitis range from 86% to 98% and 77% to 100%, respectively.[60] The edematous marrow demonstrates decreased SI on T1-weighted images and increased SI on T2-weighted and STIR images (Fig. 12).[60] It is important to differentiate these changes from normal hematopoietic marrow in children. In osteomyelitis, in general the SI on T1-weighted images is lower than that of red marrow, and on T2-weighted and STIR images the SI tends to be higher than for red marrow. Complications of osteomyelitis, such as chronic osteomyelitis and growth arrest caused by formation of a bony bridge across the physis, can be readily evaluated with MR imaging.[62]

Septic Arthritis

Septic arthritis may be caused by hematogenous seeding or by direct extension into the joint space in children with osteomyelitis and/or an adjacent soft tissue infection. In neonates, a septic joint is most often seen in the shoulder or hips, followed by the knee, elbow, and ankle. In the very young patient, multifocal joint involvement is common.[63] Septic arthritis of the shoulder is relatively uncommon in children, accounting for approximately 4% of all septic joints.[64] The diagnosis often is delayed, as the clinical diagnosis is difficult because of young patient age and lack of localizing symptoms.[65,66]

MR imaging findings of a septic shoulder joint include an effusion, enhancement of thickened

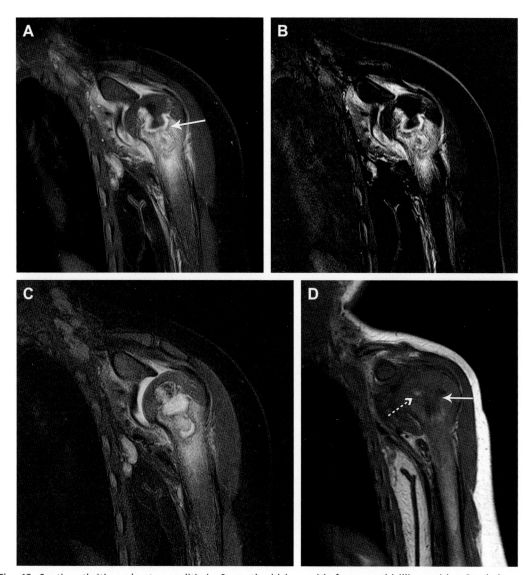

Fig. 12. Septic arthritis and osteomyelitis in 9-month-old boy with fever, methicillin-sensitive *Staphylococcus aureus* bacteremia, and pseudoparalysis of the left arm. (*A*) Coronal T1-weighted fat-suppressed postgadolinium image shows edema within the proximal humeral metaphysis and periosteal reaction consistent with osteomyelitis with an intraosseous abscess (*arrow*), which crosses the physis. There is a joint effusion with enhancement of the synovium. (*B*) Subtraction image demonstrates lack of perfusion of the humeral epiphysis. The patient underwent irrigation and debridement. Purulent joint fluid was present. (*C*) Coronal T2-weighted fat-suppressed image demonstrates edema within the proximal humeral secondary ossification center. (*D*) Follow-up coronal T1-weighted image 6 months later shows early bony bridging (*solid arrow*) with osteolysis of the secondary ossification center (*dashed arrow*).

synovium, and reactive edema within the adjacent bone. Joint infections of the shoulder may result in subluxation and avascular necrosis of the proximal humeral epiphysis. Subtraction postgadolinium T1-weighted images are useful for depiction of subtle changes in blood flow in the adjacent epiphysis (**Fig. 13**). Imaging findings can help direct clinical management and aid in planning open

debridement. To limit long-term complications, appropriate intervention should be initiated as soon as possible.

The sequelae of septic arthritis of the shoulder is variable and is affected by the age of the patient at diagnosis, virulence of the organism, prematurity, and time from the onset of symptoms to treatment.[67] Suppurative arthritis that occurs before

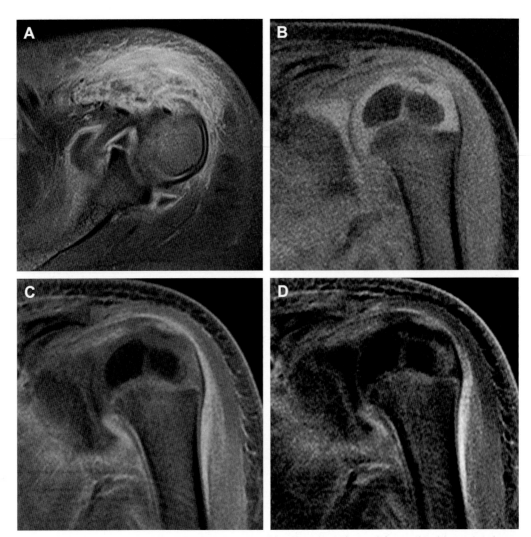

Fig. 13. Pyomyositis and secondary arthritis in 2-year-old girl with prolonged fever, shoulder pain, decreased motion, and *Salmonella* bacteremia. (*A*) Axial T1-weighted fat-suppressed postgadolinium image of the shoulder demonstrates marked soft tissue edema and diffuse enhancement anteriorly. There is mild synovitis. Coronal T1-weighted fat-suppressed (*B*) pregadolinium, (*C*) postgadolinium, and (*D*) subtraction views demonstrate lack of enhancement of the proximal humeral epiphyseal ossification centers. The patient underwent arthrotomy with incision and drainage; the joint fluid was not purulent.

the appearance of the proximal humeral epiphyseal secondary ossification centers generally delays their radiographic appearance by months, often resulting in irregular and small ossific nuclei and, ultimately, a deformed humeral head. If the joint infection occurs after the ossific nuclei are present, the ossific nuclei may undergo osteolysis, gradually redeveloping as small and irregular ossification centers with subsequent humeral head deformity.[68] A late diagnosis of septic arthritis may cause damage to the proximal humeral secondary ossification centers and physis, leading to growth arrest. There also may be functional

impairment caused by development of retroversion and the resultant restriction of external rotation. In a retrospective review of 46 septic shoulders (mean age 63 days) by Lejman and colleagues[68] with follow-up at 6 to 10 years, the discrepancy in humeral length varied from 0 to 9 cm, with an average of 2.4 cm. Long-term follow-up studies have demonstrated that those children with 3 cm or more of humeral shortening have a higher incidence of inferior shoulder subluxation with related shoulder dysfunction. Surgical procedures such as derotational osteotomy of the humeral shaft are reserved for those patients with extreme rotational deformities of the humerus.

INFLAMMATION
Juvenile Idiopathic Arthritis

Juvenile idiopathic arthritis (JIA) is the most common chronic musculoskeletal disease in children, and plays an important role in short-term and long-term morbidity.[69,70] In North America, the prevalence of JIA ranges between 0.5 and 1 in every 1000 children.[71] JIA is defined as an arthritis that begins before the age of 16 years, persists for at least 6 weeks, and has no known cause; it is therefore a diagnosis of exclusion.[72] The International League of Associations for Rheumatology has provided a recent classification of JIA into 7 disease categories based on the clinical features present within the first 6 months of illness, particularly the number of affected joints and whether systemic features are present.[70]

Arthritis of the shoulder is generally seen later in the course of ongoing systemic or polyarticular JIA, with an incidence of approximately 13% at 15 years from the onset of the illness.[73] In the immature shoulder, persistent arthritis produces deformity of the proximal humerus and glenoid cavity. With ongoing inflammation, erosion of the cartilage and bone may cause medial migration and superior subluxation of the humeral head. Basic functions of daily living become challenging, and if other joints in the upper limbs are affected, particularly the elbow, functionality of the shoulder declines.[74]

The aim of imaging is to assist in the initial diagnosis of arthritis, to detect disease complications at an early stage, and to evaluate response to treatment and diagnosis complications with the aim of optimizing clinical management.[75] MR imaging plays an important role in detecting early signs of synovitis and erosions, severity of joint involvement, evaluating for associated internal derangement and rice bodies, and monitoring disease progression (**Fig. 14**).[76] MR imaging shows loss of articular cartilage, subarticular erosions, and edema of the adjacent marrow (**Fig. 15**). Fat-suppressed intermediate-weighted and GRE sequences can best evaluate glenohumeral cartilage abnormalities. More advanced techniques such as cartilage T2 mapping with postprocessing quantitative techniques can also be used to allow for assessment of early biochemical and biophysical changes in the extracellular cartilage.[77]

The inflamed synovium will appear thickened and irregular, with low to intermediate SI on T1-weighted and high SI on T2-weighted sequences.

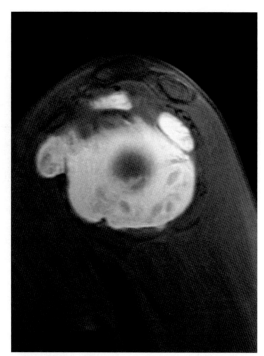

Fig. 14. Rice bodies in a 9-month-old boy with olioarticular JIA. Sagittal T1-weighted fat-suppressed MR arthrogram image depicts multiple hypointense ovoid intra-articular fragments consistent with rice bodies.

It rapidly enhances after gadolinium administration; differentiating hypervascular synovium from inactive, fibrous synovium, or from joint effusion. Normal synovium will demonstrate some degree of enhancement, but it should not be more than 2 mm thick. Postgadolinium imaging should be performed within 5 minutes after the intravenous injection of the contrast, as synovial tissue has no tight junction or basement membrane and contrast will diffuse into the joint space, gradually increasing the SI of the adjacent fluid.[75] MR imaging is not sensitive for the diagnosis of osteopenia.[76]

Chronic Recurrent Multifocal Osteomyelitis

Chronic recurrent multifocal osteomyelitis (CRMO) is an idiopathic inflammatory disorder of bone, which affects predominately children and young adults.[78] The disease is seen more commonly in girls, and patients present with slowly progressive pain and swelling affecting multiple bones. The disease course may persist for many years, plagued with remissions and relapses at previously affected sites, or can involve new areas.[79] Although there is no known causative agent,

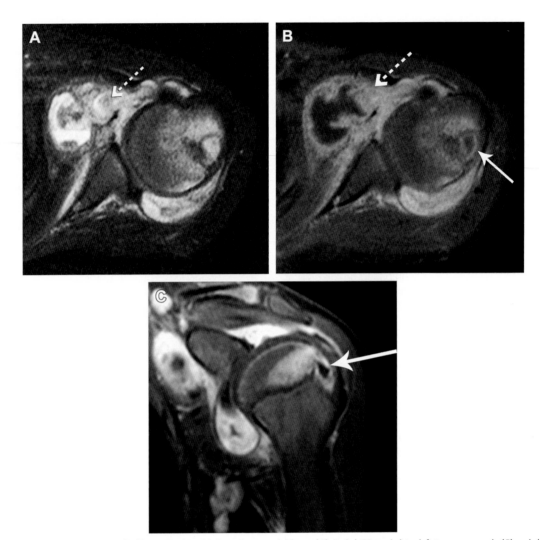

Fig. 15. Newly diagnosed oligoarticular JIA in a 5-year-old boy. (*A*) Axial T2-weighted fat-suppressed, (*B*) axial, and (*C*) coronal T1-weighted fat-suppressed postgadolinium images demonstrate a joint effusion with diffuse thickening and proliferation of the synovium (*dashed arrows*) with brisk enhancement consistent with synovitis and pannus. There is a rounded, focal, subcortical region of high T2 SI with surrounding edema, which demonstrates peripheral enhancement, consistent with an erosion (*solid arrow*).

a genetic susceptibility and autoimmune etiology has been theorized because of the association of CRMO with dermatologic disorders (such as psoriasis) and inflammatory bowel disease, as well as its favorable response to steroids.[80,81] The diagnosis of CRMO can be based on clinical features, imaging appearances, and nonspecific histopathology and laboratory findings. Biopsy specimens of affected bones will demonstrate nonspecific inflammatory change with granulocytic infiltration, often with mixed acute, subacute, and chronic changes within the same sample.[80]

Imaging has an important role in the diagnosis of CRMO. MR imaging is extremely useful for evaluating the extent of marrow edema, as it often is greater than suspected on conventional radiography.[79] In the active phase of the lesions, periostitis, soft tissue inflammation, and clinically occult joint effusions may also be present.[80] The presence of a large fluid collection, a fistulous tract, or a sequestrum makes the diagnosis of infectious osteomyelitis more likely than a diagnosis of CRMO. The lower extremities are 3 times more affected than the upper extremities.[80,81] Symmetric bilateral disease is common; however, active lesions often lack clinical temporal symmetry. CRMO lesions are located predominantly within the metaphyses of long bones, followed by the clavicle and spine.[82] Up to 30% of all CRMO lesions are located in the clavicle.[83]

CRMO is the most common nonneoplastic process of the clavicle in patients younger than 20 years.[84] Clavicular disease typically presents with local swelling, pain, or impairment of shoulder motion. The clavicle undergoes a lytic medullary process, typically within the medial third, generating surrounding periosteal reaction, which may have a worrisome onion-skin appearance. With each exacerbation, the disease tends to progress laterally. In children, typically the sternoclavicular joint is not involved, which is in contradistinction to clavicular involvement in adults.[80] Early in the disease, MR imaging will reveal bone marrow edema with periosteal reaction. With ongoing inflammation there is increased sclerosis and hyperostosis, which will appear as hypointense areas on both T1-weighted and T2-weighted images (**Fig. 16**). This sclerotic and hyperostotic phenomenon of the clavicle may persist for years and can cause thoracic outlet obstruction.[80]

BONE TUMORS
Benign Tumors

Simple (unicameral) bone cysts (UBC) represent 3% of all primary bone tumors; however, approximately half occur in the proximal humerus.[85] This lesion generally arises centrally within the proximal humeral metaphysis. UBCs are the most frequent cause of pathologic fractures in long bones. The proximal upper extremity, despite being a non–weight-bearing joint, is prone to pathologic fractures because of considerable lever-arm load and torque. In young patients, despite operative treatment, the proximal humerus has the highest recurrence rate for cysts in comparison with any other body site.[85] On MR imaging, the intramedullary fluid-filled cyst shows high SI on T2-weighted images and intermediate SI on T1-weighted images.[86] UBCs do not display a fluid-fluid level unless complicated by fracture (**Fig. 17**). However, because pathologic fractures are common, most UBCs at presentation have a complicated appearance, showing heterogeneous fluid on fluid-sensitive images and nodular and thick peripheral enhancement on images following intravenous contrast administration.[87]

Chondroblastoma, a benign cartilaginous lesion, represents 1% to 2% of all primary bone tumors and most commonly occurs during childhood or adolescence. Chondroblastomas arise from secondary centers of ossification, namely epiphyses and apophyses. The most common sites of involvement include proximal humeral epiphyses and proximal tibial epiphyses.[88,89] MR imaging shows an intraosseous lobulated mass with a hypointense rim, and low or intermediate SI on T1-weighted and T2-weighted sequences (**Fig. 18**). Characteristic associated marrow edema is common and may be extensive.[90,91] Other frequent findings include periosteal reaction, soft tissue edema pattern, and synovitis.[92] Fluid levels can be seen when there are associated changes of aneurysmal bone cyst formation. Other benign tumors that can be seen with a preference to the proximal humerus include osteochondromas and aneurysmal bone cysts.

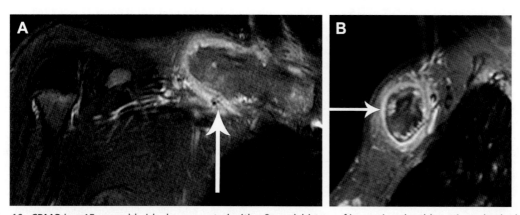

Fig. 16. CRMO in a 15-year-old girl who presented with a 3-week history of increasing shoulder pain and palpable mass. She had similar episodes of pain approximately 2 years prior. (*A*) Coronal T2-weighted fat-suppressed image shows marked hyperostosis of the clavicle with peripheral foci of increased SI and surrounding inflammatory change (*arrow*). (*B*) Sagittal T1-weighted fat-suppressed postgadolinium image shows peripheral bone enhancement (*arrow*) consistent with active inflammation, as well as surrounding inflammatory change. Additional findings in other bones were seen on whole-body MR imaging (not pictured).

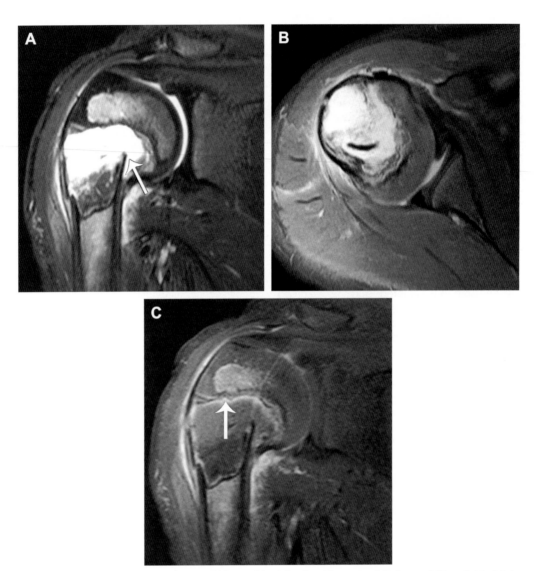

Fig. 17. Unicameral bone cyst in a 6-year-old boy with right shoulder pain. (*A*) Coronal T2-weighted fat-suppressed image shows an expansile intramedullary cystic lesion within the proximal humerus, which abuts the physis. A pathologic fracture (*arrow*) can be seen in the medial aspect of the metaphysis. (*B*) Axial intermediate-weighted fat-suppressed image shows heterogeneous SI within the cyst. (*C*) Coronal T1-weighted fat-suppressed postgadolinium image demonstrates enhancement (*arrow*) along the cyst wall.

Malignant Tumors

The most common malignant bone tumors in children are osteosarcoma and Ewing sarcoma, which comprise approximately 6% all of childhood malignancies.[86] Osteosarcoma is the most common primary bone malignancy in children. The proximal humerus is the third most common site of occurrence.[93] Sixty percent of cases of Ewing sarcoma occur in the lower extremities and pelvic girdle, and the humerus is the next most commonly affected site.[94] Soft tissue tumor components generally demonstrate high SI on fluid-sensitive sequences, low SI on T1-weighted images, and avid enhancement following the administration of gadolinium. The neoplastic bone is dark on all imaging sequences, and associated marrow edema can be massive.[86] The involved humerus should be imaged from the shoulder to the elbow to evaluate for skip lesions.

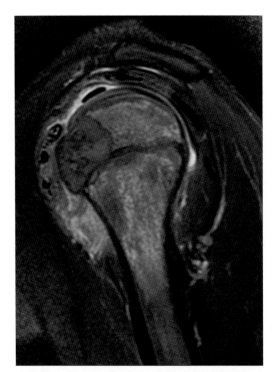

Fig. 18. Chondroblastoma of the proximal humeral epiphysis in a 9-year-old girl. Sagittal T2-weighted image shows a well-delineated oval lesion of the epiphysis, extending through the anterior cortex and traversing the proximal humeral physis. There is abundant surrounding soft tissue and adjacent bone marrow edema pattern. A small amount of joint fluid also is present.

Although uncommon, Ewing sarcoma also can affect the clavicle.[95]

REFERENCES

1. Rockwood CA. The shoulder. 4th edition. Philadelphia: Saunders/Elsevier; 2009.
2. Gray DJ, Gardner E. The prenatal development of the human humerus. Am J Anat 1969;124(4):431–45.
3. Gardner E, Gray DJ. Prenatal development of the human shoulder and acromioclavicular joints. Am J Anat 1953;92(2):219–76.
4. Fealy S, Rodeo SA, Dicarlo EF, et al. The developmental anatomy of the neonatal glenohumeral joint. J Shoulder Elbow Surg 2000;9(3):217–22.
5. Dwek JR. The periosteum: what is it, where is it, and what mimics it in its absence? Skeletal Radiol 2010; 39(4):319–23.
6. Laor T, Jaramillo D. MR imaging insights into skeletal maturation: what is normal? Radiology 2009;250(1): 28–38.
7. Rivas R, Shapiro F. Structural stages in the development of the long bones and epiphyses: a study in the New Zealand white rabbit. J Bone Joint Surg Am 2002;84(1):85–100.
8. Jaramillo D, Connolly SA, Mulkern RV, et al. Developing epiphysis: MR imaging characteristics and histologic correlation in the newborn lamb. Radiology 1998;207(3):637–45.
9. Gupta P, Babyn PS, Shammas A, et al. Brown fat distribution in the chest wall of infants-normal appearance, distribution and evolution on CT scans of the chest. Pediatr Radiol 2011;41(8):1020–7.
10. Jaramillo D, Laor T. Pediatric musculoskeletal MRI: basic principles to optimize success. Pediatr Radiol 2008;38(4):379–91.
11. Zawin JK, Jaramillo D. Conversion of bone marrow in the humerus, sternum, and clavicle: changes with age on MR images. Radiology 1993;188(1):159–64.
12. Jaramillo D, Laor T, Hoffer FA, et al. Epiphyseal marrow in infancy: MR imaging. Radiology 1991; 180(3):809–12.
13. Mirowitz SA. Hematopoietic bone marrow within the proximal humeral epiphysis in normal adults: investigation with MR imaging. Radiology 1993;188(3): 689–93.
14. Jaramillo D, Shapiro F. Growth cartilage: normal appearance, variants and abnormalities. Magn Reson Imaging Clin N Am 1998;6(3):455–71.
15. Ecklund K, Jaramillo D. Imaging of growth disturbance in children. Radiol Clin North Am 2001; 39(4):823–41.
16. Kuhns LR, Sherman MP, Poznanski AK, et al. Humeral-head and coracoid ossification in the newborn. Radiology 1973;107(1):145–9.
17. Odita JC, Ugbodaga CI, Omene JA, et al. Humeral head and coracoid ossification in Nigerian newborn infants. Pediatr Radiol 1983;13(5):276–8.
18. Clarke SE, Chafetz RS, Kozin SH. Ossification of the proximal humerus in children with residual brachial plexus birth palsy: a magnetic resonance imaging study. J Pediatr Orthop 2010;30(1):60–6.
19. Cardoso HF. Age estimation of adolescent and young adult male and female skeletons II, epiphyseal union at the upper limb and scapular girdle in a modern Portuguese skeletal sample. Am J Phys Anthropol 2008;137(1):97–105.
20. Baxter MP, Wiley JJ. Fractures of the proximal humeral epiphysis. Their influence on humeral growth. J Bone Joint Surg Br 1986;68(4):570–3.
21. Ogden JA, Phillips SB. Radiology of postnatal skeletal development. VII. The scapula. Skeletal Radiol 1983;9(3):157–69.
22. Macalister A. Notes on acromion. J Anat Physiol 1893;27(Pt 2):244, 241–51.
23. Sammarco VJ. Os acromiale: frequency, anatomy, and clinical implications. J Bone Joint Surg Am 2000;82(3):394–400.
24. Sahajpal D, Strauss EJ, Ishak C, et al. Surgical management of os acromiale: a case report and

review of the literature. Bull NYU Hosp Jt Dis 2007; 65(4):312–6.

25. Kleinman PK, Spevak MR. Variations in acromial ossification simulating infant abuse in victims of sudden infant death syndrome. Radiology 1991;180(1):185–7.

26. Kim HK, Emery KH, Salisbury SR. Bare spot of the glenoid fossa in children: incidence and MRI features. Pediatr Radiol 2010;40(7):1190–6.

27. Mintzer CM, Waters PM, Brown DJ. Glenoid version in children. J Pediatr Orthop 1996;16(5):563–6.

28. Foad SL, Mehlman CT, Ying J. The epidemiology of neonatal brachial plexus palsy in the United States. J Bone Joint Surg Am 2008;90(6):1258–64.

29. Alfonso DT. Causes of neonatal brachial plexus palsy. Bull NYU Hosp Jt Dis 2011;69(1):11–6.

30. Waters PM, Smith GR, Jaramillo D. Glenohumeral deformity secondary to brachial plexus birth palsy. J Bone Joint Surg Am 1998;80(5):668–77.

31. Hogendoorn S, van Overvest KL, Watt I, et al. Structural changes in muscle and glenohumeral joint deformity in neonatal brachial plexus palsy. J Bone Joint Surg Am 2010;92(4):935–42.

32. Pollock AN, Reed MH. Shoulder deformities from obstetrical brachial plexus paralysis. Skeletal Radiol 1989;18(4):295–7.

33. Ruchelsman DE, Grossman JA, Price AE. Glenohumeral deformity in children with brachial plexus birth injuries. Bull NYU Hosp Jt Dis 2011;69(1):36–43.

34. Emery KH. MR imaging in congenital and acquired disorders of the pediatric upper extremity. Magn Reson Imaging Clin N Am 2009;17(3):549–70, vii.

35. Poyhia TH, Lamminen AE, Peltonen JI, et al. Brachial plexus birth injury: US screening for glenohumeral joint instability. Radiology 2010;254(1):253–60.

36. Gudinchet F, Maeder P, Oberson JC, et al. Magnetic resonance imaging of the shoulder in children with brachial plexus birth palsy. Pediatr Radiol 1995; 25(Suppl 1):S125–8.

37. Poyhia TH, Nietosvaara YA, Remes VM, et al. MRI of rotator cuff muscle atrophy in relation to glenohumeral joint incongruence in brachial plexus birth injury. Pediatr Radiol 2005;35(4):402–9.

38. Jaramillo D, Shapiro F. Musculoskeletal trauma in children. Magn Reson Imaging Clin N Am 1998; 6(3):521–36.

39. Schalamon J, Dampf S, Singer G, et al. Evaluation of fractures in children and adolescents in a level I trauma center in Austria. J Trauma 2011;71(2):E19–25.

40. Caine D, Caine C, Maffulli N. Incidence and distribution of pediatric sport-related injuries. Clin J Sport Med 2006;16(6):500–13.

41. Guo JB, Zhang JD, Zhao YM, et al. Fracture separation of the proximal humeral epiphyses in neonate: a case report and literature review. Chin J Traumatol 2010;13(1):62–4.

42. Pahlavan S, Baldwin KD, Pandya NK, et al. Proximal humerus fractures in the pediatric population:

a systematic review. J Child Orthop 2011;5(3): 187–94.

43. Broker FH, Burbach T. Ultrasonic diagnosis of separation of the proximal humeral epiphysis in the newborn. J Bone Joint Surg Am 1990;72(2):187–91.

44. Neer CS 2nd, Horwitz BS. Fractures of the proximal humeral epiphysial plate. Clin Orthop Relat Res 1965;41:24–31.

45. Binder H, Schurz M, Aldrian S, et al. Physeal injuries of the proximal humerus: long-term results in seventy two patients. Int Orthop 2011;35(10):1497–502.

46. Cleeman E, Flatow EL. Shoulder dislocations in the young patient. Orthop Clin North Am 2000;31(2): 217–29.

47. Marans HJ, Angel KR, Schemitsch EH, et al. The fate of traumatic anterior dislocation of the shoulder in children. J Bone Joint Surg Am 1992;74(8):1242–4.

48. MacKenzie JD. MR arthrography made simple: indications and techniques. Pediatr Radiol 2008; 38(Suppl 2):S240–2.

49. Carson WG Jr, Gasser SI. Little Leaguer's shoulder. A report of 23 cases. Am J Sports Med 1998; 26(4):575–80.

50. Laor T, Wall EJ, Vu LP. Physeal widening in the knee due to stress injury in child athletes. AJR Am J Roentgenol 2006;186(5):1260–4.

51. Hebert KJ, Laor T, Divine JG, et al. MRI appearance of chronic stress injury of the iliac crest apophysis in adolescent athletes. AJR Am J Roentgenol 2008; 190(6):1487–91.

52. Alberty A, Peltonen J. Proliferation of the hypertrophic chondrocytes of the growth plate after physeal distraction. An experimental study in rabbits. Clin Orthop Relat Res 1993;(297):7–11.

53. Obembe OO, Gaskin CM, Taffoni MJ, et al. Little Leaguer's shoulder (proximal humeral epiphysiolysis): MRI findings in four boys. Pediatr Radiol 2007;37(9):885–9.

54. Gafur OA, Copley LA, Hollmig ST, et al. The impact of the current epidemiology of pediatric musculoskeletal infection on evaluation and treatment guidelines. J Pediatr Orthop 2008;28(7):777–85.

55. Browne LP, Mason EO, Kaplan SL, et al. Optimal imaging strategy for community-acquired *Staphylococcus aureus* musculoskeletal infections in children. Pediatr Radiol 2008;38(8):841–7.

56. Pineda C, Vargas A, Rodriguez AV. Imaging of osteomyelitis: current concepts. Infect Dis Clin North Am 2006;20(4):789–825.

57. Offiah AC. Acute osteomyelitis, septic arthritis and discitis: differences between neonates and older children. Eur J Radiol 2006;60(2):221–32.

58. Ceroni D, Cherkaoui A, Ferey S, et al. *Kingella kingae* osteoarticular infections in young children: clinical features and contribution of a new specific real-time PCR assay to the diagnosis. J Pediatr Orthop 2010;30(3):301–4.

59. Kanavaki A, Ceroni D, Tchernin D, et al. Can early MRI distinguish between *Kingella kingae* and Gram-positive cocci in osteoarticular infections in young children? Pediatr Radiol 2012;42(1):57–62.

60. Kothari NA, Pelchovitz DJ, Meyer JS. Imaging of musculoskeletal infections. Radiol Clin North Am 2001;39(4):653–71.

61. Jaramillo D. Infection: musculoskeletal. Pediatr Radiol 2011;41(Suppl 1):S127–34.

62. Oudjhane K, Azouz EM. Imaging of osteomyelitis in children. Radiol Clin North Am 2001;39(2):251–66.

63. Blickman JG, van Die CE, de Rooy JW. Current imaging concepts in pediatric osteomyelitis. Eur Radiol 2004;14(Suppl 4):L55–64.

64. Nelson JD. The bacterial etiology and antibiotic management of septic arthritis in infants and children. Pediatrics 1972;50(3):437–40.

65. Saisu T, Kawashima A, Kamegaya M, et al. Humeral shortening and inferior subluxation as sequelae of septic arthritis of the shoulder in neonates and infants. J Bone Joint Surg Am 2007;89(8):1784–93.

66. Obeidat MM, Omari A. Osteomyelitis of the scapula with secondary septic arthritis of the shoulder joint. Singapore Med J 2010;51(1):e1–2.

67. Bos CF, Mol LJ, Obermann WR, et al. Late sequelae of neonatal septic arthritis of the shoulder. J Bone Joint Surg Br 1998;80(4):645–50.

68. Lejman T, Strong M, Michno P, et al. Septic arthritis of the shoulder during the first 18 months of life. J Pediatr Orthop 1995;15(2):172–5.

69. Miller E, Uleryk E, Doria AS. Evidence-based outcomes of studies addressing diagnostic accuracy of MRI of juvenile idiopathic arthritis. AJR Am J Roentgenol 2009;192(5):1209–18.

70. Davidson J. Juvenile idiopathic arthritis: a clinical overview. Eur J Radiol 2000;33(2):128–34.

71. Oen K, Malleson PN, Cabral DA, et al. Disease course and outcome of juvenile rheumatoid arthritis in a multicenter cohort. J Rheumatol 2002;29(9):1989–99.

72. Ravelli A, Martini A. Juvenile idiopathic arthritis. Lancet 2007;369(9563):767–78.

73. Dabrowski W, Fonseka N, Ansell BM, et al. Shoulder problems in juvenile chronic polyarthritis. Scand J Rheumatol 1979;8(1):49–53.

74. Thomas S, Price AJ, Sankey RA, et al. Shoulder hemiarthroplasty in patients with juvenile idiopathic arthritis. J Bone Joint Surg Br 2005;87(5):672–6.

75. Johnson K. Imaging of juvenile idiopathic arthritis. Pediatr Radiol 2006;36(8):743–58.

76. Daldrup-Link HE, Steinbach L. MR imaging of pediatric arthritis. Magn Reson Imaging Clin N Am 2009;17(3):451–67, vi.

77. Gold GE, Reeder SB, Beaulieu CF. Advanced MR imaging of the shoulder: dedicated cartilage techniques. Magn Reson Imaging Clin N Am 2004;12(1):143–59, vii.

78. Giedion A, Holthusen W, Masel LF, et al. Subacute and chronic "symmetrical" osteomyelitis. Ann Radiol (Paris) 1972;15(3):329–42 [in Multiple languages].

79. Iyer RS, Thapa MM, Chew FS. Chronic recurrent multifocal osteomyelitis: review. AJR Am J Roentgenol 2011;196(Suppl 6):S87–91.

80. Khanna G, Sato TS, Ferguson P. Imaging of chronic recurrent multifocal osteomyelitis. Radiographics 2009;29(4):1159–77.

81. Fritz J, Tzaribatchev N, Claussen CD, et al. Chronic recurrent multifocal osteomyelitis: comparison of whole-body MR imaging with radiography and correlation with clinical and laboratory data. Radiology 2009;252(3):842–51.

82. Cyrlak D, Pais MJ. Chronic recurrent multifocal osteomyelitis. Skeletal Radiol 1986;15(1):32–9.

83. Beretta-Piccoli BC, Sauvain MJ, Gal I, et al. Synovitis, acne, pustulosis, hyperostosis, osteitis (SAPHO) syndrome in childhood: a report of ten cases and review of the literature. Eur J Pediatr 2000;159(8):594–601.

84. Suresh S, Saifuddin A. Unveiling the 'unique bone': a study of the distribution of focal clavicular lesions. Skeletal Radiol 2008;37(8):749–56.

85. Teoh KH, Watts AC, Chee YH, et al. Predictive factors for recurrence of simple bone cyst of the proximal humerus. J Orthop Surg (Hong Kong) 2010;18(2):215–9.

86. Wootton-Gorges SL. MR imaging of primary bone tumors and tumor-like conditions in children. Magn Reson Imaging Clin N Am 2009;17(3):469–87, vi.

87. Margau R, Babyn P, Cole W, et al. MR imaging of simple bone cysts in children: not so simple. Pediatr Radiol 2000;30(8):551–7.

88. Sailhan F, Chotel F, Parot R. Chondroblastoma of bone in a pediatric population. J Bone Joint Surg Am 2009;91(9):2159–68.

89. Ramappa AJ, Lee FY, Tang P, et al. Chondroblastoma of bone. J Bone Joint Surg Am 2000;82(8):1140–5.

90. Azouz EM. Magnetic resonance imaging of benign bone lesions: cysts and tumors. Top Magn Reson Imaging 2002;13(4):219–29.

91. James SL, Panicek DM, Davies AM. Bone marrow oedema associated with benign and malignant bone tumours. Eur J Radiol 2008;67(1):11–21.

92. Kaim AH, Hugli R, Bonel HM, et al. Chondroblastoma and clear cell chondrosarcoma: radiological and MRI characteristics with histopathological correlation. Skeletal Radiol 2002;31(2):88–95.

93. Yaw KM. Pediatric bone tumors. Semin Surg Oncol 1999;16(2):173–83.

94. Peersman B, Vanhoenacker FM, Heyman S, et al. Ewing's sarcoma: imaging features. JBR-BTR 2007;90(5):368–76.

95. Rodriguez Martin J, Pretell Mazzini J, Vina Fernandez R, et al. Ewing sarcoma of clavicle in children: report of 5 cases. J Pediatr Hematol Oncol 2009;31(11):820–4.

Magnetic Resonance Imaging of Shoulder Arthropathies

A. Ross Sussmann, MD[a],*, Jodi Cohen, MD[a],
George C. Nomikos, MD[b,†], Mark E. Schweitzer, MD[c]

KEYWORDS

- Septic arthritis • Rheumatoid arthritis
- Calcium pyrophosphate dihydrate • Hydroxyapatite

Magnetic resonance (MR) imaging is well established for assessment of the shoulder. The integrity and morphology of the rotator cuff tendons, musculature, and capsular structures, and any associated findings, help the orthopedist to determine the appropriateness and type of any surgical intervention that may be necessary after injury. In cases of osseous or soft tissue neoplasm, the sensitivity of MR imaging for marrow changes and soft tissue contrast can direct biopsy planning and help determine appropriate surgical resection margins. The role of MR imaging in the assessment of various shoulder arthropathies is less defined and is evolving. In this review, the clinical and MR imaging features of 4 of the major shoulder arthropathies are addressed: septic arthritis, rheumatoid arthritis (RA), calcium pyrophosphate dihydrate (CPPD) deposition disease–related arthropathy, and hydroxyapatite disease (HAD).

Septic arthritis remains primarily a clinical diagnosis based on symptoms, physical examination findings, and laboratory analysis of joint fluid aspirate. A missed or delayed diagnosis can lead to articular destruction, concomitant osteomyelitis, and eventually sepsis. Conventional radiographic manifestations of disease occur late and once they are present, often only salvage procedures can be performed. The much greater sensitivity of MR imaging for early joint infection, although not a replacement for fluid sampling or operative management, helps narrow the clinical differential diagnosis, determine the extent of infection, and assess for associated osteomyelitis and soft tissue or intraosseous abscesses. Findings also provide a baseline for assessment of treatment response.

This sensitivity of MR imaging for even subtle levels of inflammatory activity is also of benefit in the case of RA. The classic features of periarticular osteoporosis, soft tissue swelling, osseous erosions, and loss of joint space are well assessed on radiography, which rightfully remains a fundamental part of disease surveillance. However, as RA begins with inflammatory changes at the synovial level, MR imaging offers a unique opportunity to identify disease at its earliest stages. Similar to the situation with septic arthritis, it has become a clinical necessity to assess for changes before there is articular destruction. Enhancement patterns of synovium and associated changes in bone marrow can distinguish between different levels of disease activity. Proper timing in the initiation of newer

Disclosures: A.R.S., J.C. and G.C.N. have nothing to disclose. M.E.S. is a financial consultant for Pfizer, Inc and Paradigm Spine, LLC.
[a] Radiology, Hospital for Joint Diseases/Orthopedic Institute, 6th Floor, 301 East 17th Street, New York, NY 10003, USA
[b] Department of Radiology, Georgetown University Medical Center, 3800 Reservoir Road Northwest, CCC Building, Washington, DC 20007, USA
[c] Department of Diagnostic Imaging, The Ottawa Hospital, University of Ottawa, 501 Smyth Road, Ottawa, ON K1H 8L6, Canada
[†] Deceased March 5, 2011.
* Corresponding author.
E-mail address: amado.sussmann@nyumc.org

disease-modifying drugs is critical to obtain a good therapeutic response, and the ability to identify RA stage and activity is therefore invaluable. Perhaps even more important is to assess, by functional musculoskeletal MR imaging, the effectiveness of these expensive and often toxic medications.

CPPD disease and HAD are usually readily identified on conventional radiography, as the soft tissue calcifications typical of each entity are the cardinal finding. With the increased use of advanced imaging for other indications, however, these entities may be encountered on MR imaging and can be confused with other arthropathies such as RA or primary osteoarthrosis. In the case of HAD especially, reactive bursitis and regional inflammation related to resorbing intratendinous calcifications can be confused for infection or rotator cuff tear. Although such confusion can often be resolved by correlation with radiography, films are not always available at the time of interpretation.

SEPTIC ARTHRITIS
Background, Demographics, and Presentation

The shoulder is a relatively uncommon site of septic arthritis. In one retrospective review, Leslie and colleagues[1] reported on 18 cases over 18 years based on all records from 2 large North American hospitals. Another earlier study by Lossos and colleagues[2] identified 11 cases from 6 major hospitals in Israel over a 9-year period. More recent reviews from both Europe and the United States have reported similarly low incidence among their patient populations, with rates such as 21, 17, and 23 cases over 8-, 11-, and 15-year periods, respectively.[3–5] As the shoulder is the second largest joint in the body, with commensurately large synovium, it seems peculiar that infection is infrequent. The incidence is higher if infection in the setting of joint arthroplasty is included. For instance, during a 5-year prospective study of consecutive patients with or without arthroplasty and with a diagnosis of septic glenohumeral arthritis, Kirchhoff and colleagues[6] enrolled 43 patients.

However, the incidence may be increasing because of the increasing longevity of the population, resulting in more individuals with comorbid risk factors for infection being exposed for longer periods. Multiple studies have observed at least one major comorbidity in 80% or more of patients.[5,6] In general, septic shoulder occurs in older adults, with a mean age of 60 to 65 years.[1,3]

Septic shoulder is quite uncommon in neonates as well as in healthy adults, but septic arthritis (of any joint) is very rare between later infancy and young adulthood. This process is thought to relate to changes in vascularity within developing bone. Diaphyseal vessels in the newborn traverse the physis, allowing hematogenous agents ready access to the epiphysis and joint. Beginning at approximately 8 to 18 months of age, the diaphyseal vessels instead terminate in sinusoidal lakes situated in the metaphysis, effectively obliterating any hematogenous pathway to the epiphysis. This condition accounts for the metaphyseal predilection of infections such as Brodie abscesses in adolescence. After closure of the growth plate in adulthood, infection can again more easily extend to the epiphysis and joint. Even in the neonatal age group, incidentally, the knee and hip are much more common sites of infection than is the shoulder.

As with any septic arthritis, there are 3 major routes of seeding: hematogenous spread, direct inoculation, and contiguous spread. Hematogenous seeding is the most common route, and may occur with bacteremia of any cause.[7–9] Direct routes include intraarticular injection, joint surgery, and penetrating trauma; contiguous routes include regional infection such as osteomyelitis, tenosynovitis, soft tissue abscess, cellulitis, and septic bursitis. Of the direct routes, intraarticular injection is most common, typically when performed therapeutically (corticosteroid injection). Because contrast is bacteriostatic, septic arthritis after diagnostic injection for arthrography is exceptionally rare. Postinjection septic arthritis occurs in approximately 1 per 1000 cases according to some reports; other studies report lower rates such as 1 per 3500, all joints included.[10,11] Postsurgical septic arthritis has been reported in as many as 2% of constrained arthroplasties and fewer than 1% of unconstrained systems.[10,12] Infection may present anywhere from months to years after the surgery. In the last 2 decades, with improvements in operative technique and infection control, acute postarthroplasty infections have significantly decreased; however, the rate of delayed infections has remained stubbornly constant.

By far the most common causative agent is *Staphylococcus aureus*, accounting for 40% to 70% in some series.[1,3–6,10] In Kirchhoff's study, the next most common agents were *Staphylococcus epidermidis* and *Staphylococcus agalactiae*.[6] In recent years, an increasing number of *S aureus* infections have been attributable to methicillin-resistant *S aureus* (MRSA) strains. In Cleeman and colleagues'[5] series of 23 cases of glenohumeral infection, for instance, 70% of cases were due to *S aureus* and of these 17% were MRSA. Gram-negative bacilli (*Escherichia coli*,

Klebsiella pneumoniae, Proteus mirabilis) have accounted for up to 20% of infections in some series. *Streptococcus* (*S pyogenes, S pneumoniae*) and *Gonococcus* are other potential agents. Specific types of patients have a greater susceptibility to otherwise rare causative agents. In particular, patients with sickle cell anemia are prone to *Salmonella* infection and immunocompromised patients (AIDS, immunosuppressive therapy) are at increased risk for *Mycobacterium tuberculosis*. However, in both these groups *Staphylococcus* is still the most common causative organism.

As already noted, one of the major risk factors for infection is the presence of comorbidities. Preexistent arthritis is a significant risk factor, and the risk of secondary septic arthritis increases with the severity of the primary arthropathy.[13] The arthropathy with the highest secondary risk of infection is rheumatoid, followed by gout and even osteoarthritis. Theoretically, this is related to the hyperemia these arthropathies engender, increasing the risk of bacterial emboli. Diabetes mellitus is another major risk factor for septic arthritis, usually from focal spread. Additional factors include underlying malignancy, cirrhosis, immunosuppression (human immunodeficiency virus/AIDS, chemotherapy, stem cell/solid organ transplant recipients), obesity, chronic obstructive pulmonary disease, alcoholism, hyperuricemia (even in the absence of gout), and intravenous drug use.[1,2]

On clinical examination, no finding is specific for septic arthritis. The initial presentation of septic arthritis can mimic that of any inflammatory arthropathy. Pain and limited range of motion are common presenting findings.[6,10] Patients may also refer warmth, erythema, and swelling, but these are less reliable indicators. In a study by Ambacher and colleagues,[14] these 3 findings were observed in only 60% of patients. The presence of fever and malaise is inconsistent. Evident signs of inflammation do not rule in infection, nor does their absence rule it out. Furthermore, preexisting joint abnormalities, especially concurrent arthropathies, can mimic or mask infectious symptoms. Adjacent inflammatory conditions such as bursitis and calcific tendinitis can also mimic septic arthritis.[1] Immune status is also important, as compromised patients may not be able to mount an appropriate clinical response. Also, the precise causative agent must be considered. Tuberculous infection, in particular, most often has a more indolent course with subclinical manifestations for months to years, especially in older patients. Incomplete treatment with antibiotics, all too common in clinical care, can leave smoldering levels of infection while partially masking

or blunting corresponding signs and symptoms. The nonspecific and variable presentations of septic arthritis can considerably delay diagnosis and treatment. The relative difficulty in palpating the shoulder joint because of its deep situation further limits assessment. In Leslie and colleagues'[1] series, diagnosis was delayed by more than 6 months in one-third of cases. In Kirchhoff and colleagues'[6] study population, only 44% of the patients were diagnosed or treated within 10 days of symptom onset. The remaining 56% were diagnosed or treated at a mean of 57 days from onset. In both of these studies, a longer delay in diagnosis correlated with poorer outcomes.[1,6]

Laboratory analysis can imperfectly aid in the diagnosis of septic arthritis. Leukocytosis is an unreliable indicator, as it may be absent even in immunocompetent patients who are infected. The erythrocyte sedimentation rate (ESR) may also be increased. Several series have reported that 90% to 100% of subjects have increased C-reactive protein (CRP).[4,6,15] However, increased levels are probably not sufficiently specific, as other inflammatory conditions such as RA would still need to be considered. A normal CRP may help to exclude infection.

Imaging Findings

Septic arthritis is ultimately a clinical diagnosis that hinges on appropriate synovial fluid analysis. Direct sampling of joint fluid is the single most important diagnostic step, and can be accomplished either by image-guided needle aspiration or intraoperative collection during irrigation. Nevertheless, imaging can offer significant information for both diagnosing and assessing the extent of infection. Furthermore, the posttreatment course can be monitored, albeit in a delayed fashion, with the aid of serial studies.

Radiographs are neither sensitive nor specific for early septic arthritis, but still offer useful information. Preexistent conditions such as osteoarthrosis and inflammatory arthropathy may be identified. The radiograph also offers a baseline by which the long-term treatment outcome may be monitored. In more advanced stages of infection, radiographs will show narrowing of joint space secondary to cartilage destruction, marginal erosions at the bare areas of the joint, or, rarely, periostitis and bone destruction if there is associated osteomyelitis. Inadequately treated disease may also demonstrate secondary arthrosis and/or bone destruction. Ankylosis, subchondral bone loss with reactive sclerosis, and periarticular calcifications may also be seen, the latter being more common in nonpyogenic infections.

Ultrasonography has a growing role in the evaluation of the septic shoulder. Both effusions and synovial hypertrophy can be well visualized, the latter typically appearing as hypoechoic intraarticular material that lacks compressibility and mobility and often demonstrates flow on Doppler analysis.[9] The dynamic nature of sonography allows the entire glenohumeral joint to be scrutinized, which is useful, because an effusion may distribute unevenly. In one review of 30 glenohumeral joint effusions, fluid was consistently identified by ultrasonography in the posterior joint recess in 100% of the patients and in the biceps tendon sheath in 97%.[16] Ultrasonography may also be used in this way to facilitate aspiration for diagnostic and therapeutic purposes. Accessing the joint without image guidance can be considerably less reliable. In one study, Sethi and colleagues[17] found that only 26% of landmark-guided anterior glenohumeral joint injections by orthopedic surgeons were ultimately successful in reaching the intraarticular space.

Although the role for conventional radiography in evaluating and following septic arthritis should not be understated, MR imaging offers many advantages that make it a useful and important imaging step in assessing for joint infection.[18–20] The presence and amount of joint effusion can be established, which may help direct aspiration. In the normal glenohumeral joint, almost no fluid should be present. In a review of 20 shoulder MR imaging studies from 12 asymptomatic patients,

Recht and colleagues[21] found joint fluid in 14 shoulders, but not exceeding 2 mL in any case. Furthermore, MR imaging allows at least a general grading of fluid volume in the abnormal joint. The following criteria have been proposed: grade 0 reflects scant fluid not distending any joint recesses; grade 1 demonstrates a small amount of fluid in the subscapularis recess, axillary recess (marked by a U-shaped inferior capsule), or biceps tendon sheath on at least 2 coronal-oblique images; grade 2 demonstrates distention of at least 2 of these recesses; and grade 3 demonstrates fluid in all 3 recesses.[22]

The overall extent of soft tissue and osseous involvement in septic arthritis may also be assessed by MR imaging. Conversely, given the exquisite sensitivity for soft tissue and marrow changes that MR provides, the absence of joint effusion and of any other typical early findings for infection can exclude the diagnosis of septic shoulder in a way that radiography cannot.

T2-weighted and/or short-tau inversion recovery (STIR) sequences are particularly useful in identifying early stages of disease. Initial manifestations include glenohumeral effusion and synovitis. Reactive marrow edema is often present as well, within both the humeral head and the apposing portion of the glenoid. Postcontrast fat-suppressed T1-weighted images are helpful in demonstrating thick and/or frondlike rim-enhancing synovium (**Fig. 1**). The authors recommend that these be done dynamically to quantify the extent of articular

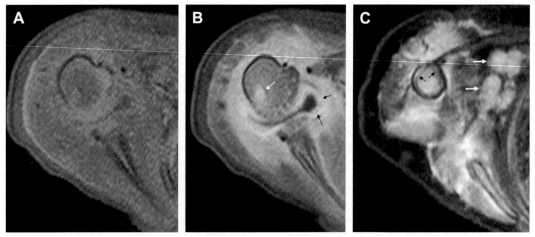

Fig. 1. Septic glenohumeral arthritis and osteomyelitis in a 4-month-old infant. Fat-suppressed T1-weighted axial images before (*A*) and after (*B*) administration of intravenous contrast material demonstrate thick synovial enhancement (*black arrows*) and periarticular soft tissue enhancement, as well as humeral head marrow enhancement (*white arrow*) compatible with secondary osteomyelitis. Fat-suppressed T2-weighted axial image (*C*) demonstrates extensive deep soft tissue edema, as well as marrow hyperintensity and cortical/pericortical hyperintensity (*black arrows*) felt to represent osteomyelitis with associated periostitis. Scapular edema and large reactive axillary lymph nodes (*thick white arrows*) are also seen.

hyperemia. On postcontrast images, the acromio-clavicular joint can be used as a standard of reference for normal enhancement in the absence of complete communicating rotator cuff tears. A periarticular abscess, if present, may be distinguished by characteristic thick-walled peripheral enhancement.

As infection progresses beyond mere synovitis and effusion, marginal erosions form at the bare areas of the joint and cartilage degradation may occur within days, leading to narrowing of the joint space.[23] With protracted chondral loss, the infection may progress into the subacute phase, when subchondral edema and subchondral cyst formation occur. Patients are also at increased risk for rotator cuff tear at this time, as extension of joint fluid into the subscapularis recess facilitates invasion of the cuff tendons by inflamed outpouchings of synovium. In the setting of a cuff defect, a secondary acromioclavicular septic arthritis can develop. Acromioclavicular joint sepsis can also occur in the absence of any preexisting glenohumeral infection. However, this a rare occurrence; one recent review from France reported 5 cases over a 6-year period.[24] The same review noted only about 20 reported cases in the literature.

In the chronic stages of glenohumeral septic arthritis, joint destruction progresses and ultimately can lead to ankylosis. Osteomyelitis may also occur, and can be difficult at times to distinguish from reactive marrow edema caused by the joint infection. One of the more reliable indicators of osteomyelitis is more confluent T1 hypointensity within the marrow, more overt than that usually seen in the setting of reactive edema. In neonates, incomplete red to yellow marrow conversion limits the usefulness of T1-weighted images for osteomyelitis detection, and in these cases the distinction between reactive edema and true osteomyelitis may be more challenging (see **Fig. 1**). The temporal and anatomic progression of red to yellow marrow conversion during normal maturation has been elaborated.[25] Knowledge of these conversion patterns may help prevent false-positive and false-negative interpretations in the neonatal population. Also, if the contralateral joint is within the field of view, assessing the degree of marrow T1 hypointensity or T2 hyperintensity relative to the normal joint may be helpful.

Overall, the findings reported to correlate most strongly with septic arthritis are synovial enhancement, perisynovial edema, and joint effusion (**Fig. 2**). Karchevsky and colleagues[26] reported the presence of these findings in 98%, 84%, and 70%, respectively, of 50 consecutive subjects with joint infection (the study was not restricted to glenohumeral infection). Still, no one MR sign reliably confirms septic arthritis while excluding aseptic inflammatory arthritis. Graif and colleagues[20] had demonstrated this in their assessment of multiple MR findings: joint effusion, fluid outpouching, fluid heterogeneity, synovial thickening, synovial periedema, synovial enhancement, cartilage loss, bone erosions, bone erosion enhancement, bone marrow edema, bone marrow enhancement, soft tissue edema, soft tissue enhancement, and periosteal edema.[27] Their study did, however, demonstrate a strong trend toward significance for erosions indicating joint infection, as well as for erosions combined with bone marrow edema, synovial thickening, synovial periedema, bone marrow enhancement, or soft tissue edema.

When considering septic shoulder arthritis, it is important also to be mindful of nonpyogenic infections, especially those caused by *Mycobacterium tuberculosis* and other mycobacteria, as they can present with quite different clinical and imaging features. Skeletal tuberculosis (TB) is encountered in 1% to 3% of extrapulmonary cases of TB, and of these skeletal cases 1% to 10% involve the shoulder.[28] Fever, erythema, and warmth around the joint are highly unreliable indicators on examination, as nonpyogenic infection can smolder in the joint for years. Richter and colleagues[29] found an average 15-month delay from time of symptom onset to correct diagnosis of TB of the shoulder. Although MR imaging and radiography lack specificity for tuberculous shoulder infection, they demonstrate certain helpful findings. Generally, the cardinal features of mycobacterial infection are osteoporosis, marginal subchondral erosions (usually occurring later), and gradual rather than rapid cartilage destruction: the triad of Phemister.[30] An appearance somewhat similar to chronic pyogenic osteomyelitis also can sometimes be seen, including sclerosis, periostitis, and synovial membrane thickening.[28] Large effusion and osteolysis are other associated features. Even T2-intermediate intraosseous tubercles are sometimes encountered.[28] Tuberculous bursitis has also been well described, having been encountered most commonly in bursae of the shoulder, hands, ischia, and gluteal muscles.[30] Although also nonspecific, intrabursal rice bodies may be shed in the setting of TB or any chronic bursitis, appearing subcentimeric and isointense to muscle on both T1-weighted and T2-weighted images.[31] Like pyogenic septic arthritis, nonpyogenic disease can result in significant bone and joint destruction in advanced stages of infection.

Assessment for potential infection of the postoperative shoulder poses unique challenges.

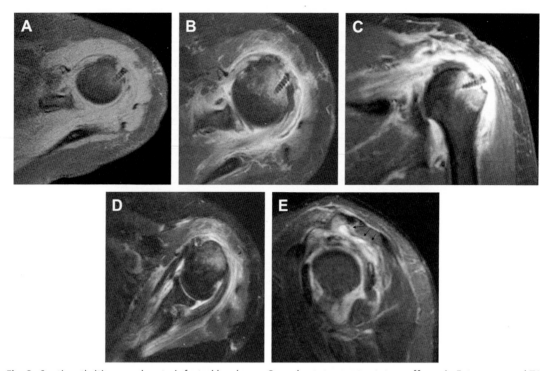

Fig. 2. Septic arthritis secondary to infected hardware, 3 weeks status post rotator cuff repair. Fat-suppressed T1-weighted images before (*A*) and after (*B, C*) intravenous contrast material administration demonstrate extensive synovitis, periarticular soft tissue inflammation, and subacromial-subdeltoid bursitis. The plastic suture anchor is partially backed out of the greater tuberosity. Fat-suppressed T2-weighted axial (*D*) and sagittal-oblique (*E*) images demonstrate, respectively, a small glenohumeral joint effusion and an abscess (*arrows*) thought to be in communication with the acromioclavicular joint.

Susceptibility artifact related to metallic hardware or to cement has been the major limitation to using MR imaging for diagnosing acute joint infection, as areas of interest may easily be obscured. Computed tomography (CT) is also subject to metal-related artifacts, which compounds the inherent low sensitivity of this modality for detecting subtle or early soft tissue changes. Radionuclide imaging has been the mainstay for evaluating the instrumented shoulder for septic arthritis, as it does not show deleterious artifacts from the presence of hardware and can be targeted for visualization of either soft tissue–centered or osseous-centered inflammation. Bone scintigraphy, although lacking in specificity, can almost entirely exclude osteomyelitis via a completely normal scan. By coupling bone scintigraphy with gallium 67 imaging, soft tissue inflammation that may occur in the earlier stages of septic arthritis can be detected, even before any associated osteomyelitis has developed. Accuracy for diagnosing or excluding joint infection in the setting of arthroplasty may be increased even further, to 90%, through the combination of bone scintigraphy with labeled-leukocyte imaging, as leukocytes demonstrate the highest sensitivity for detecting neutrophil-mediated processes.[32] Some studies have reported on positron emission tomography (PET) imaging for diagnosing infection, but the clinical usefulness of this application remains unsettled.

Regardless of its limitations, MR imaging is still of value in the setting of joint arthroplasty with potential infection. Field distortion can be minimized by using lower field strength, wider bandwidths, smaller voxels, and/or higher gradients. Frequency-selective fat suppression and gradient echo techniques should be avoided. STIR and water excitation show less distortion. Although not yet widely used in clinical practice, there are also rapid advances in further minimizing artifacts through the use of fast spin echo (FSE) metal artifact reduction sequences (MARS), and newer multi-acquisition variable-resonance image combination (MAVRIC) and slice-encoding metal artifact reduction (SEMAC) sequences. Initial studies on patients undergoing shoulder, hip, and knee arthroplasty have demonstrated improved visualization of synovitis, periprosthetic bone, supraspinatus tendon fibers, and supraspinatus tendon tears with MAVRIC sequences.[27,33,34]

RA

Background, Demographics, and Imaging Findings

RA is an inflammatory arthritis that begins at the synovial level. Certain autoimmune factors are important in the pathogenesis of RA. Naive B cells accumulate in synovium where select clones seem to be continuously activated.[35] Synovial tissue T cells express transcription factors also important for maintaining an inflammatory response. The synovium, now congested with immune cells, becomes progressively more inflamed under the influence of monocyte and macrophage-secreted cytokines such as interleukins (IL)-1, IL-6, and IL-17, and tumor necrosis factor alpha (TNFα).[35–37] Several of these cytokines also upregulate osteoclast activity and production of chondrolytic factors. The inflamed synovium can either return to a normal state or continue to hypertrophy into pannus that destroys articular cartilage, periarticular soft tissues, and bone under the influence of these inflammatory factors. Recent studies have also emphasized the importance of fibroblastlike synoviocytes (FLSs) that predominate in the synovium of patients with RA, especially as these may be the cell type most responsible for the spread of RA from one joint to another. Many studies have implicated the oral cavity bacterium *Porphyromonas gingivalis* in the pathogenesis of the disease, noting that patients with RA have high antibodies to the organism.[35] It is thought that the bacterium's ability to citrullinate enolase molecules at a site slightly different from that which is citrullinated physiologically may produce the autoantigen central to the inception of RA. Anticitrullinated protein antibodies (ACPAs) have been found in the serum of patients with RA and are thus considered a fundamental part of the disease pathway.[38]

Recent epidemiologic summaries cite an approximate 1% prevalence of RA in the United States, England, and much of mainland Europe.[39,40] Rates are slightly to considerably lower among the world's remaining populations, with the exception of some Native American groups in which as many as 6% of individuals may be affected. The incidence rate of RA for the United States is approximately 0.02% to 0.07%. RA has a 3:1 female-to-male predominance, and a median age at onset of 30 to 50 years. Genetics and heavy smoking are additional risk factors.

RA can affect any synovial joint in the appendicular or axial skeleton, but favors the metacarpophalangeal, metatarsophalangeal, and proximal interphalangeal joints of the hands and feet, as well as the radiocarpal and radioulnar joints. However, the glenohumeral and acromioclavicular joints are frequently involved as well. Shoulder symptoms have been reported in 50% of patients within 2 years of disease and 83% within 14 years.[41] Radiographic changes at the shoulder have been seen within 6 years of disease in more than 50% of patients and in 64% of patients within 19 years.

As opposed to septic arthritis, which rarely involves the acromioclavicular joint in isolation, RA of the shoulder frequently affects the acromioclavicular joint. In a study of 148 shoulders at 15 years of follow-up, Lehtinen and colleagues[42] found erosive change in the acromioclavicular joint alone in 17% of the shoulders, in the glenohumeral joint alone in 6%, and in both joints in 42%.

RA can involve the bursae, especially the subacromial-subdeltoid bursa, resulting in marked, masslike distention that may be mistaken for a soft tissue neoplasm. The pain that results may prompt patients to limit motion, leading in the long term to tightening of the joint capsule, ie, adhesive capsulitis. Although ultimately a clinical diagnosis, adhesive capsulitis may be suggested by certain MR imaging findings in the appropriate patient population for which pretest probability is already increased. Classically, rigidity of the coracohumeral and superior glenohumeral ligaments may present as thickening on MR imaging. Concomitant findings include obliteration of the normal fatty signal intensity within the rotator interval and thickening of the joint capsule at the axillary recess. The tightened joint capsule makes motion even more uncomfortable, prompting chronic diminished use of the shoulder, which in turn leads to atrophy of the rotator cuff muscles. Then, gradual superior migration of the humeral head results in a narrowed outlet with rotator cuff impingement, leading to tear. Up to 80% of patients with RA have significant thinning of the rotator cuff; and up to 20% have full-thickness tears.[43,44] Although cuff repair is an option, benefits are limited. One review of 23 repairs performed on RA shoulders over a 15-year period demonstrated significant improvements in pain and patient satisfaction after repair, but functional gains (defined as an increased range of abduction) were only obtained in the partial-thickness tear group.[45]

Radiography remains a critical component in monitoring progression of joint compromise and destruction in RA. Osteoporosis, marginal erosions, narrowing of joint space, subchondral sclerosis and cyst formation, and soft tissue swelling are cardinal features seen in varying combinations depending on the stage of disease. As joint space is lost to destruction by synovial pannus, bone is also eroded, classically in a periarticular distribution. At the shoulder, this typically manifests at the superolateral aspect of the humerus, adjacent to the greater tuberosity, corresponding to the humeral bare area between the articular cartilage of the humeral head and the reflection of the joint capsule. An erosion may also develop opposite this site, in the medial aspect of the surgical neck of the humerus secondary to pressure from the glenoid. As the erosive process progresses, the greater tuberosity, anatomic neck, and apposing glenoid are destroyed and the resulting arthropathy can mimic a neuroarthropathy or crystal-associated arthropathy.

Such destructive changes are well assessed by conventional radiography and are part of the meter by which disease severity is scored. The low cost of radiographs, their widespread availability, the relative ease of establishing reproducible interpretations and assessment algorithms, and the ability to correlate findings with standardized scoring criteria are major benefits.[46] For these reasons, radiographic findings are included in the American College of Rheumatology (ACR) classification criteria for RA and radiographs are recommended in clinical trials with duration of 1 year or longer.[47]

MR imaging offers several advantages over conventional radiography. Because RA begins at the synovium, an isolated finding of subtle synovitis can suggest early disease in the appropriate clinical context. Standardized methods of scoring disease have been developed; most notably the rheumatoid arthritis MRI scoring (RAMRIS) system, developed as part of the Outcome Measures in Rheumatoid Arthritis Clinical Trials (OMERACT) international initiative.[48] Generally, this uses standard field strength (1.5 T) contrast-enhanced MR imaging of the wrist and metacarpophalangeal joints to assign numeric scores for the severity of each of 3 findings: synovitis, marrow edema, and erosions. Studies have demonstrated good intrareader variability but less reliable interreader performance with this method. Other newer efforts include quantification of synovitis volume through segmentation and dynamic contrast-enhanced (DCE) MR imaging. DCE MR imaging has been particularly promising. A gadolinium dose of 0.05 to 0.3 mmol/kg is used and, typically, short repetition time, short echo time T1-weighted gradient echo images are acquired every few seconds over a period of minutes.

DCE MR imaging of the knees and wrist joints has yielded promising results. Cimmino and colleagues[49] demonstrated that the enhancement rate of wrist synovium can be used to distinguish between active and inactive disease. Although the correlation with disease activity is probably the strongest advantage of DCE MR imaging at this point, other studies have shown that the early (within approximately the first 60 seconds after injection) enhancement rate of synovium correlates with erosions, pain, ESR levels, erosive progression, and treatment effects. DCE MR imaging findings have also correlated well with histopathologic findings. Active research is focusing on the potential role for DCE MR imaging in monitoring and helping to appropriately time RA treatment with newer disease-modifying antirheumatoid drugs (DMARDs) such as anti-TNFα. Response to more established agents such as corticosteroids and methotrexate are also under investigation.[48,50] Because the shoulder tends to be affected later and less commonly than the hands and wrists in RA, these more recent MR scoring methods and dynamic enhancement protocols have not yet, to our knowledge, been scientifically applied to the glenohumeral and acromioclavicular joints. Similarly, no standardized protocols to assess treatment response via shoulder imaging have been developed. As RA tends to produce more pronounced changes in the dominant hand and wrist, multiple studies monitoring response to therapy use MR imaging of the dominant hand and wrist only.[51,52] It would seem reasonable, then, to image the dominant shoulder if clinically indicated for treatment monitoring. Perhaps not surprisingly, whereas most of the sequelae of RA favor the dominant limb, adhesive capsulitis more commonly affects the nondominant shoulder.

Although dynamic and other advanced MR techniques are not in widespread use for the shoulder, conventional MR imaging is already a powerful tool for evaluating the extent of both early and late disease. The earliest findings of RA, namely, synovitis and joint effusion, are soon followed by erosions, all well demonstrated by MR imaging. As in the case of septic arthritis, synovitis can be appreciated by avid or thick enhancement, sometimes with a frondlike morphology as a more masslike pannus begins to develop. Even in the absence of intravenous contrast, synovitis can often be appreciated, especially if well outlined by a joint effusion. Over time, as RA reaches its advanced stages, portions of the synovium may even fail to enhance or may demonstrate relative hypoenhancement and T2 intermediate to low signal intensity, reflecting fibrous synovitis, although small amounts of fibrotic pannus can even be seen earlier in the disease course.[53] Later on, the synovium will turn fatty. As with radiography, marginal erosions are found at the posterolateral aspect of the humeral head, and are often well-marginated T1-hypointense, T2-hyperintense foci within the bone, sometimes quite large (**Fig. 3**). In Lehtinen and colleagues[54] series of 148 glenohumeral joints, MR imaging revealed erosive changes in 71(48%) of the joints; and erosions were seen on the superolateral articular surface of the humeral head in 61 of these 71 joints. Glenoid involvement was only found in 28. Alasaarela and colleagues[55] demonstrated the superiority of MR imaging for visualizing humeral head erosions. In their prospective multimodality study of 26 shoulders in 26 symptomatic patients with RA, MR imaging revealed humeral erosions in 25 shoulders, ultrasonography in 24, CT in 20, and conventional radiography in 19. All erosions were on the posterolateral aspect of the humeral head at the insertion of the rotator cuff. It was thus concluded that MR imaging is superior to other modalities in detecting small erosions of the humeral head.

MR imaging is also useful for assessing cartilage but this can be considerably more challenging than evaluating erosions and synovitis given that the mean widths of humeral head cartilage (1.24 mm) and glenoid cartilage (1.88 mm) are near the limit of spatial resolution for most MR imaging scanners.[56] Nevertheless, focal regions of wear and destruction can often be appreciated, and visualization improves with high field strength (3T) scanners. Advances in structural and biochemical-based cartilage imaging in other parts of the body, particularly the hip and knee, could theoretically provide a more detailed picture of chondral compromise and areas of impending joint space loss in the shoulder. Recent advances include rotating frame T1 (T1 rho) mapping, Na mapping, T2 mapping, and delayed gadolinium-enhanced MR imaging of cartilage (dGEMRIC). However, these methods are not yet in widespread clinical use even for other joints.[56,57]

As noted earlier, the prevalence of thinning and tearing within the rotator cuff tendons is substantial in the setting of RA (**Figs. 4 and 5**).[43,44] This may be related partly to the destructive effects of synovitis at and near the supraspinatus-infraspinatus footprints. MR imaging allows for characterization of the extent of tearing, facilitating surgical planning for repair. In more longstanding cases, identification of fatty muscle atrophy has important prognostic implications for the potential success of a primary repair.[58] Multiple studies suggest that patients with advanced rheumatoid arthropathy benefit from either hemiarthroplasty or reverse shoulder arthroplasty, provided that either the rotator cuff is intact or can be well repaired at the time of arthroplasty.[59,60] MR imaging is useful in assessing the integrity of the deltoid muscle, a key consideration when determining appropriateness for reverse shoulder arthroplasty. Results of a recent Cochrane review, however, highlight a relative paucity of research evidence to support decision-making about arthroplasty in patients with RA.[61] At least one study by Soini and colleagues[62] concluded that MR imaging before arthroplasty was of only minor importance in cases of severely destroyed rheumatoid shoulder. The investigators observed that the extent of scar tissue and inflammation in their series of 31 patients limited the accuracy of soft tissue analysis. However, these were advanced

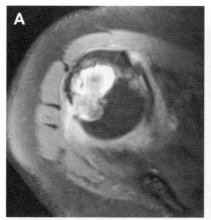 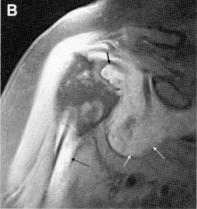

Fig. 3. RA. Fat-suppressed T2-weighted axial (*A*) image demonstrates classic superolateral location of a large humeral head erosion, in association with synovitis and large effusion. Fat-suppressed T2-weighted coronal-oblique (*B*) image better demonstrates the joint effusion, which extends distally within the biceps tendon sheath (*black arrow*) and medially into the subscapularis recess (*white arrows*). Smaller erosions are also present in the superomedial humeral head (*thick black arrow*).

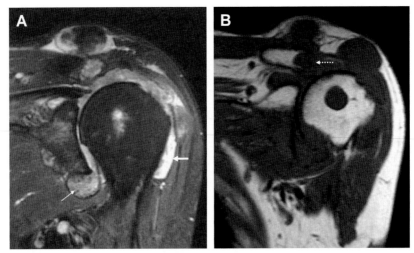

Fig. 4. RA in a 52-year-old woman. Coronal-oblique fat-suppressed fluid-sensitive weighted (A) and T1-weighted (B) images demonstrate a retracted full-thickness tear of the supraspinatus tendon with superior migration of the humeral head. Additional findings include subacromial-subdeltoid bursitis (*thick white arrow*) and glenohumeral joint effusion with tiny presumed rice bodies (*thin white arrow*) in the axillary pouch. Erosive changes are appreciated at the distal clavicle (*dashed white arrow*), and the protuberant subcutaneous lesions overlying the acromioclavicular joint and humeral head were thought to be rheumatoid nodules (these diminished in size on follow-up studies).

cases of disease and the same study demonstrated that an accurate determination of cuff damage and surrounding anatomy was difficult even during open inspection at time of surgery.

Beyond assessment of the cuff, analysis of surrounding soft tissue and osseous structures is important. The acromioclavicular joint, for instance, is of particular significance. In a review of 66 patients with RA with total shoulder arthroplasty and 75 patients with RA with hemiarthroplasty, erosions and cysts at the acromioclavicular joint were found to be associated with poorer

postoperative scores on the Clinical Hospital for Special Surgery Inventory.[60,63] Also, the status of the rotator cuff, and its repair at time of surgery, were predictive of the degree of postoperative improvement. Careful assessment of acromioclavicular joint integrity is therefore advisable, alongside characterization of any rotator cuff compromise when using MR imaging to examine the patient with RA preoperatively.

In a series of 49 patients with RA, Petersson[64] assessed clinical and radiographic findings and noted radiographic changes to the acromioclavicular joint

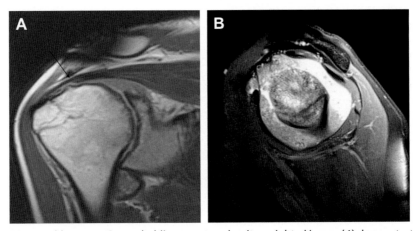

Fig. 5. RA in a 31-year-old woman. Coronal-oblique proton-density weighted image (A) demonstrates attenuated caliber of the supraspinatus tendon (*arrow*). Fat-suppressed fluid-sensitive sagittal-oblique (B) image demonstrates a large glenohumeral joint effusion containing numerous small rice bodies.

in 85% of cases. Pain and tenderness on examination were observed in one-third of the cases. Early in the course of disease, the acromioclavicular joint may demonstrate subchondral osteoporosis on radiographs, followed by erosions at the undersurface of the clavicle. On MR imaging, distention of the acromioclavicular joint capsule with extension of pannus into the joint may be seen at any stage of disease. As involvement progresses to the early stages of distal clavicular osteolysis, the distal end of the clavicle demonstrates subchondral marrow edema disproportionate to the acromion. Erosions enlarge over time to produce eventual osteolysis of the distal clavicle and even possible erosion of the distal acromion (see **Fig. 4**). Erosive changes often remain more pronounced at the caudal aspect of the distal clavicle. Radiographs and MR imaging demonstrate associated joint space widening, but dislocation and subluxation are uncommon.[65] Lehtinen and colleagues[66] reviewed 148 shoulders in 74 patients with RA after 15 years of follow-up. These investigators found a mean acromioclavicular joint distance (defined as the average of the joint distances measured from the cranial and caudal edges of the distal clavicle to the acromion) of more than 7 mm in 31% of the male shoulders and more than 5 mm in 15% of the female shoulders.

Although it is traditionally taught that the acromioclavicular joint is affected earlier and more severely than the glenohumeral joint in RA, this has not been our experience. However, as RA and septic arthritis can appear similar on many imaging modalities, when the acromioclavicular joint is involved as well, regardless of severity, it makes the diagnosis of RA more likely.

Synovial cyst formation is another complication of RA commonly encountered. The cysts develop within immediately surrounding soft tissues and frequently will dissect along tendon sheaths. Extension along the biceps tendon sheath is characteristic. This synovitis may dissect more than half way down the humerus (see **Fig. 3**). Synovial cysts may also develop under the subscapularis or around the axillary recess. However, the latter 2 locations are more common with septic arthritis. MR imaging allows enumeration and location of these cysts, which are of course not usually appreciable with conventional radiography. Rarely, a cyst may grow large enough to be masslike.[67] MR also identifies subacromial-subdeltoid bursitis, which may manifest on physical examination as swelling about the shoulder in patients with longstanding RA. Regions of proliferative synovium can, over time, infarct and shed into the bursae or joint, appearing as small nodules of varying signal intensity (although generally isointense to muscle) known as rice bodies (see **Figs. 4** and **5**).

Gandjbakhch and colleagues[68] recently published their analysis of 6 cohorts from 5 international medical centers, confirming that synovitis and marrow edema in patients with RA can still be appreciated on MR imaging even in patients who have achieved clinical remission. Thus, MR imaging, even without dynamic enhancement, provides a better gauge of disease activity than conventional radiography by demonstrating subclinical inflammation. This subclinical state of activity accounts for the observation that sometimes radiographic signs of RA progress despite a patient's being in remission.

CPPD DISEASE AND RELATED ARTHROPATHIES
Background

CPPD disease comprises a spectrum of entities with varying clinical and imaging manifestations. At the cellular level, CPPD disease is defined by the accumulation of CPPD crystals in soft tissues, most commonly within the extracellular matrix of midzonal articular cartilage.[69] It is thought that the initial insult may be a derangement in chondrocyte function that impairs maintenance of the extracellular matrix. The result is a buildup of excess adenosine triphosphate (ATP) and, subsequently, of the inorganic extracellular pyrophosphate (ePPi) that results from its cleavage.[70] The ePPi in turn binds calcium, producing crystals. Numerous factors contribute to the initial pyrophosphate imbalance, and their enumeration is beyond the scope of this review. Ultimately, they affect molecular transport, degradation, and cell signaling, and the more important contributors include molecules such as ANK (a transmembrane pyrophosphate transporter), PC-1 (a pyrophosphate generating hydrolase), and TGF-β (an upregulator of ANK and PC-1).[70,71] The symptomatic forms of CPPD disease (and other crystal diseases) reflect complex inflammatory cascades that are triggered by these chemical imbalances. These cascades occur usually at the synovial and chondral levels and are mediated by matrix metalloproteinases, prostaglandins, toll-like receptors, and ILs, among other factors.[70]

It has not been established to what extent, or even whether, calcium-containing crystals themselves actually promote cartilage destruction. Nor is it clear whether CPPD crystals can cause osteoarthrosis (OA) or are themselves secondary to chondral damage that occurs from OA. Results from at least 2 studies by Neogi and colleagues[72] have even suggested that chondrocalcinosis may stall cartilage loss, or at least be associated with delayed cartilage loss. In another study,

Viriyavejkul and colleagues[73] found knee arthroplasties were needed at a later age in patients with osteoarthrosis and CPPD disease compared with patients with osteoarthrosis alone. Nevertheless, many studies also support the more intuitive hypothesis that CPPD crystals, once shed into the joint cavity, incite an inflammatory response, especially within the synovium, with mediators such as those noted earlier being most strongly implicated. In vitro studies demonstrate the ability of CPPD crystals to induce IL and TNF expression by monocytes, as well as expression of an inflammasome important to IL-1β production.[74,75] Although details are lacking, most of the literature supports a strong correlation between calcium-containing crystals and arthritis. Rosenthal[69] cites that almost all tissue samples obtained from patients with severe osteoarthrosis have included calcium-containing crystals and that in one study investigating cartilage removed from joints undergoing arthroplasty, the prevalence of intracartilaginous CPPD crystals was 20%. Synovial inflammation has been found in more than half of osteoarthritic joints.

Accepting that there is some uncertainty about the exact manner in which CPPD crystals and arthritis relate to each other, the authors nevertheless acknowledge that there are well-characterized clinical and radiologic presentations of CPPD disease, and special attention is paid in this review to its MR imaging manifestations within the shoulder.

Demographics, Presentation, and Imaging Findings

CPPD disease has classically been divided into 2 major radiologic presentations: chondrocalcinosis and pyrophosphate arthropathy. In a recent review of the epidemiology of CPPD disease, Richette and colleagues[76] offered the following useful definitions: "chondrocalcinosis refers to radiographically visible chondral calcifications; pyrophosphate arthropathy refers to structural changes of cartilage and bone in the setting of CPPD deposition."

Age is the strongest risk factor for chondrocalcinosis. In the same review, Richette and colleagues noted that chondrocalcinosis has been reported in 7% to 10% of individuals around age 60 years; other studies have found it in up to 60% of individuals over the age of 85 years.[77,78] There is no strong gender predilection. Most cases occur idiopathically, although metabolic causes (such as hemochromatosis and ochronosis) and heritable genetic mutations also account for some cases and should be considered in patients less than 55 years of age and in patients with dramatic polyarticular involvement. In patients more than 55 years of age, hyperparathyroidism warrants some consideration when chondrocalcinosis is seen.[76] At least one study has found significantly lower prevalence of chondrocalcinosis in Chinese individuals who live in China compared with Caucasians living in the United States.[79]

Classically encountered as a radiographic finding, CPPD presents as thin, usually linear calcification within soft tissues (most often hyaline cartilage although it can also deposit in fibrocartilage), synovial tissue, ligaments (especially in the spine), tendons, and capsular structures. In the shoulder, it may be found within the labrum as linear density paralleling the glenoid contour or within the humeral articular cartilage paralleling the humeral head. Chondrocalcinosis may also present at the acromioclavicular joint, within the acromioclavicular joint articular meniscus, or within the tissue of the joint capsule itself. MR imaging, although not routinely used for screening in suspected cases of CPPD disease, can be surprisingly sensitive for chondrocalcinosis. It is seen as linear or punctate hypointensities on spin echo, FSE, and STIR images (**Fig. 6**).[80] The blooming effect may make deposits even more conspicuous than they would be on radiographs if gradient echo sequences are obtained (with an echo time greater than 5 milliseconds), as a result of the inhomogeneity between the magnetic susceptibility of crystals and that of hyaline cartilage.

Pyrophosphate arthropathy is more common in elderly women. The knee, radiocarpal, and first and second metacarpophalangeal joints are the most common sites of involvement, but shoulder involvement is not uncommon. Pyrophosphate arthropathy has been further divided into 5 clinical presentations by Canhao and colleagues[81] based on a study of 50 patients with confirmed CPPD disease: pseudogout, pseudo-osteoarthritis, pseudo-osteoarthritis with synovitis, monoarthropathy, and pseudo-RA.

Pseudogout accounts for roughly one-quarter of CPPD arthropathies and presents as acute onset pain, similar to but often not as intense as that experienced in gouty arthritis flares. Generally, the diagnosis is made based on symptoms and timing in patients already known to have CPPD disease. It is believed that shedding of CPPD crystals into joint fluid induces an inflammatory response. Episodes of pseudogout can be extremely painful and can imitate septic infection on physical examination. Potential triggers include joint lavage, granulocyte colony-stimulating factor therapy, bisphosphonates, and intraarticular hyaluronic acid injections.[76]

The pseudo-osteoarthritic patterns account for approximately half of pyrophosphate arthropathy

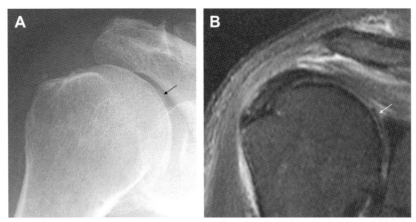

Fig. 6. Chondrocalcinosis in a 76-year-old man with confirmed history of pseudogout. Anteroposterior radiograph (*A*) demonstrates thin curvilinear chondrocalcinosis paralleling the central-medial portion of the humeral head (*black arrow*). Fat-suppressed, fluid-sensitive, coronal-oblique image (*B*) demonstrates linear hypointensity along the superomedial humeral head cartilage, corresponding to the chondrocalcinosis on radiograph (*white arrow*). Subacromial-subdeltoid bursitis had raised concern for infection versus pseudogout. Acromioclavicular joint aspirate (albeit obtained after antibiotic initiation) yielded CPPD crystals and no definite organisms.

cases. Like primary osteoarthrosis, they may present with narrowing of joint space and subchondral sclerosis. Although it may be difficult to differentiate pyrophosphate arthropathy from osteoarthrosis based on these findings alone, several clues favor the diagnosis of CPPD disease. Involvement of the shoulder is itself somewhat atypical of primary osteoarthrosis, given that the glenohumeral and acromioclavicular joints are not weight bearing. A combination of pronounced narrowing of joint space and chondrocalcinosis, either on radiography or MR imaging, suggests pyrophosphate arthropathy (**Fig. 7**). Primary shoulder osteoarthrosis is worse posteriorly on an axillary view, whereas pyrophosphate arthropathy, when there is associated secondary cuff arthropathy, may be worse anteriorly. Also, because shoulder osteoarthrosis may be a sequela

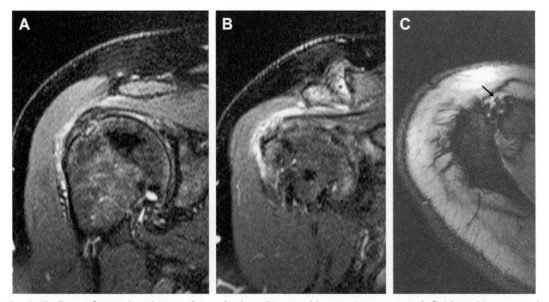

Fig. 7. Findings of pyrophosphate arthropathy in a 74-year-old man. Fat-suppressed, fluid-sensitive, coronal-oblique images (*A, B*) demonstrate pronounced glenohumeral and acromioclavicular joint arthrosis. Axial gradient echo image (*C*) through the acromioclavicular joint demonstrates arthrosis and irregularly curvilinear hypointensity within the joint (*arrow*), thought to represent chondrocalcinosis.

of remote trauma, asymmetric bilaterality of articular disease should also raise consideration of an alternate process such as CPPD disease. Concomitant involvement of other non–weight-bearing joints also favors pyrophosphate arthropathy. Osteophytosis occurs less frequently in pyrophosphate arthropathy than in usual osteoarthrosis.[82] Also, although subchondral cysts are found in both processes, those of CPPD disease tend to be greater in size and number and more widespread and confluent in distribution (**Fig. 8**). As opposed to the situation in primary osteoarthrosis, whereby cyst formation tends to follow narrowing of joint space, in pyrophosphate arthropathy the cysts may precede it. Large subchondral cysts can rupture, resulting in osseous fragmentation and formation of intraarticular, intracartilaginous, and instrasynovial bodies.[82,83] On MR imaging, therefore, relative preservation of the glenohumeral cartilage may be seen in the face of dramatic osseous and synovial cystic change. Indeed, destructive features of CPPD arthropathy are more commonly encountered in larger joints, particularly the shoulder, hip, and knee.

Less commonly, CPPD deposits can be seen within periarticular structures such as rotator cuff and biceps tendons, or embedded within the synovium or joint capsule. Gerster and colleagues[84] demonstrated tendinous involvement by CPPD crystals in 13.5% of all joints containing chondrocalcinosis. In contrast to hydroxyapatite disease, CPPD deposits tend to be linear rather than homogeneous or nodular, and can extend into the tendon far proximal to the insertion. The supraspinatus is commonly involved, and crystal disease should always be a consideration in cases of full-thickness and massive rotator cuff tears amongst the younger population. In the study by Canhao and colleagues,[81] 26 of the 50 patients demonstrated symptoms of periarthritis and 10 of these cases were within the shoulder. This finding suggests that crystal disease of the periarticular structures of the shoulder may be more prevalent than one might expect, even if deposits are not always visible on imaging. It has been established that pyrophosphate arthropathy can occur even in the absence of radiologically detectable crystals. CPPD crystals have also been found within acromioclavicular joint cyst aspirates in the setting of chronic, massive rotator cuff tears.

CPPD crystals that accumulate in bursal linings may trigger or exacerbate a bursitis. In the synovium, they may mimic other deposition or synovial-based processes. Extensive crystal disease can resemble pigmented villonodular synovitis, synovial osteochondromatosis, hemophilia, posttraumatic blood products, gas, and postsurgical susceptibility artifact from micrometallic debris.[82]

Pseudorheumatic arthropathy accounts for 5% to 8% of pyrophosphate arthropathies and, like RA, may present with fatigue, flexion contractures, and bilateral shoulder stiffness, often worse in the morning.[81,85] Laboratory analysis often reveals an increased ESR. Up to 1% of patients with true RA also have CPPD disease. Resnick and colleagues[86] observed that a key radiographic distinction between pseudo-RA and true RA in the setting of coexistent CPPD disease is that the former lacks erosions.

Although chondrocalcinosis and pyrophosphate arthropathy are the 2 predominant presentations of CPPD disease, less common presentations

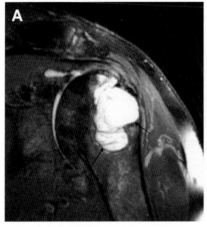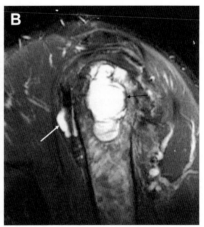

Fig. 8. Features of crystal-related arthropathy in a 59-year-old man. Coronal-oblique (*A*) and sagittal-oblique (*B*) fat-suppressed, fluid-sensitive weighted images demonstrate large, confluent, humeral head cysts (*black arrows*) in association with glenohumeral joint arthrosis. Synovial cystic change is appreciated around a segment of the extraarticular long head of the biceps tendon (*white arrow*).

exist as well, including tophaceous pseudogout, wherein tumoral deposits of CPPD are found, often at smaller joints (such as the acromioclavicular and temporomandibular joints), and a neuropathic-type arthropathy, wherein prominent osseous fragmentation, sclerosis, and disorganization are seen. In the case of tumoral pseudogout of the shoulder, deposits demonstrating low T1 and low to high T2 signal intensities have been described, often with pressure erosion or frank destruction of subjacent bone.[87] Although deposits can grow large with time, they are generally smaller than 10 cm. Lobulated margins and location near a joint without frank intraarticular invasion are additional characteristic features.

HAD
Background

HAD refers to deposition of hydroxyapatite, the most common of the basic calcium phosphate crystals, in the periarticular or, less commonly, intraarticular soft tissues. The precise cause of HAD is unknown. Like CPPD deposition disease, it depends at least in part on balances between extracellular and intracellular PPi. In distinction to CPPD disease, it has been suggested by some sources that deficient rather than excessive extracellular quantities of PPi play a large role in pathogenesis.[88–90] Hydroxyapatite is prevalent in other pathologic processes besides HAD. It is the primary constituent of the deposits found in tumoral calcinosis, end-stage renal disease, and hypervitaminosis D.[91] Although the most recognized manifestation of HAD is calcific tendinitis, some prefer the more inclusive phrase, calcific periarthritis, because crystals can deposit in any periarticular tissue, not just tendons.

The pathophysiology of periarticular HAD has been extensively studied, with most research having focused on its most common site, the rotator cuff tendons. One of the main questions has been whether calcifications preferentially deposit in degenerated tendons or in healthy tendons. Earlier theories favored the former, degenerative hypothesis, which holds that calcifications arise within necrotic and dystrophic tendon fibers that occur naturally with aging. This proposal was originally championed by Codman.[92] The newer, reactive hypothesis proffered by Uhthoff and colleagues[93,94] proposes that hydroxyapatite deposits in healthy tissue via cell-mediated processes and that the calcifications of HAD pass through 3 distinct stages. The first, or precalcific, stage is marked by fibrocartilaginous metaplasia of tenocytes into chondrocytes. The stimulus for this metaplasia may be decreased

local oxygen tension, which in turn may be secondary to repetitive compression of tendon fibers. The second, calcific, stage is divided into formative, resting, and resorptive phases. Chalky deposits develop during the formative phase, and then are bordered by fibrocollagenous tissues during the resting phase when calcium hydroxyapatite accumulation ceases. In the resorptive phase, vascular channels form around the deposit and provide access to macrophages and multinucleated giant cells that phagocytose and remove the calcium. Uhthoff and Loehr[93] note that, during this resorptive phase, the calcification has a toothpaste like, creamy quality and is often under pressure. The third, postcalcific, stage is marked by fibroblast proliferation and partial or complete tendon reconstitution.

Demographics, Presentation, and Imaging Findings

HAD peaks in the fifth decade of life, and has a slight male predilection. Bosworth[95] reviewed more than 6000 shoulders and found HAD deposits in 2.7%; but of these only 30% were symptomatic. Half of the affected cases showed bilateral calcifications. The shoulder is the most commonly affected joint in the body, in contrast to its much less common involvement by CPPD deposition disease. Also distinguishing HAD is its tendency toward unilaterality and monoarticularity, and the preferential presence of calcifications within the periarticular rather than intraarticular structures.[96] However, clinical findings in both HAD and CPPD can be similar, with local pain, decreased range of motion, erythema, and sometimes increased ESR being fairly common features.

The most symptomatic of the HAD stages is the calcific stage, specifically during its resorptive phase. Patients may present with acute onset, severe pain. The pain often mimics subacromial impingement, being elicited or exacerbated by recurrent or prolonged abduction. It is also during the resorptive phase that the deposits, being more pastelike, can extrude into the subacromial-subdeltoid bursa and incite a vigorous inflammatory response. In this situation, inflammatory corresponding symptoms, almost septiclike, can occur. Although the other stages of HAD can be symptomatic as well, they tend to produce a more chronic, dull pain.

The radiographic morphologies of HAD have been well characterized. De Palma and Kruper[97] identified 2 main types: Type I has a fluffy, fleecy appearance that corresponds to the resorptive phase. Sometimes it is accompanied by crescentic, streaky density overlying the main deposit; this crescent suggests extrusion into the overlying bursa. Type II deposits correspond often to the late formative stage, and are marked by homogeneous, circumscribed, discrete densities. Morphology is usually ovoid, but triangular and linear configurations are possible as well.

Considerably less has been written about the MR imaging characteristics of HAD deposits. At times it can be difficult to distinguish the hypointense deposit of HAD from native normal portions of tendon on MR imaging, because both are hypointense on most sequences. Less commonly, HAD deposits may be isointense to muscle, making them sometimes effectively invisible on MR imaging. Zubler and colleagues[98] concluded from a study of 62 MR arthrograms that MR imaging alone is unreliable for diagnosis of HAD. Still, several MR features of HAD may be sought out to make or at least suggest the diagnosis in the absence of radiographic correlation. For instance, the predilection for HAD to assume an ovoid shape may be helpful in the nonresorptive phases. In the resorptive phase, one can look for reactive edema. In the case of rupture, the finding of subacromial bursitis provides dramatic evidence of HAD (**Fig. 9**). Intrabursal HAD sometimes assumes a dumbbell-shaped configuration.[99]

At least one study has classified different morphologies of HAD on MR imaging. Loew and colleagues[100] attempted to determine whether the MR imaging appearances of calcific tendinitis in 76 patients correlated with features of osseous subacromial impingement. The investigators concluded there was no significant correlation, but did observe 3 distinct MR imaging morphologies of rotator cuff HAD in 71 of their patients. Type A (54%) appeared as a compact, homogenous, single deposit with a defined outline. Type B (38%) deposits were subdivided rather than solitary but remained homogeneous and well defined. Type C (7%) presented as diffuse low signal intensity without a defined outline. In 45 of their patients, a band of T2 signal hyperintensity surrounded the calcification and was thought to represent perifocal edema (see **Fig. 9**). Others have also reported this associated finding.[101] To our knowledge, no definitive correlation between MR and radiographic morphologies has yet been published. It seems probable, however, that the more fluffy, cloudlike radiographic appearance of Type I deposits in the resorptive phase are more likely to correlate with the Type C and perhaps sometimes Type B deposits on MR imaging.

Although the supraspinatus tendon is the most common site of involvement by HAD, any of the rotator cuff tendons can be affected. In order of decreasing frequency, the infraspinatus, teres minor, and subscapularis may be affected.[102] However, in Loew and colleagues' study,[100] the site with the highest incidence of HAD deposits was broadened to include not only the supraspinatus tendon but also the adjoining, cranial portion of the subscapularis. The study further noted that most supraspinatus deposits lay in the midportion of the tendon or just subjacent to its acromial surface. Uhthoff and Loehr[93] observed that it is uncommon for intratendinous HAD deposits to contact the bone surface because they are generally 1.5 to 2.0 cm away from it. In the case of the supraspinatus, this corresponds to the critical zone thought to be the region most susceptible to tears because of its relatively diminished vascularity and/or lower oxygen tension. Despite this, rotator cuff tears are not common in the setting of calcific periarthritis. In Loew and colleagues'[100] study population, only 1 patient had a coexistent partial-thickness supraspinatus tendon tear; none had a full-thickness tear; and only 1 had intraosseous extension of calcification. Multiple other studies have corroborated this lack of correlation between HAD and tears. When tears do occur, they are more often seen in the setting of small rather than large deposits.[101] The characteristic location of calcification within the critical zone provides a further useful means to distinguish HAD from degenerative calcifications on radiographs, as the latter tend to be smaller and are much more likely to lie immediately adjacent to the greater tuberosity. On MR imaging, degenerative calcifications are typically not appreciated because of their small size.

Erosions within the humerus are also rare when HAD involves the rotator cuff, although it seems to be a more prominent feature in rare cases of pectoralis calcific tendinitis. Despite its rarity, HAD of the pectoralis has been reported with certain characteristic features.[103] Hypointense calcification lies at or near the lateral lip of the distal aspect of the bicipital groove. Varying amounts of reactive edema may be seen: within surrounding musculature, around the tendon itself, and/or within the subjacent marrow. Cortical erosion at the tendinous insertion may occur, and the juxtaposition of the erosive change and the insertional HAD deposit can radiographically mimic a destructive juxtacortical, partially mineralized mass. The few reported cases in the literature have noted that the HAD deposit spontaneously resolved over 6 to 10 weeks.[103–105] However, for more ambiguous or worrisome cases, biopsy may be performed, with the finding of psammomatous bodies confirming HAD rather than neoplasm. In addition to the pectoralis, other rare sites of calcific tendinitis

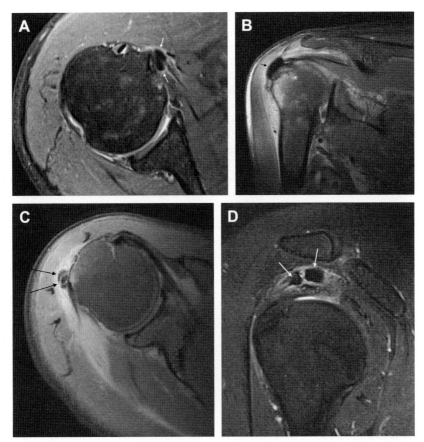

Fig. 9. Calcific tendinitis. Transaxial, fat-suppressed, fluid-sensitive weighted image (*A*) demonstrates 2 circumscribed HAD deposits in the subscapularis, each with a thin rim of signal hyperintensity (*white arrows*) compatible with perifocal edema. Coronal-oblique (*B*) and transaxial (*C*) fat-suppressed, fluid-sensitive weighted images from a second patient demonstrate a large circumscribed HAD deposit within the infraspinatus tendon (*short arrow*) as well as subacromial-subdeltoid bursitis secondary to additional deposits (*long arrows*) that had ruptured into the bursa. Sagittal-oblique, fat-suppressed, fluid-sensitive, weighted image (*D*) from a third patient demonstrates HAD deposits near the supraspinatus myotendinous junction (*white arrows*), just beneath the acromial surface of the tendon.

include beside the supraglenoid tubercle and beside the coracoid process, corresponding to the insertions of the long and short heads of the biceps tendon, respectively.[106]

Treatment of calcific tendinitis is most often conservative, relying on nonsteroidal antiinflammatory drugs.[107] In more difficult cases, ultrasound-guided lavage and aspiration followed by subacromial steroid injection offers a minimally invasive alternative to surgery. Extracorporeal shockwave therapy has been advocated by some, and a recent meta-analysis by Lee and colleagues[108] concluded level B support for this technique in recalcitrant cases.[109] Surgical debridement remains the definitive treatment for refractory calcific tendinitis, with postoperative physical therapy identified as a critical component expediting return to baseline activity levels. Concomitant

subacromial decompression has fallen out of favor because of longer recovery times and no demonstrable added benefit on 5-year outcome analysis.[110]

Milwaukee Shoulder

In contrast to calcific periarthritis, Milwaukee shoulder is a destructive arthropathy that results from the less common intraarticular accumulation of hydroxyapatite crystals. There is some contention about whether the entity purely involves HA crystals or also involves coexistent intraarticular CPPD deposition.[82] The classic features, described by McCarty[111,112] include pain, loss of joint function, and effusion. In their original series of 30 patients and through their analysis of 42 additional patients who had been reported in other studies, they noted Milwaukee shoulder favored female patients with a 4:1 ratio, and occurred predominated in the elderly, with a mean age of 72 years. Bilaterality of involvement was observed in 82%. The dominant arm was always involved and the nondominant arm, when involved, often demonstrated less dramatic changes. However, this pattern is common in most arthropathies. In their series, pain tended to be mild or intermittent, but restricted range of motion was universal. Potential predisposing factors were previous trauma (9 patients), CPPD disease (8 patients), neuroarthropathy (3 patients), dialysis-associated arthropathy (1 patient), and idiopathic (10 patients). Roughly half of patients with Milwaukee shoulder have been found to have a pyrophosphate-like arthropathy of the knee.[113]

As with periarticular HAD, the precise cause of Milwaukee shoulder is unknown. However, as in the case of pyrophosphate arthropathy, intraarticular HA crystals are thought to incite a chronic synovitis that eventually triggers release of proteases and collagenases. In turn, these are suspected to degrade both cartilage and bone. Secondary destabilization of the joint resulting from these processes may promote subclinical recurrent trauma that exacerbates the degree of destruction.[96] Periarticular calcifications frequently accumulate as well over the course of the disease, and in time the periarticular tissues can also undergo significant destruction.

Imaging features of Milwaukee shoulder therefore overlap with those of other arthropathies. Loss of joint space progressing to destruction is

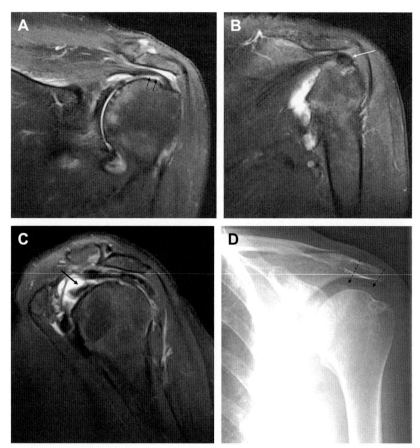

Fig. 10. Findings indicating Milwaukee shoulder in a 69-year-old woman. Fat-suppressed, fluid-sensitive weighted coronal-oblique (*A, B*) and sagittal-oblique (*C*) images demonstrate glenohumeral joint arthrosis, joint effusion, and articular surface tearing of the supraspinatus tendon (*thin black arrows*) in association with hypointense deposits in the infraspinatus (*white arrow*), on a background of more diffuse rotator cuff degeneration as well as attenuation and irregularity of the intraarticular biceps tendon (*thick black arrow* in *C*). The constellation of findings was thought to be most compatible with a HAD-associated arthropathy (Milwaukee shoulder). Radiograph from 2 years earlier (*D*) demonstrates rotator cuff calcific deposits (*dashed black arrows*) that likely represent HAD, possibly with coexistent CPPD given their elongated morphology.

the hallmark; and periarticular calcifications, occasionally appreciable as hypointense signal foci on MR imaging, have been described in approximately 40% of cases (**Fig. 10**).[91] Joint effusion is a cardinal feature and tends to be large or massive. In contrast to calcific periarthritis, Milwaukee shoulder commonly includes full-thickness tears of the supraspinatus and/or other cuff tendons. McCarty[111] even noted that original descriptions of HAD dating to the mid-nineteenth century identified loss of the intraarticular segment of the long head of the biceps tendon as another typical feature. Superior migration of the humeral head is not uncommon, and may in turn scallop the undersurface of the acromion, forming a pseudoarticulation. This feature can be seen with all causes of chronic rotator cuff tears in the setting of rotator cuff arthropathy, and is termed acetabularization of the acromion; the changes in the humeral head are called femurization.

Severe and focal osteoporosis of the humeral head is typical. Glenohumeral osteophytes tend to be small or absent. Subchondral cysts are not as prominent a feature as in pure pyrophosphate arthropathy. Although there is no definitive management for Milwaukee shoulder beyond conservative care in milder cases and arthroplasty in severe cases, more recent studies have suggested some benefit from tidal irrigation.[114]

SUMMARY

MR imaging is a powerful tool for evaluating shoulder involvement by RA, CPPD disease, and HAD, which have traditionally been monitored through conventional radiography, and within the setting of a septic shoulder, which remains a clinical diagnosis but can be difficult to evaluate thoroughly on only symptoms and examination findings. With attention to the characteristic features of each entity, the radiologist may be able to differentiate these processes from each other, as well as from primary degenerative disease or posttraumatic changes that can mimic them. With its sensitivity for the soft tissue and marrow changes that typify not only the more dramatic but also the earliest manifestations of these disease entities, MR imaging greatly facilitates timely diagnosis and can help direct management.

REFERENCES

1. Leslie BM, Harris JM 3rd, Driscoll D. Septic arthritis of the shoulder in adults. J Bone Joint Surg Am 1989;71(10):1516–22.
2. Lossos IS, Yossepowitch O, Kandel L, et al. Septic arthritis of the glenohumeral joint. A report of 11 cases and review of the literature. Medicine 1998; 77(3):177–87.
3. Klinger HM, Baums MH, Freche S, et al. Septic arthritis of the shoulder joint: an analysis of management and outcome. Acta Orthop Belg 2010;76(5):598–603.
4. Mehta P, Schnall SB, Zalavras CG. Septic arthritis of the shoulder, elbow, and wrist. Clin Orthop Relat Res 2006;451:42–5.
5. Cleeman E, Auerbach JD, Klingenstein GG, et al. Septic arthritis of the glenohumeral joint: a review of 23 cases. J Surg Orthop Adv 2005;14(2):102–7.
6. Kirchhoff C, Braunstein V, Buhmann Kirchhoff S, et al. Stage-dependant management of septic arthritis of the shoulder in adults. Int Orthop 2009; 33(4):1015–24.
7. Morgan DS, Fisher D, Merianos A, et al. An 18 year clinical review of septic arthritis from tropical Australia. Epidemiol Infect 1996;117(3):423–8.
8. Shirtliff ME, Mader JT. Acute septic arthritis. Clin Microbiol Rev 2002;15(4):527–44.
9. Garcia-De La Torre I. Advances in the management of septic arthritis. Infect Dis Clin North Am 2006; 20(4):773–88.
10. Cofield RH. The shoulder: results of complications. In: Morey BF, Cooney WP, editors. Joint replacement arthroplasty. New York: Churchill Livingstone; 1991. p. 437–53.
11. Geirsson AJ, Statkevicius S, Vikingsson A. Septic arthritis in Iceland 1990-2002: increasing incidence due to iatrogenic infections. Ann Rheum Dis 2008; 67(5):638–43.
12. Silliman JF, Hawkins RJ. Complications following shoulder arthroplasty. In: Friedman RJ, editor. Arthroplasty of the shoulder. New York: Thieme; 1994. p. 242–53.
13. Ho G Jr. Bacterial arthritis. Curr Opin Rheumatol 2001;13(4):310–4.
14. Ambacher T, Esenwein S, Kollig E, et al. The diagnostic concept of acute infection of the shoulder joint. Chirurg 2001;72(1):54–60 [in German].
15. Hariharan P, Kabrhel C. Sensitivity of erythrocyte sedimentation rate and C-reactive protein for the exclusion of septic arthritis in emergency department patients. J Emerg Med 2011;40(4):428–31.
16. Zubler V, Mamisch-Saupe N, Pfirrmann CW, et al. Detection and quantification of glenohumeral joint effusion: reliability of ultrasound. Eur Radiol 2011; 21(9):1858–64.
17. Sethi PM, Kingston S, Elattrache N. Accuracy of anterior intra-articular injection of the glenohumeral joint. Arthroscopy 2005;21(1):77–80.
18. Learch TJ, Farooki S. Magnetic resonance imaging of septic arthritis. Clin Imaging 2000; 24(4):236–42.
19. Learch TJ. Imaging of infectious arthritis. Semin Musculoskelet Radiol 2003;7(2):137–42.

20. Graif M, Schweitzer ME, Deely D, et al. The septic versus nonseptic inflamed joint: MRI characteristics. Skeletal Radiol 1999;28(11):616–20.

21. Recht MP, Kramer J, Petersilge CA, et al. Distribution of normal and abnormal fluid collections in the glenohumeral joint: implications for MR arthrography. J Magn Reson Imaging 1994;4(2):173–7.

22. Schweitzer ME, Magbalon MJ, Fenlin JM, et al. Effusion criteria and clinical importance of glenohumeral joint fluid: MR imaging evaluation. Radiology 1995;194(3):821–4.

23. Bremell T, Abdelnour A, Tarkowski A. Histopathological and serological progression of experimental *Staphylococcus aureus* arthritis. Infect Immun 1992;60(7):2976–85.

24. Bossert M, Prati C, Bertolini E, et al. Septic arthritis of the acromioclavicular joint. Joint Bone Spine 2010;77(5):466–9.

25. Laor T, Jaramillo D. MR imaging insights into skeletal maturation: what is normal? Radiology 2009; 250(1):28–38.

26. Karchevsky M, Schweitzer ME, Morrison WB, et al. MRI findings of septic arthritis and associated osteomyelitis in adults. AJR Am J Roentgenol 2004; 182(1):119–22.

27. Hayter CL, Koff MF, Shah P, et al. MRI after arthroplasty: comparison of MAVRIC and conventional fast spin-echo techniques. AJR Am J Roentgenol 2011;197(3):W405–11.

28. Kapukaya A, Subasi M, Bukte Y, et al. Tuberculosis of the shoulder joint. Joint Bone Spine 2006;73(2): 177–81.

29. Richter R, Hahn H, Nubling W, et al. Shoulder girdle and shoulder joint tuberculosis. Z Rheumatol 1985; 44(2):87–92 [in German].

30. Rutten MJ, van den Berg JC, van den Hoogen FH, et al. Nontuberculous mycobacterial bursitis and arthritis of the shoulder. Skeletal Radiol 1998; 27(1):33–5.

31. Griffith JF, Peh WC, Evans NS, et al. Multiple rice body formation in chronic subacromial/subdeltoid bursitis: MR appearances. Clin Radiol 1996;51(7): 511–4.

32. Love C, Tomas MB, Marwin SE, et al. Role of nuclear medicine in diagnosis of the infected joint replacement. Radiographics 2001;21(5): 1229–38.

33. Chen CA, Chen W, Goodman SB, et al. New MR imaging methods for metallic implants in the knee: artifact correction and clinical impact. J Magn Reson Imaging 2011;33(5):1121–7.

34. Koch KM, Brau AC, Chen W, et al. Imaging near metal with a MAVRIC-SEMAC hybrid. Magn Reson Med 2011;65(1):71–82.

35. Cooles FA, Isaacs JD. Pathophysiology of rheumatoid arthritis. Curr Opin Rheumatol 2011;23(3): 233–40.

36. van den Berg WB. Lessons from animal models of osteoarthritis. Curr Opin Rheumatol 2001;13(5): 452–6.

37. Tak PP, Bresnihan B. The pathogenesis and prevention of joint damage in rheumatoid arthritis: advances from synovial biopsy and tissue analysis. Arthritis Rheum 2000;43(12):2619–33.

38. Hitchon CA, Chandad F, Ferucci ED, et al. Antibodies to porphyromonas gingivalis are associated with anticitrullinated protein antibodies in patients with rheumatoid arthritis and their relatives. J Rheumatol 2010;37(6):1105–12.

39. Alamanos Y, Drosos AA. Epidemiology of adult rheumatoid arthritis. Autoimmun Rev 2005;4(3): 130–6.

40. Alamanos Y, Voulgari PV, Drosos AA. Incidence and prevalence of rheumatoid arthritis, based on the 1987 American College of Rheumatology criteria: a systematic review. Semin Arthritis Rheum 2006;36(3):182–8.

41. Hamalainen N. Epidemiology of upper limb joint affections in rheumatoid arthritis. In: Baumgartner H, Dvorak J, Grob D, et al, editors. Rheumatoid arthritis: current trends in diagnostics, conservative treatment, and surgical reconstruction. Stuttgart (Germany): Georg Thieme Verlag; 1995. p. 158–61.

42. Lehtinen JT, Kaarela K, Belt EA, et al. Relation of glenohumeral and acromioclavicular joint destruction in rheumatoid shoulder. A 15 year follow up study. Ann Rheum Dis 2000;59(2):158–60.

43. Cruess RL. Corticosteroid-induced osteonecrosis of the humeral head. Orthop Clin North Am 1985; 16(4):789–96.

44. Ennevaara K. Painful shoulder joint in rheumatoid arthritis. A clinical and radiological study of 200 cases, with special reference to arthrography of the glenohumeral joint. Acta Rheumatol Scand 1967;(Suppl 11):11–116.

45. Smith AM, Sperling JW, Cofield RH. Arthroscopic rotator cuff debridement in patients with rheumatoid arthritis. J Shoulder Elbow Surg 2007;16(1): 31–6.

46. van der Heijde DM. Plain X-rays in rheumatoid arthritis: overview of scoring methods, their reliability and applicability. Baillieres Clin Rheumatol 1996;10(3):435–53.

47. Tugwell P, Boers M. OMERACT conference on outcome measures in rheumatoid arthritis clinical trials: introduction. J Rheumatol 1993;20(3): 528–30.

48. Conaghan PG, McQueen FM, Bird P, et al. Update on research and future directions of the OMERACT MRI inflammatory arthritis group. J Rheumatol 2011;38(9):2031–3.

49. Cimmino MA, Innocenti S, Livrone F, et al. Dynamic gadolinium-enhanced magnetic resonance imaging

of the wrist in patients with rheumatoid arthritis can discriminate active from inactive disease. Arthritis Rheum 2003;48(5):1207–13.

50. Hodgson RJ, O'Connor P, Moots R. MRI of rheumatoid arthritis image quantitation for the assessment of disease activity, progression and response to therapy. Rheumatology (Oxford) 2008;47(1):13–21.

51. Zikou AK, Argyropoulou MI, Voulgari PV, et al. Magnetic resonance imaging quantification of hand synovitis in patients with rheumatoid arthritis treated with adalimumab. J Rheumatol 2006; 33(2):219–23.

52. Argyropoulou MI, Glatzouni A, Voulgari PV, et al. Magnetic resonance imaging quantification of hand synovitis in patients with rheumatoid arthritis treated with infliximab. Joint Bone Spine 2005; 72(6):557–61.

53. Narvaez JA, Narvaez J, De Lama E, et al. MR imaging of early rheumatoid arthritis. Radiographics 2010;30(1):143–63 [discussion: 163–5].

54. Lehtinen JT, Kaarela K, Belt EA, et al. Incidence of glenohumeral joint involvement in seropositive rheumatoid arthritis. A 15 year endpoint study. J Rheumatol 2000;27(2):347–50.

55. Alasaarela E, Suramo I, Tervonen O, et al. Evaluation of humeral head erosions in rheumatoid arthritis: a comparison of ultrasonography, magnetic resonance imaging, computed tomography and plain radiography. Br J Rheumatol 1998;37(11):1152–6.

56. Yeh LR, Kwak S, Kim YS, et al. Evaluation of articular cartilage thickness of the humeral head and the glenoid fossa by MR arthrography: anatomic correlation in cadavers. Skeletal Radiol 1998; 27(9):500–4.

57. Jazrawi LM, Alaia MJ, Chang G, et al. Advances in magnetic resonance imaging of articular cartilage. J Am Acad Orthop Surg 2011;19(7):420–9.

58. Gladstone JN, Bishop JY, Lo IK, et al. Fatty infiltration and atrophy of the rotator cuff do not improve after rotator cuff repair and correlate with poor functional outcome. Am J Sports Med 2007;35(5): 719–28.

59. Ekelund A, Nyberg R. Can reverse shoulder arthroplasty be used with few complications in rheumatoid arthritis? Clin Orthop Relat Res 2011;469(9): 2483–8.

60. Rozing PM, Nagels J, Rozing MP. Prognostic factors in arthroplasty in the rheumatoid shoulder. HSS J 2011;7(1):29–36.

61. Christie A, Dagfinrud H, Ringen HO, et al. Beneficial and harmful effects of shoulder arthroplasty in patients with rheumatoid arthritis: results from a Cochrane review. Rheumatology (Oxford) 2011; 50(3):598–602.

62. Soini I, Belt EA, Niemitukia L, et al. Magnetic resonance imaging of the rotator cuff in destroyed rheumatoid shoulder: comparison with findings during shoulder replacement. Acta Radiol 2004;45(4): 434–9.

63. Sperling JW, Cofield RH, Schleck CD, et al. Total shoulder arthroplasty versus hemiarthroplasty for rheumatoid arthritis of the shoulder: results of 303 consecutive cases. J Shoulder Elbow Surg 2007; 16(6):683–90.

64. Petersson CJ. The acromioclavicular joint in rheumatoid arthritis. Clin Orthop Relat Res 1987;(223): 86–93.

65. Lehtinen JT, Lehto MU, Kaarela K, et al. Acromioclavicular joint subluxation is rare in rheumatoid arthritis. A radiographic 15-year study. Rev Rhum Engl Ed 1999;66(10):462–6.

66. Lehtinen JT, Lehto MU, Kaarela K, et al. Radiographic joint space in rheumatoid acromioclavicular joints: a 15 year prospective follow-up study in 74 patients. Rheumatology (Oxford) 1999;38(11): 1104–7.

67. Cuende E, Vesga JC, Barrenengoa E, et al. Synovial cyst as differential diagnosis of supraclavicular mass in rheumatoid arthritis. J Rheumatol 1996; 23(8):1432–4.

68. Gandjbakhch F, Conaghan PG, Ejbjerg B, et al. Synovitis and osteitis are very frequent in rheumatoid arthritis clinical remission: results from an MRI study of 294 patients in clinical remission or low disease activity state. J Rheumatol 2011;38(9):2039–44.

69. Rosenthal AK. Crystals, inflammation, and osteoarthritis. Curr Opin Rheumatol 2011;23(2):170–3.

70. Ea HK, Liote F. Advances in understanding calcium-containing crystal disease. Curr Opin Rheumatol 2009;21(2):150–7.

71. Bencardino JT, Hassankhani A. Calcium pyrophosphate dihydrate crystal deposition disease. Semin Musculoskelet Radiol 2003;7(3):175–85.

72. Neogi T, Nevitt M, Niu J, et al. Lack of association between chondrocalcinosis and increased risk of cartilage loss in knees with osteoarthritis: results of two prospective longitudinal magnetic resonance imaging studies. Arthritis Rheum 2006; 54(6):1822–8.

73. Viriyavejkul P, Wilairatana V, Tanavalee A, et al. Comparison of characteristics of patients with and without calcium pyrophosphate dihydrate crystal deposition disease who underwent total knee replacement surgery for osteoarthritis. Osteoarthritis Cartilage 2007;15(2):232–5.

74. Liu R, O'Connell M, Johnson K, et al. Extracellular signal-regulated kinase 1/extracellular signal-regulated kinase 2 mitogen-activated protein kinase signaling and activation of activator protein 1 and nuclear factor kappaB transcription factors play central roles in interleukin-8 expression stimulated by monosodium urate monohydrate and calcium pyrophosphate crystals in monocytic cells. Arthritis Rheum 2000;43(5):1145–55.

75. Martinon F, Petrilli V, Mayor A, et al. Gout-associated uric acid crystals activate the NALP3 inflammasome. Nature 2006;440(7081):237–41.

76. Richette P, Bardin T, Doherty M. An update on the epidemiology of calcium pyrophosphate dihydrate crystal deposition disease. Rheumatology (Oxford) 2009;48(7):711–5.

77. McCarty DJ. Calcium pyrophosphate dihydrate crystal deposition disease—1975. Arthritis Rheum 1976;19(Suppl 3):275–85.

78. Doherty M, Dieppe P. Clinical aspects of calcium pyrophosphate dihydrate crystal deposition. Rheum Dis Clin North Am 1988;14(2):395–414.

79. Zhang Y, Terkeltaub R, Nevitt M, et al. Lower prevalence of chondrocalcinosis in Chinese subjects in Beijing than in white subjects in the United States: the Beijing Osteoarthritis Study. Arthritis Rheum 2006;54(11):3508–12.

80. Beltran J, Marty-Delfaut E, Bencardino J, et al. Chondrocalcinosis of the hyaline cartilage of the knee: MRI manifestations. Skeletal Radiol 1998; 27(7):369–74.

81. Canhao H, Fonseca JE, Leandro MJ, et al. Cross-sectional study of 50 patients with calcium pyrophosphate dihydrate crystal arthropathy. Clin Rheumatol 2001;20(2):119–22.

82. Steinbach LS. Calcium pyrophosphate dihydrate and calcium hydroxyapatite crystal deposition diseases: imaging perspectives. Radiol Clin North Am 2004;42(1):185–205, vii.

83. Ellman MH, Krieger MI, Brown N. Pseudogout mimicking synovial chondromatosis. J Bone Joint Surg Am 1975;57(6):863–5.

84. Gerster JC, Baud CA, Lagier R, et al. Tendon calcifications in chondrocalcinosis. A clinical, radiologic, histologic, and crystallographic study. Arthritis Rheum 1977;20(2):717–22.

85. Schumacher HR Jr, Klippel JH, Koopman WJ. Calcium pyrophosphate dihydrate crystal deposition disease. In: Schumacher HR Jr, Klippel JH, Koopman WJ, editors. Primer on the rheumatic diseases. Atlanta (GA): Arthritis Foundation; 1993. p. 219–22.

86. Resnick D, Williams G, Weisman MH, et al. Rheumatoid arthritis and pseudo-rheumatoid arthritis in calcium pyrophosphate dihydrate crystal deposition disease. Radiology 1981;140(3):615–21.

87. Mizutani H, Ohba S, Mizutani M, et al. Tumoral calcium pyrophosphate dihydrate deposition disease with bone destruction in the shoulder. CT and MR findings in two cases. Acta Radiol 1998; 39(3):269–72.

88. Hessle L, Johnson KA, Anderson HC, et al. Tissue-nonspecific alkaline phosphatase and plasma cell membrane glycoprotein-1 are central antagonistic regulators of bone mineralization. Proc Natl Acad Sci U S A 2002;99(14):9445–9.

89. Ho AM, Johnson MD, Kingsley DM. Role of the mouse ank gene in control of tissue calcification and arthritis. Science 2000;289(5477):265–70.

90. Okawa A, Nakamura I, Goto S, et al. Mutation in Npps in a mouse model of ossification of the posterior longitudinal ligament of the spine. Nat Genet 1998;19(3):271–3.

91. Hayes CW, Conway WF. Calcium hydroxyapatite deposition disease. Radiographics 1990;10(6): 1031–48.

92. Codman EA. The shoulder. Boston: Todd; 1934.

93. Uhthoff HK, Loehr JW. Calcific tendinopathy of the rotator cuff: pathogenesis, diagnosis, and management. J Am Acad Orthop Surg 1997;5(4):183–91.

94. Uhthoff HK, Sarkar K, Maynard JA. Calcifying tendinitis: a new concept of its pathogenesis. Clin Orthop Relat Res 1976;(118):164–8.

95. Bosworth BM. Calcium deposits in the shoulder and subacromial bursitis: a survey of 12,122 shoulders. JAMA 1941;116:2477–82.

96. Garcia GM, McCord GC, Kumar R. Hydroxyapatite crystal deposition disease. Semin Musculoskelet Radiol 2003;7(3):187–93.

97. Depalma AF, Kruper JS. Long-term study of shoulder joints afflicted with and treated for calcific tendinitis. Clin Orthop 1961;20:61–72.

98. Zubler C, Mengiardi B, Schmid MR, et al. MR arthrography in calcific tendinitis of the shoulder: diagnostic performance and pitfalls. Eur Radiol 2007;17(6):1603–10.

99. Moseley HF. Shoulder lesions. 3rd edition. Baltimore (MD): Williams & Wilkins; 1969.

100. Loew M, Sabo D, Wehrle M, et al. Relationship between calcifying tendinitis and subacromial impingement: a prospective radiography and magnetic resonance imaging study. J Shoulder Elbow Surg 1996;5(4):314–9.

101. Hurt G, Baker CL Jr. Calcific tendinitis of the shoulder. Orthop Clin North Am 2003;34(4):567–75.

102. Wainner RS, Hasz M. Management of acute calcific tendinitis of the shoulder. J Orthop Sports Phys Ther 1998;27(3):231–7.

103. Cahir J, Saifuddin A. Calcific tendonitis of pectoralis major: CT and MRI findings. Skeletal Radiol 2005;34(4):234–8.

104. Durr HR, Lienemann A, Silbernagl H, et al. Acute calcific tendinitis of the pectoralis major insertion associated with cortical bone erosion. Eur Radiol 1997;7(8):1215–7.

105. Ikegawa S. Calcific tendinitis of the pectoralis major insertion. A report of two cases. Arch Orthop Trauma Surg 1996;115(2):118–9.

106. Ji JH, Shafi M, Kim WY. Calcific tendinitis of the biceps-labral complex: a rare cause of acute shoulder pain. Acta Orthop Belg 2008;74(3):401–4.

107. Cho NS, Lee BG, Rhee YG. Radiologic course of the calcific deposits in calcific tendinitis of the

shoulder: does the initial radiologic aspect affect the final results? J Shoulder Elbow Surg 2010; 19(2):267–72.

108. Lee SY, Cheng B, Grimmer-Somers K. The midterm effectiveness of extracorporeal shockwave therapy in the management of chronic calcific shoulder tendinitis. J Shoulder Elbow Surg 2011;20(5): 845–54.

109. Mouzopoulos G, Stamatakos M, Mouzopoulos D, et al. Extracorporeal shock wave treatment for shoulder calcific tendonitis: a systematic review. Skeletal Radiol 2007;36(9):803–11.

110. Marder RA, Heiden EA, Kim S. Calcific tendonitis of the shoulder: is subacromial decompression in combination with removal of the calcific deposit

beneficial? J Shoulder Elbow Surg 2011;20(6): 955–60.

111. McCarty DJ. Arthritis associated with crystals containing calcium. Med Clin North Am 1986;70(2):437–54.

112. McCarty DJ. Milwaukee shoulder syndrome. Trans Am Clin Climatol Assoc 1991;102:271–83 [discussion: 283–4].

113. Halverson PB, McCarty DJ, Cheung HS, et al. Milwaukee shoulder syndrome: eleven additional cases with involvement of the knee in seven (basic calcium phosphate crystal deposition disease). Semin Arthritis Rheum 1984;14(1):36–44.

114. Epis O, Caporali R, Scire CA, et al. Efficacy of tidal irrigation in Milwaukee shoulder syndrome. J Rheumatol 2007;34(7):1545–50.

Entrapment Neuropathies of the Shoulder

Jean-François Budzik, MD, MSc[a,b,c],
Guillaume Wavreille, MD, MSc[d,e], Vittorio Pansini, MD[f,g],
Antoine Moraux, MD[f], Xavier Demondion, MD, PhD[e,f],
Anne Cotten, MD, PhD[f,g],*

KEYWORDS

- Entrapment neuropathy • Shoulder • MR imaging
- Scapular winging

Entrapment neuropathies are reported to be responsible for 2% of shoulder pain or painful instability.[1] However, this frequency is likely to be underestimated because these conditions have been overlooked in the past.[2] The main reasons for this are an ill-defined clinical presentation and a lack of specific clinical signs, whatever the nerve involved. The common feature is nerve damage, caused either by extrinsic compression or by stretching secondary to repeated movements. Electrodiagnostic studies are classically considered to be the gold standard for the diagnosis of entrapment neuropathies.[1] However, the referring clinician must have considered this diagnosis to prescribe this test. Moreover, patients suffering from shoulder pain or weakness are often referred to the radiologist for a magnetic resonance (MR) examination. Because some lesional patterns are evocative of the diagnosis, the radiologist needs to know in what situations this diagnosis must be suggested, especially before concluding that the result of an MR imaging scan of the shoulder is normal.

To understand these conditions, and especially their imaging features, it is essential to recall some key anatomic points. The author then tackles the 2 different clinical situations a radiologist can encounter: either patients present with an abnormality of the position of the scapula, known as scapular winging, or they complain of nonspecific shoulder pain, which is the most frequent situation. After explaining the common imaging features, the distribution of the abnormalities proper to each type of nerve entrapment and their differential diagnoses are discussed.

ANATOMIC STRUCTURES AND LANDMARKS
Suprascapular Nerve

The suprascapular nerve generally originates from the upper trunk of the brachial plexus, with fibers from the C5 and C6 nerve roots and partially the

[a] Service d'Imagerie Médicale, Groupe Hospitalier de l'Institut Catholique de Lille/Faculté Libre de Médecine, F-59000 Lille, France
[b] UCLille, F-59000 Lille, France
[c] Univ Nord de France, F-59000 Lille, France
[d] Service de Chirurgie de la main et du Membre Supérieur, Centre de Consultations et d'Imagerie de l'Appareil Locomoteur, Univ Nord de France, 59037 Lille Cedex, France
[e] Faculté de Médecine, Laboratoire d'Anatomie et d'Organogénèse, Université de Lille2, Univ Nord de France, 59045 Lille, France
[f] Service de Radiologie et Imagerie Musculosquelettique, Centre de Consultation et d'Imagerie de l'Appareil Locomoteur, CHRU de Lille, 59037 Lille, France
[g] Université Lille Nord de France, EA 4490 PMOI, F-59000 Lille, France
* Corresponding author. Service de Radiologie et Imagerie Musculosquelettique, Centre de Consultations et d'Imagerie de l'Appareil Locomoteur, Rue du Pr. Emile Laine, 59037 Lille Cedex, France.
E-mail address: acotten@gmail.com

Magn Reson Imaging Clin N Am 20 (2012) 373–391
doi:10.1016/j.mric.2012.01.013
1064-9689/12/$ – see front matter © 2012 Published by Elsevier Inc.

C4 nerve root. It runs posterolaterally from its origin and passes through the suprascapular notch (**Fig. 1**). This notch, immediately medial to the root of the coracoid process, is highly variable in shape; 6 types have been reported (**Fig. 2**).[3] The transverse scapular ligament, which closes this notch, may be bifid and partially or completely ossified, and its thickness is variable.[4] The suprascapular vessels also cross the superior edge of the scapula but remain above the suprascapular ligament.

Following its course in the posterior scapular region, the nerve passes under the supraspinatus muscle, which it innervates, and then through the spinoglenoid notch, situated between the root of the spine of the scapula and the glenoid cavity. This notch is inconsistently closed by the spinoglenoid ligament,[5] which connects the scapular spine to the posterior glenohumeral capsule, turning the notch in a second osteofibrous tunnel. The suprascapular nerve terminates in and innervates the infraspinatus muscle.

The course of the nerve therefore presents 3 fixed points: the cervical origin, the suprascapular notch, and the spinoglenoid notch. The nerve also receives sensory branches from the glenohumeral and acromioclavicular joints and from the subacromial-deltoid bursa. Cadaver and clinical studies[6–8] suggest that this nerve may be responsible for much of the sensation of the shoulder (up to 70%) and report that suprascapular nerve block is effective for the management of postoperative pain after shoulder surgery.

Axillary Nerve

The axillary nerve originates from the posterior cord of the brachial plexus, with fibers from the C5 and C6 nerve roots. It exits the axilla by passing through the quadrangular space together with the posterior circumflex humeral artery and vein. This space is limited superiorly by the inferior edge of the teres minor, inferiorly by the superior edge of the teres major, medially by the lateral edge of the long head of the triceps brachii, and laterally by the surgical neck of the humerus (see **Fig. 1A**). Then the axillary nerve runs posterolaterally around the surgical neck of the humerus on the deep surface of the deltoid muscle. It provides

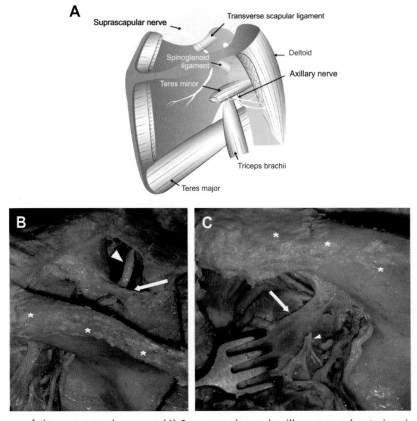

Fig. 1. Anatomy of the suprascapular nerve. (*A*) Suprascapular and axillary nerves (posterior view). Anatomic dissection of the course of the suprascapular nerve around the scapula (posterior view), showing the suprascapular notch (*B*) and the spinoglenoid notch. (*C*) Suprascapular nerve (*arrowhead*), spinous process of the scapula (*asterisks*), suprascapular ligament (*arrow in B*), and spinoglenoid ligament (*arrow in C*).

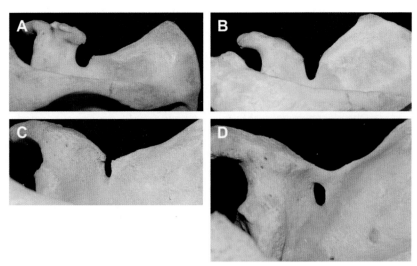

Fig. 2. Posterior view of 4 cadaveric left scapula morphologic variants of the suprascapular notch. (*A*) Large round notch. (*B*) V-shaped notch. (*C*) Narrow notch. (*D*) Ossified suprascapular ligament forming a suprascapular foramen.

motor innervation to the teres minor and deltoid muscles. It also has a cutaneous branch, which is sensory for the skin over the superior part of the deltoid muscle.

Long Thoracic Nerve

The long thoracic nerve arises from the C5 to C7 nerve roots. It runs downward, passing through the scalenus medius muscle. It descends behind the brachial plexus and the axillary vessels, resting on the outer surface of the serratus anterior muscle. It extends along the side of the thorax to the lower border of that muscle, supplying each of its digitations (**Fig. 3**). Two fixed points are recognized: the scalenus medius muscle and the serratus anterior muscle at the level of the second rib.

Accessory Nerve

The accessory nerve, the eleventh cranial nerve, exits the skull through the nervous part of the jugular foramen. It descends obliquely in a posteroinferior direction and innervates the sternocleidomastoid and trapezius muscles from their deep surfaces, passing through the posterior triangle of the neck.

Dorsal Scapular Nerve

The dorsal scapular nerve arises from the brachial plexus, usually from the C5 root. It courses down posterior to the ribs and provides motor innervation to the rhomboid muscles and levator scapulae muscle.

PATHOPHYSIOLOGY

Broadly speaking, nerves can be affected in 2 different situations: either by direct compression or by repeated microtrauma consecutive to particular movements (during sports or occupational activities).

Compressed Nerves

Direct compression occurs mainly because a space-occupying lesion develops in the vicinity of the nerve; this can also occur if the local anatomy

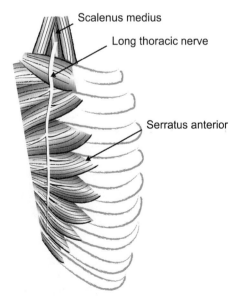

Fig. 3. The long thoracic nerve (lateral view of the thoracic wall).

has been modified by a fracture. The nerve is therefore affected by ischemic conditions, resulting in denervation lesions of the muscles, which it innervates. Any bony or soft tissue lesion can cause this. However, the most frequent situation is compression of the suprascapular nerve occurring at the suprascapular or spinoglenoid notch because of a cyst extending from the glenohumeral joint.[9]

Nerve Stretching

There are fixed points along the course of each nerve, as described previously. Therefore, certain repetitive movements are thought to generate excess traction, thus entailing strain injuries at one or another of the fixed points. Inflammation occurs within the nerve, impairing its functioning. Additional elements, such as fibrous bands or small arterial branches crossing a nerve, can create additional fixed points. This can be responsible for an authentic entrapment situation (Fig. 4). In the specific case of axillary neuropathy, entrapment occurs in the quadrilateral space, where fibrous bands linking the teres major and the long head of the triceps have been described.[10] These points are not discussed because these structures cannot be precisely identified by imaging techniques.

Sensory impairment is responsible for pain and/or paresthesia, whereas motor impairment involves loss of strength and muscular atrophy.

Multiple factors may be incriminated. In an overhead throwing position, the spinoglenoid ligament has been shown to tighten the suprascapular nerve,[11] resulting in strain stress. Anatomic variants have also been reported to increase the risk of lesions; this is true for instances of variations in the morphology of the suprascapular notch (see Fig. 2).[2–4] Another suggested mechanism of suprascapular neuropathy is arterial damage, leading to microemboli in the vasa nervorum and thus ischemic damage.[12] Entrapment situations have been well described in overhead athletes[13,14] and also in occupational situations,[15,16] because repetitive movements are frequent in both situations.

Iatrogenic Lesions

Iatrogenic lesions (due to surgical procedures) can also be encountered. The accessory nerve may be injured after biopsies of the cervical lymph node. However, these situations are less diagnostically challenging and thus fall outside the scope of this discussion.

CLINICAL PRESENTATION

The author has intentionally distinguished 2 different clinical presentations: the patient will present either with nonspecific shoulder pain or with a scapular prominence known as scapular

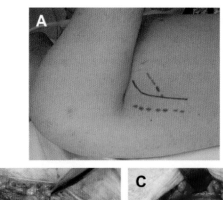

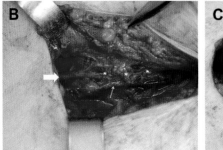
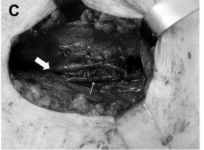

Fig. 4. Example of long thoracic nerve entrapment caused by small arterial branches. After an anterolateral and proximal thoracic approach (A), the long thoracic nerve is identified ([B], *thick arrow*). Branches (*asterisks*) of the dorsal thoracic artery (*thin arrow*) can be seen crossing over the nerve. After surgical resection of these branches (C), the patient fully recovered in 3 months.

winging. Although the latter presentation is more characteristic, it is far less frequent than that of shoulder pain associated with suprascapular or axillary nerve involvement.

These 2 situations must be distinguished by the radiologist because they require different MR imaging protocols. Although the sequences are the same, the field of view (FOV) needs to be adjusted. This adjusting is discussed later.

Nonspecific Shoulder Pain: Suprascapular and Axillary Nerve Entrapment

This condition is the most frequent situation in entrapment neuropathies of the shoulder. The supraspinatus, infraspinatus, or teres minor muscle is involved, thus mimicking other shoulder ailments, mainly tearing of the rotator cuff, and making for a difficult diagnosis.

Suprascapular neuropathy

Overhead athletes are typically affected by this disease, not only volleyball, baseball, handball, and tennis players but also swimmers. Patients usually complain of an insidious onset of dull aching pain in the superior or posterolateral aspects of the shoulder. Complaints of shoulder weakness and fatigue on exercise are common. Functional impairment is variable. At physical examination, infraspinatus or supraspinatus atrophy can be seen after several weeks. Functional impairment is possible, particularly in abduction and external rotation, depending on the level of compression; strength is more likely to be impaired in the case of proximal lesions (in regard to the infraspinatus and supraspinatus muscles) than that of distal lesions, where an isolated deficit of the infraspinatus muscle can be compensated by the surrounding muscles.[17]

Axillary neuropathy: quadrilateral space syndrome

Axillary neuropathy affects young (25–35 years old) throwing athletes complaining of poorly localized anterolateral pain with paresthesia of the shoulder, overlying the deltoid muscle. Sustained flexion, abduction, and external rotation of the arm make the pain worse. On clinical examination, tenderness is found over the lateral aspect of the scapula, at the site of insertion of the teres minor.[18]

Differential diagnosis: Parsonage-Turner syndrome

Also referred to as neuralgic amyotrophy or acute brachial neuritis, Parsonage-Turner syndrome is a rare (incidence estimated at 2–3 per 100,000[19]) condition, characterized by sudden onset of shoulder pain associated with progressive weakness of the shoulder girdle muscles. The age of

the patients varies widely, ranging from the third to the seventh decades.[20,21] Men are predominantly affected, and a bilateral asymmetric[22] presentation has been reported in up to one-third of the cases.[23,24] Involvement of nerves outside the brachial plexus is reported in 17% of the patients.[22] A history of recent viral infection,[24] immunization,[25] exercise, or surgery[22] is sometimes reported. An autoimmune mechanism is suspected.[26] The clinical symptoms are variable[22] because patients present with isolated pain, weakness, or numbness or a combination of the 3, the most common presentations being associated pain and weakness followed by isolated pain. No asymptomatic presentation has been reported.[21] However, the most typical presentation is an attack of severe relentless neuropathic pain involving 1 arm and worsening at night.[22] The clinical diagnosis may be challenging because the symptoms are nonspecific and may mimic other shoulder girdle conditions such as labral tear, rotator cuff tear, impingement, and adhesive capsulitis.[21]

Gaskin and Helms[27] reported that the suprascapular nerve was almost invariably involved in patients with Parsonage-Turner syndrome (97% of cases); axillary nerve involvement was also commonly observed (in 50% of shoulders). However, any other nerve derived from the brachial plexus may be affected. The prognosis is poor, with 75% of the patients still experiencing pain and 25% still unable to work after 3 years, with a recurrence rate of 25% in the idiopathic form and 75% in the hereditary form of the condition.[22]

Winging Scapula

On the other hand, entrapments of the long thoracic, accessory, or dorsal scapular nerves directly impede scapular movements because of the muscles involved. These entrapments are responsible for the static or dynamic scapular prominence known as scapular winging.

This clinical situation is different from suprascapular and axillary nerve entrapment because there is a clinical abnormality evocative of it, which can be detected on physical examination. The patient is likely to be referred for the exploration of this abnormality.

Long thoracic nerve neuropathy

This condition is responsible for medial scapular winging, which is more frequent than the lateral form. The scapular asymmetry (objectivized by comparing the distance between the spinal processes and the medial edge of the scapula on both sides) may be clinically obvious on physical examination (**Fig. 5A**). It can be exacerbated still

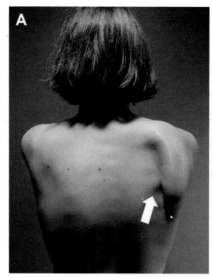
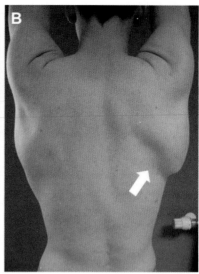

Fig. 5. Scapular winging caused by entrapment of the long thoracic nerve in 2 different patients. (*A*) At rest, the right scapula is prominent, elevated, and displaced laterally. The gap between the spine and the medial border of the scapula (*arrow*) is increased. (*B*) In more subtle cases, forward flexion of both arms can be required to reveal the asymmetry of the scapulas, with a visible depression medial to the right scapula (*arrow*).

more on forward flexion of both arms (see **Fig. 5B**) or by the wall push-up test. In the most severe cases, full elevation of the arm may be impossible.[28]

Accessory nerve neuropathy

Lateral scapular winging is always present.[29] However, it is only in the more severe forms that the droopy shoulder aspect may be seen, associating trapezius atrophy, shoulder drop, and lateral winging. Abduction and external rotation against resistance exacerbate the scapular displacement, whereas forward flexion lessens the deformation because of serratus anterior contraction. As described earlier, this nerve is wounded mainly because of biopsies of the cervical lymph node.[30]

Dorsal scapular nerve neuropathy

Dorsal scapular nerve neuropathy is a very rare condition, responsible for levator scapulae and rhomboid muscle denervation. Pain in this area may be encountered and may be the only symptom. Mild scapular winging is encountered. The functional impact is negligible.

IMAGING ENTRAPMENT NEUROPATHIES

Identifying muscular denervation (muscular edema, atrophy, and fatty degeneration) in a neural distribution pattern is key to the diagnosis of entrapment neuropathies. The MR imaging protocol needs to be adapted to each situation: in case of suspected suprascapular or axillary entrapment, the FOV needs to be centered on

the glenohumeral joint, whereas in case of scapular winging, the FOV has to be enlarged to include both scapulas, covering the posterior and medial muscles attaching to them. Apart from this difference, the semiology and reasoning are the same. In this article, the author successively discusses the prevailing role of MR imaging among other imaging modalities, the MR imaging protocol required for each clinical situation, the abnormalities to be sought, and the systematic analysis to be performed when exploring these conditions.

Imaging Modalities: the Prevalent Role of MR Imaging

The author focuses on MR imaging because it is the only imaging modality that allows the detection of muscular edema, which is the earliest abnormality to appear. MR imaging also allows an evaluation of the severity of the disease and the search for a cause. It is also very efficient in excluding several differential diagnoses. Once radiologists understand what to look for and how to do it in MR imaging, they will be able to reproduce this scheme with other imaging modalities, each of which has its own limitations.

Other imaging modalities perform less well. Plain radiographs are useful to appreciate the gross morphology of the scapula, especially the suprascapular notch, by using dedicated views.[2] A fracture, an osteolytic lesion, or calcifications of the surrounding soft tissues can also be detected. Computed tomographic (CT) scan does the same job in a more accurate way and allows

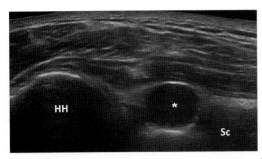

Fig. 6. This axial US image of the posterior aspect of the glenohumeral joint shows a mucoid cyst (*asterisk*) occupying the spinoglenoid notch. HH, humeral head; Sc, scapula.

the identification of muscular fatty degeneration and atrophy. CT arthrography helps identify some paralabral cysts and differential diagnoses such as rotator cuff tears.

Shoulder ultrasonography (US) is not the best method for the exploration of these conditions because it cannot identify muscular edema. However, the technique's role should not be neglected. It is routinely used as a first-intention modality for shoulder pain. Although the initially suspected diagnosis is often a rotator cuff tendon tear, the radiologist must not overlook differential diagnoses, especially when no cuff tendon abnormality has been identified. For this reason, we suggest that the reader systematically includes the following items in a US shoulder examination[31]:

- The suprascapular and spinoglenoid notches, in search of a space-occupying lesion (**Fig. 6**). A paralabral or mucoid cyst can be easily differentiated from dilated suprascapular veins by combining color Doppler and compression of the structure; veins are filled with colored flow signal and collapse under pressure, whereas cysts do not.

- The bodies of the supraspinatus and infraspinatus muscles as compared with the contralateral side. Muscular atrophy can be easily identified (asymmetry of the muscular bulk), as well as fatty degeneration (increased echogenicity) (**Fig. 7**).

This can be done very quickly in the late stage of a US shoulder examination while assessing the posterior aspect of the glenohumeral joint. Any suggestive abnormality should be explored by complementary MR examination.

Only suprascapular neuropathy can be explored with this scheme, but it counts for 97% of entrapment neuropathies of the shoulder. A search for other muscle and nerve courses could be done but would require a great deal of experience and prove time consuming, with very few positive results expected.[30]

Thanks to this method, the radiologist may play a key role by being the first to suggest the diagnosis of shoulder nerve entrapment.

Building Your MR Imaging Protocol

The key sequence is fast-spin echo T2-weighted imaging associated with fat suppression, performed in the axial plane. This imaging allows the identification of muscular edema. Echo time should be long enough ($\geq$45 ms) for sufficient T2 weighting.[1] T1-weighted sequences without fat suppression are indicated because they make the identification of fatty degeneration easier. Acquisition in the sagittal plane may be complementary to allow better comparisons between the different muscles, especially if the signal abnormalities are subtle.

It may be advisable to increase the gap between the slices to cover the whole volume of the muscles, because partial damage may occur (depending on the site of entrapment), even though

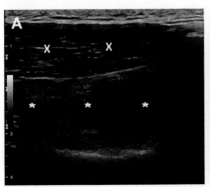
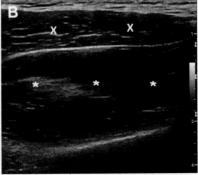

Fig. 7. Comparative sagittal US sections focused on the middle of the supraspinous fossa. The left supraspinatus muscle (*asterisks*) is hyperechoic and atrophied (*A*) compared with the contralateral muscle (*B*). The trapezius is normal on both sides (*crosses*).

this is rare. The gap and number of slices need to be adjusted to the morphology of the patient.

No gadolinium injection is necessary because gadolinium-enhanced T1-weighted sequences provide results similar to those of T2-weighted sequences associated with fat suppression, with T1 sequences revealing hypervascularization and the T2 sequences showing hyperintensities. It is, however, crucial to note that denervated muscles frequently demonstrate contrast enhancement.[32] This must be kept in mind to avoid misinterpreting this feature, particularly indicating neoplastic or infectious disease (**Fig. 8**).

Suspected suprascapular or axillary neuropathy
The exploration of the rotator cuff tendons and glenohumeral joint is mandatory within the framework of the differential diagnosis. The use of a dedicated shoulder coil is advisable. Fat-suppressed T2-weighted sequences must be performed in the axial plane and in oblique sagittal and coronal planes (in regard to the body of the scapula). The imaging must be centered on the glenohumeral joint because this enables the study of the rotator cuff. Sagittal and axial T1-weighted sequences must be performed in the axial and oblique sagittal planes.

Winging scapula
Extended coverage is required in this situation; the serratus anterior, the rhomboid muscles, and the trapezius need to be explored. Because this coverage is beyond the reach of a dedicated shoulder coil, a multichannel phased array body coil should be used for the exploration of scapular winging. The entire width of the scapular girdle must be covered. Craniocaudally, the exploration must range from the upper edge of the shoulder to the tip of the scapula. This allows a comparison between both sides, which can be useful when dealing with subtle abnormalities. T2-weighted sequences associated with fat suppression and T1-weighted sequences are performed in the axial and sagittal planes.

What Must One Look For

The exploration of a suspected entrapment neuropathy involves 4 steps:

1. Looking for signs of muscular denervation: edema, atrophy, and fatty degeneration
2. Topographic analysis: linking up the denervation pattern with the corresponding nerve

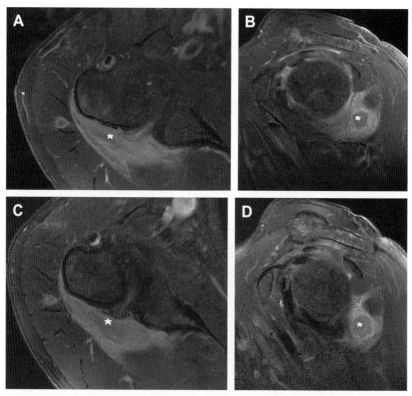

Fig. 8. Contrast-enhanced T1-weighted images with fat suppression (*A*: axial plane; *B*: sagittal plane). The enhancement is intense within the teres minor muscle (*asterisk*). A pseudo-tumoral aspect on sagittal images can be misleading, but axial images help avoid misinterpretation. The aspect of the lesions is exactly the same on the corresponding T2-weighted images with fat suppression (*C*: axial plane; *D*: sagittal plane).

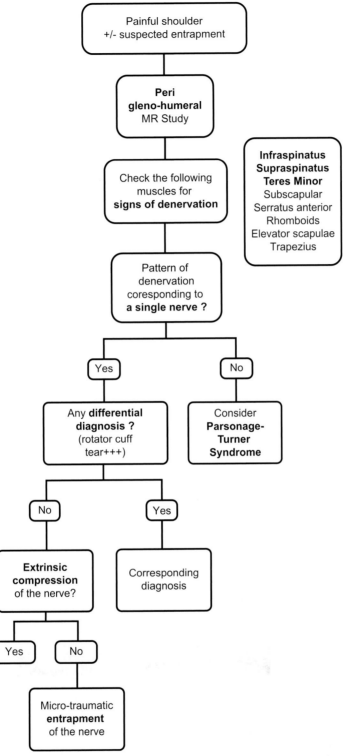

Fig. 9. Decision tree for nonspecific painful shoulders or suspected entrapment neuropathy of the suprascapular or axillary nerves.

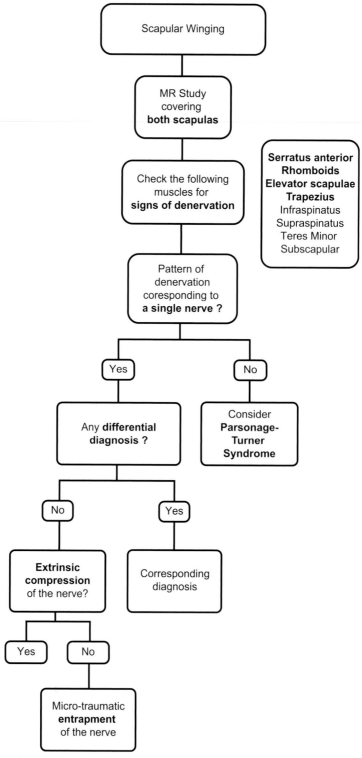

Fig. 10. Decision tree for winging scapulas.

3. Etiologic analysis: is there a space-occupying lesion compressing the nerve
4. Ruling out a differential diagnosis (essentially rotator cuff tears and Parsonage-Turner syndrome).

These steps are summed up in **Fig. 9** (nonspecific shoulder pain) and **Fig. 10** (winging scapula).

Muscular denervation

Muscular denervation is the indirect sign of neuropathy. Three abnormalities can be encountered, depending on the severity and the duration of the disease course. This is often described as involving an acute phase lasting from a few days to a month, a subacute phase lasting between 1 and 6 months, and a chronic phase after 6 months.[32] However, these stages are not always precisely defined.[1,33] Yet it is important to place this "calendar" in perspective, because this vocabulary has been mainly based on animal or clinical studies in which an acute nerve trauma was considered.[34,35] Although this information is valuable, it must be extrapolated with care when dealing with entrapment neuropathies in which long-term nerve compression or stretching occurs. With this in mind, these terms are used for the sake of convenience.

Muscular edema is the earliest abnormality to appear in denervated muscles. It is present in the acute and subacute phases and corresponds to a hyperintensity of the muscular fibers on T2-weighted images. It is not specific because it is reported in various pathologic conditions such as trauma, tumors, or infections.[36] However, the edema seen in entrapment neuropathies has several specific features[1]: it affects denervated muscles only, and, in these, it is homogenous in intensity and affects the whole muscular body (**Figs. 11** and **12**). Rare exceptions such as partial forms occur, but an obvious compressive lesion is then seen. Muscular edema occurs early; in fact, it has been reported a few days after trauma in experimental studies.[37] The same reference reports that its intensity and duration are related to the severity of the neuropathy.

Fatty replacement and atrophy appear during the subacute phase and are the only persistent abnormalities during the chronic phase.[33]

Atrophy of the muscle can be best appreciated on sagittal T1-weighted images (see **Fig. 12**; **Fig. 13**). T1-weighted images offer the best contrast between the muscles and the surrounding fat. The sagittal plane allows a comparison with the periscapular muscles also. The muscles are mainly studied along their short axis, which best allows an assessment of their bulk. The atrophy may be

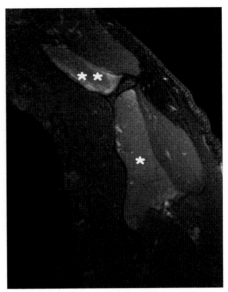

Fig. 11. Both supraspinatus (*double asterisk*) and infraspinatus (*asterisk*) muscles show signs of denervation in this case of suprascapular entrapment occurring in a volleyball player. Muscular edema is homogenous in the affected muscles on this oblique sagittal fat-suppressed T2-weighted image.

graded by studying the surface of the muscles. This surface is normally convex, but when atrophy occurs it tends to become flat and finally concaves in the late stages.[38] Denervation pseudohypertrophy has been reported; the affected muscle paradoxically enlarges in response to the denervation.[32] However, unlike true muscle hypertrophy in which the signal is normal on all MR sequences, the enlarged muscle loses its normal signal intensity because of edema and fatty replacement (see **Fig. 12**).

Fatty replacement can be evaluated in the same way as when assessing rotator cuff tendon tears (see **Figs. 12** and **13**). The proportion of fat within the muscle body is described according to the following features: no fat; some fatty streaks; fat accounting for less than 50% of the muscle, 50% of the muscle, or more than 50% of the muscle; and total fatty conversion.[39] Severe fatty degeneration reflects the irreversibility of the lesions.

At the end of the analysis stage, the radiologist knows which muscles are concerned by the abnormalities and how severe the lesions appear and has an idea of whether the pathology is rather recent (isolated edema), semirecent (edema associated with atrophy and/or fatty degeneration), or chronic (atrophy and severe fatty degeneration).

Topographic analysis

The distribution of the lesions may incriminate a nerve (**Table 1**). **Figs. 14** and **15** show typical

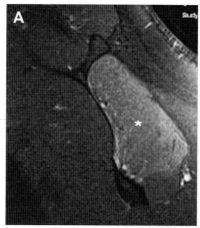
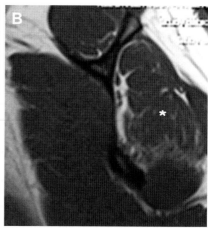

Fig. 12. In this case of suprascapular entrapment neuropathy, edema and fatty degeneration (of <50% of the muscular body) coexist in the infraspinatus muscle (*asterisk*) (sagittal fat-suppressed T2-weighted [A] and T1-weighted [B] images). Pseudohypertrophy of the infraspinatus muscle is also seen. Although the muscle is increased in size, pseudohypertrophy may be recognized because signal abnormalities exist both in T2-weighted (A) and T1-weighted (B) images.

cases in which isolated unilateral involvement of the serratus anterior muscle is diagnostic of a neuropathy of the long thoracic nerve. If the distribution of the lesion does not correspond to any of these situations, differential diagnoses must be considered. Once the affected nerve is identified, the next step consists in studying the nerve throughout its course, mainly focusing on the classical entrapment sites.

Is there a space-occupying lesion

Although any compressive lesion can occur anywhere, some lesions and some compression sites are far more frequent than others.

In suprascapular neuropathies, the suprascapular and spinoglenoid notches are the key places.

Classic compressive lesions such as soft tissue or bone tumors can be seen. However, mucoid cysts are common lesions responsible for

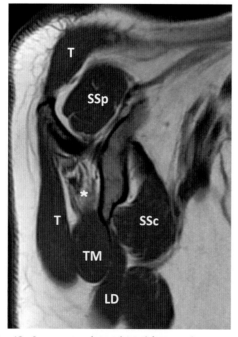

Fig. 13. Severe atrophy and total fatty replacement of the infraspinatus (*asterisk*) consecutive to a suprascapular entrapment neuropathy at a chronic stage. The supraspinatus (SSp), subscapularis (SSc), trapezius (T), teres minor (TM) and latissimus dorsi (LD) muscles have a normal bulk and do not show any signal abnormality.

Table 1
Relations between affected muscles and corresponding neuropathy

Denervated Muscles	Suspected Neuropathy
Supraspinatus and infraspinatus	Suprascapular neuropathy at or before the suprascapular notch
Isolated infraspinatus	Suprascapular neuropathy at the spinoglenoid notch
Teres minor	Axillary neuropathy (quadrilateral space entrapment)
Serratus anterior	Long thoracic nerve
Trapezius	Accessory nerve
Rhomboid and/or levator scapulae	Dorsal scapular nerve

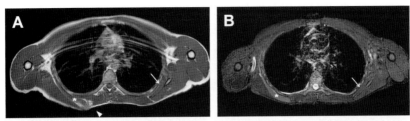

Fig. 14. The scapular asymmetry is clearly visible (*arrowhead*) in this patient complaining of right periscapular pain, with evident spontaneous scapular winging at clinical examination. The right serratus anterior (*asterisk*) shows signal abnormalities on both T1-weighted (*A*) and fat-suppressed T2-weighted (*B*) images when compared with the contralateral muscle (*arrow*), which is normal.

entrapment, especially in the spinoglenoid notch (**Fig. 16**). They communicate with the glenohumeral joint and are frequently associated with posterior labral tears, whatever their etiology (superior labrum anterior posterior lesion, posterior instability, or posterior impingement).[40,41]

In both notches, entrapment can, however, occur in the absence of any identifiable compressive lesion. The absence of obvious compressive lesions in the presence of indirect signs of neuropathy is diagnostic of a microtraumatic cause related to repeated movements. This is a diagnosis by exclusion because no imaging abnormality can be found. This movement-related condition is mainly encountered in case of regular practice of sports but has also been reported as occupational.

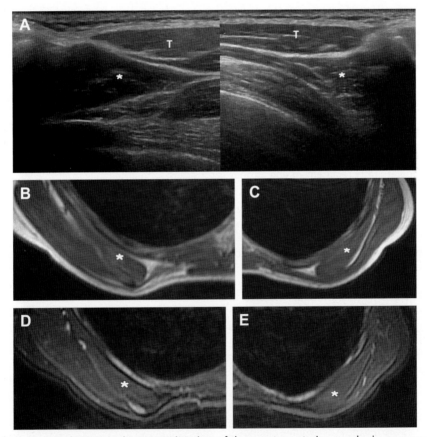

Fig. 15. (*A*) In this US axial paraspinal comparative view of the serratus anterior muscles in a young athlete with winging scapula, atrophy and fatty replacement of the right serratus anterior (*asterisk*, *right*) can be diagnosed, when compared with the contralateral muscle (*asterisk*, *left*), because the incriminated muscle is hyperechoic and shows loss of bulk. The trapezius (T) shows normal echogenicity. (*B–E*) Comparative MR examination in the same patient with T1-weighted (*B* and *C*) and T2-weighted (*D* and *E*) sequences confirms the atrophy and fatty replacement (*asterisks*, *B* and *C*), without any edema (*D* and *E*). This is consistent with a chronic-stage condition.

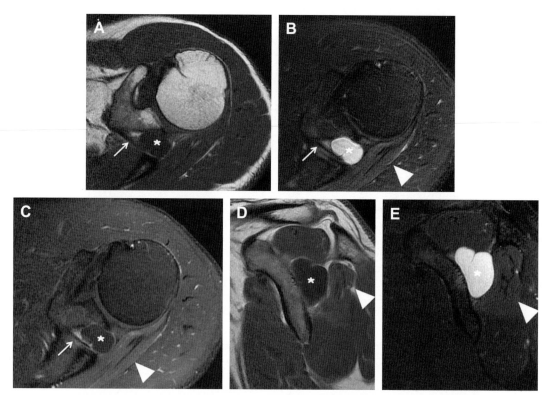

Fig. 16. Suprascapular entrapment neuropathy consecutive to a mucoid cyst (*asterisks*) of the spinoglenoid notch (*arrows* indicate the spinoglenoid ligament). The lesion is oval-shaped, polylobulated, with regular borders. The signal is low on T1 (*A*), high on T2 (*B*). In case of doubt, linear peripheral enhancement after gadolinium injection (*C*) will allow differentiation from low-grade soft tissue tumors. Denervation of the infraspinatus muscle (*arrowheads*) results in signal abnormalities: linear hyperintensities interspersed in T1 (*A, D*) corresponding to fatty replacement and overall moderate hyperintensity in T2 with fat suppression (*B, E*) corresponding to edema. The edema is homogeneous within the muscle and no other muscle is involved. Comparison with the supraspinatus is easily made on oblique sagittal images (*D, E*) and shows muscular atrophy. The association of mild-intensity edema, moderate fatty replacement and atrophy is consistent with potentially reversible lesions.

This condition can be facilitated by anatomic variants such as stenotic notches and ossified suprascapular transverse or spinoglenoid ligaments.[3,4] These abnormalities can be best identified by complementary CT scan, particularly if surgery is planned.

In many cases, no imaging modality is able to identify the structures responsible for the entrapment, which are per-operative findings. This is the rule in quadrilateral space syndrome, in which the axillary nerve is entrapped by fibrous bands developing between the muscles.

Differential diagnoses

Suprascapular and axillary neuropathies Rotator cuff tendon tears are the main differential diagnosis to consider when dealing with a painful shoulder. Yet suprascapular neuropathies secondary to rotator cuff tendon tears have been reported.[42,43] The suspected pathophysiologic mechanism is too much tension of the nerve with a bend occurring at the suprascapular notch or against the scapular spine, consecutive to a retraction of the supraspinatus or infraspinatus tendons. How much retraction is necessary to create these conditions is still debated.[2,44–46] This may be responsible for an authentic entrapment leading to supraspinatus or infraspinatus muscular edema, an abnormality that is not usual in rotator cuff tendons tears. On the contrary, muscular atrophy and fatty degeneration can be noticed in both pathologies.

Scapular winging Extraneurologic causes of scapular winging are known[47]: osseous lesions such as fractures or tumors, soft tissue abnormalities such as muscular pathologies (trauma or agenesis), or scapulothoracic bursitis, secondary scapular winging consecutive to glenohumeral conditions.

All neuropathies In Parsonage-Turner syndrome, denervation lesions are present: edema, atrophy, and fatty degeneration. The order of appearance of the abnormalities is the same as that described previously for neuropathies: edema, followed a few weeks later by atrophy and fatty infiltration, which are the only remaining abnormalities in the late stages.[32] The diagnosis is suggested when there is an abnormality of the muscles innervated by the brachial plexus in the absence of a history of trauma or excessive overhead activity.[18] Unlike what is seen in entrapment, the edema is frequently inhomogeneous within a muscle or between the different affected muscles (**Fig. 17**). The most common situation is the involvement of more than one nerve, for example, of more than one muscle group,[18,21] although a single nerve only may be affected. The suprascapular nerve is overwhelmingly affected, whether alone (**Fig. 18**) or in association with other nerves.

Therefore, the radiologist should be the first to sound the alarm in 2 conditions:

- If more than one nerve of the brachial plexus is concerned, that is, if the pattern of the lesions includes several shoulder girdle muscles

- If the clinical history is not consistent with entrapment neuropathies (no sports or occupational overuse), especially in isolated suprascapular neuropathy.

However, although this diagnosis may be suspected on MR imaging, clinicians insist that the imaging findings should be interpreted with care and only in the light of the clinical picture. These patterns cannot serve to rule out the clinical diagnosis of neuralgic amyotrophy but may be an additional argument for the confirmation of the diagnosis.[22,48]

Muscle edema Muscle edema on MR imaging is a nonspecific finding because it may be seen in various conditions such as posttraumatic conditions, infections, radiation therapy, compartment syndrome, early myositis ossificans, polymyositis and dermatomyositis, rhabdomyolysis, and sickle

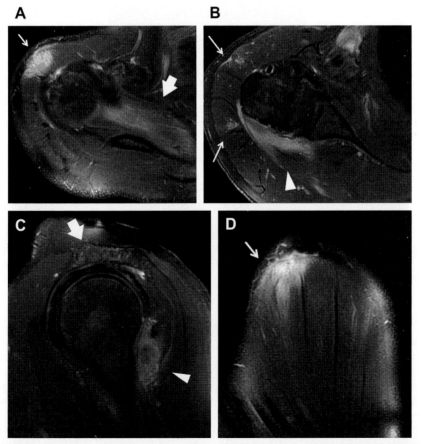

Fig. 17. T2-weighted sequences with fat suppression in a patient with Parsonage-Turner syndrome (A and B, axial plane; C and D, oblique sagittal plane). The edema affects muscles innervated by different nerves derived from the brachial plexus. The distribution of edema is inhomogeneous, whether inside a single muscle or in different muscles. The deltoid (*thin arrows*), supraspinatus (*thick arrows*), and teres minor (*arrowheads*) muscles are concerned.

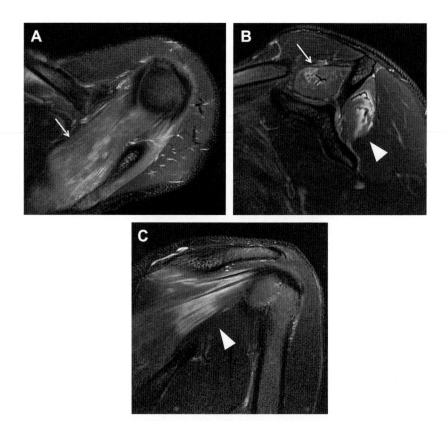

Fig. 18. Parsonage-Turner syndrome in a patient with isolated suprascapular nerve involvement. Unlike entrapment neuropathies, for which signal abnormalities are homogenous within a muscle, the pattern of lesions is heterogeneous within both the supraspinatus (*arrows*) and infraspinatus (*arrowheads*) muscles. T2-weighted sequences with fat suppression. (*A*) Axial plane, (*B*) oblique sagittal plane, and (*C*) oblique coronal plane.

cell crisis.[36] Unlike what is observed in entrapment neuropathies, the edema is likely to be heterogeneous within a muscle or between different muscles and to involve several muscles without any relation to the territory of a nerve (Fig. 19). Although the radiologist should keep these possibilities in mind, confusion may be avoided because the clinical situations are very different and because of other evocative imaging abnormalities.

TREATING ENTRAPMENT NEUROPATHIES

The initial treatment of entrapment neuropathy is typically nonoperative, consisting of physical therapy, nonsteroidal antiinflammatory drugs, and rest or moderation of activity. Open or arthroscopic surgery is primarily considered when there is extrinsic nerve compression.[1,2] It is also considered when medical treatment fails. The surgical treatment consists of decompression of the nerves and/or specific treatment of any identified shoulder abnormalities, such as labral tears. Controversy still exists among surgeons regarding these various options.[2] Surgical procedures are not

undertaken in the late stage of the disease when atrophy and fatty infiltration are present.

Mucoid cysts can benefit from percutaneous procedures, either under US or CT control, with puncture, aspiration, and steroid injection. In case of recurrence, surgery may be performed. In the event of compression of the suprascapular nerve by a mucoid cyst, healing is achieved in 50% of cases following radiologic procedures[1] and 80% to 90% after surgical intervention.[49]

Key Points

- Nerve entrapment is a rare but presumably underdiagnosed cause of shoulder pain, essentially because of nonspecific symptoms mimicking other pathologies.
- Radiologists must be aware of these conditions because they may be the first to suggest the diagnosis.
- A knowledge of the key anatomic features of the nerves is mandatory to allow a correct diagnosis.
- The MR imaging protocol must be adapted to the clinical situation, depending on

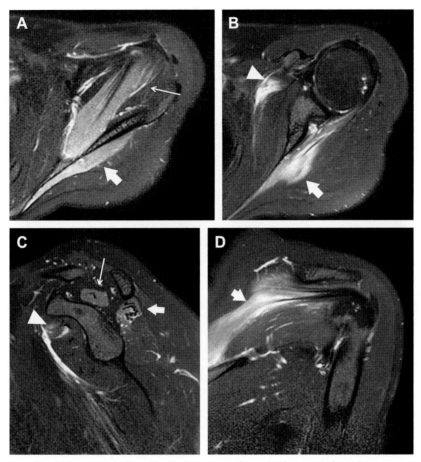

Fig. 19. Dermatopolymyositis can mimic entrapment neuropathy, as in this example. However, muscular edema is inhomogeneous in regard to both its intensity and its distribution within a single muscle. This is also true when comparing 2 affected muscles. The supraspinatus (*thin arrows*), infraspinatus (*thick arrows*), and subscapularis (*arrowheads*) muscles are involved. T2-weighted sequences with fat suppression. (*A* and *B*) Axial plane, (*C*) oblique sagittal plane, and (*D*) oblique coronal plane.

whether scapular winging or shoulder pain is explored.

- Key imaging findings are signs of denervation, muscular edema in the early stages, and atrophy and fatty replacement in the late ones. They are present in the muscles innervated by the entrapped nerve.
- Direct compression of the entrapped nerve must be sought because this can allow primary interventional (percutaneous/surgical) treatment.
- Usual causes of shoulder pain (eg, rotator cuff tendons tears) must be ruled out before considering this diagnosis.
- The involvement of different muscular groups suggests the differential diagnosis of Parsonage-Turner syndrome.
- Imaging abnormalities are not sufficient to establish the diagnosis; they must be evaluated in the light of clinical features.

REFERENCES

1. Blum A, Lecocq S, Louis M, et al. The nerves around the shoulder. Eur J Radiol 2011. [Epub ahead of print].
2. Boykin RE, Friedman DJ, Higgins LD, et al. Suprascapular neuropathy. J Bone Joint Surg Am 2010; 92(13):2348–64.
3. Rengachary SS, Burr D, Lucas S, et al. Suprascapular entrapment neuropathy: a clinical, anatomical, and comparative study. Part 2: anatomical study. Neurosurgery 1979;5(4):447–51.
4. Bayramoglu A, Demiryurek D, Tuccar E, et al. Variations in anatomy at the suprascapular notch possibly causing suprascapular nerve entrapment: an anatomical study. Knee Surg Sports Traumatol Arthrosc 2003;11(6):393–8.
5. Demirhan M, Imhoff AB, Debski RE, et al. The spinoglenoid ligament and its relationship to the suprascapular nerve. J Shoulder Elbow Surg 1998;7(3):238–43.

6. Brown DE, James DC, Roy S. Pain relief by supra-scapular nerve block in gleno-humeral arthritis. Scand J Rheumatol 1988;17(5):411–5.

7. Matsumoto D, Suenaga N, Oizumi N, et al. A new nerve block procedure for the suprascapular nerve based on a cadaveric study. J Shoulder Elbow Surg 2009;18(4):607–11.

8. Ritchie ED, Tong D, Chung F, et al. Suprascapular nerve block for postoperative pain relief in arthroscopic shoulder surgery: a new modality? Anesth Analg 1997;84(6):1306–12.

9. Zehetgruber H, Noske H, Lang T, et al. Suprascapular nerve entrapment. A meta-analysis. Int Orthop 2002;26(6):339–43.

10. McClelland D, Paxinos A. The anatomy of the quadri-lateral space with reference to quadrilateral space syndrome. J Shoulder Elbow Surg 2008;17(1):162–4.

11. Plancher KD, Luke TA, Peterson RK, et al. Posterior shoulder pain: a dynamic study of the spinoglenoid ligament and treatment with arthroscopic release of the scapular tunnel. Arthroscopy 2007;23(9):991–8.

12. Ringel SP, Treihaft M, Carry M, et al. Suprascapular neuropathy in pitchers. Am J Sports Med 1990;18(1):80–6.

13. Ferretti A, Cerullo G, Russo G. Suprascapular neuropathy in volleyball players. J Bone Joint Surg Am 1987;69(2):260–3.

14. Lajtai G, Pfirrmann CW, Aitzetmuller G, et al. The shoulders of professional beach volleyball players: high prevalence of infraspinatus muscle atrophy. Am J Sports Med 2009;37(7):1375–83.

15. Arboleya L, Garcia A. Suprascapular nerve entrap-ment of occupational etiology: clinical and electro-physiological characteristics. Clin Exp Rheumatol 1993;11(6):665–8.

16. Karatas GK, Gogus F. Suprascapular nerve entrap-ment in newsreel cameramen. Am J Phys Med Re-habil 2003;82(3):192–6.

17. Romeo AA, Rotenberg DD, Bach BR Jr. Suprascapular neuropathy. J Am Acad Orthop Surg 1999;7(6):358–67.

18. Yanny S, Toms AP. MR patterns of denervation around the shoulder. AJR Am J Roentgenol 2010;195(2):W157–63.

19. MacDonald BK, Cockerell OC, Sander JW, et al. The incidence and lifetime prevalence of neurological disorders in a prospective community-based study in the UK. Brain 2000;123(Pt 4):665–76.

20. Helms CA, Martinez S, Speer KP. Acute brachial neuritis (Parsonage-Turner syndrome): MR imaging appearance—report of three cases. Radiology 1998;207(1):255–9.

21. Scalf RE, Wenger DE, Frick MA, et al. MRI findings of 26 patients with Parsonage-Turner syndrome. AJR Am J Roentgenol 2007;189(1):W39–44.

22. van Alfen N, van Engelen BG. The clinical spectrum of neuralgic amyotrophy in 246 cases. Brain 2006;129(Pt 2):438–50.

23. Beghi E, Kurland LT, Mulder DW, et al. Brachial plexus neuropathy in the population of Rochester, Minnesota, 1970-1981. Ann Neurol 1985;18(3):320–3.

24. Tsairis P, Dyck PJ, Mulder DW. Natural history of brachial plexus neuropathy. Report on 99 patients. Arch Neurol 1972;27(2):109–17.

25. Magee KR, Dejong RN. Paralytic brachial neuritis. Discussion of clinical features with review of 23 cases. JAMA 1960;174:1258–62.

26. Suarez GA, Giannini C, Bosch EP, et al. Immune brachial plexus neuropathy: suggestive evidence for an inflammatory-immune pathogenesis. Neurology 1996;46(2):559–61.

27. Gaskin CM, Helms CA. Parsonage-Turner syndrome: MR imaging findings and clinical information of 27 patients. Radiology 2006;240(2):501–7.

28. McFarland EG, Garzon-Muvdi J, Jia X, et al. Clin-ical and diagnostic tests for shoulder disorders: a critical review. Br J Sports Med 2010;44(5):328–32.

29. Martin RM, Fish DE. Scapular winging: anatomical review, diagnosis, and treatments. Curr Rev Musculoskelet Med 2008;1(1):1–11.

30. Canella C, Demondion X, Abreu E, et al. Anatomical study of spinal accessory nerve using ultrasonography. Eur J Radiol 2011. [Epub ahead of print].

31. Bianchi S, Martinoli C. Ultrasound of the musculo-skeletal system. Germany: Springer Verlag; 2007.

32. Kamath S, Venkatanarasimha N, Walsh MA, et al. MRI appearance of muscle denervation. Skeletal Radiol 2008;37(5):397–404.

33. Kim SJ, Hong SH, Jun WS, et al. MR imaging mapping of skeletal muscle denervation in entrap-ment and compressive neuropathies. Radio-graphics 2011;31(2):319–32.

34. Bendszus M, Koltzenburg M, Wessig C, et al. Sequential MR imaging of denervated muscle: experimental study. AJNR Am J Neuroradiol 2002;23(8):1427–31.

35. West GA, Haynor DR, Goodkin R, et al. Magnetic resonance imaging signal changes in denervated muscles after peripheral nerve injury. Neurosurgery 1994;35(6):1077–85 [discussion: 1085–6].

36. May DA, Disler DG, Jones EA, et al. Abnormal signal intensity in skeletal muscle at MR imaging: patterns, pearls, and pitfalls. Radiographics 2000;20(Spec No):S295–315.

37. Yamabe E, Nakamura T, Oshio K, et al. Peripheral nerve injury: diagnosis with MR imaging of dener-vated skeletal muscle—experimental study in rats. Radiology 2008;247(2):409–17.

38. Ludig T, Walter F, Chapuis D, et al. MR imaging evaluation of suprascapular nerve entrapment. Eur Radiol 2001;11(11):2161–9.

39. Goutallier D, Postel JM, Bernageau J, et al. Fatty infiltration of disrupted rotator cuff muscles. Rev Rhum Engl Ed 1995;62(6):415–22.

40. Chen AL, Ong BC, Rose DJ. Arthroscopic management of spinoglenoid cysts associated with SLAP lesions and suprascapular neuropathy. Arthroscopy 2003;19(6):E15–21.
41. Werner CM, Nagy L, Gerber C. Combined intra- and extra-articular arthroscopic treatment of entrapment neuropathy of the infraspinatus branches of the suprascapular nerve caused by a periglenoidal ganglion cyst. Arthroscopy 2007;23(3):328.e321–3.
42. Mallon WJ, Wilson RJ, Basamania CJ. The association of suprascapular neuropathy with massive rotator cuff tears: a preliminary report. J Shoulder Elbow Surg 2006;15(4):395–8.
43. Vad VB, Southern D, Warren RF, et al. Prevalence of peripheral neurologic injuries in rotator cuff tears with atrophy. J Shoulder Elbow Surg 2003;12(4):333–6.
44. Albritton MJ, Graham RD, Richards RS 2nd, et al. An anatomic study of the effects on the suprascapular nerve due to retraction of the supraspinatus muscle after a rotator cuff tear. J Shoulder Elbow Surg 2003;12(5):497–500.
45. Greiner A, Golser K, Wambacher M, et al. The course of the suprascapular nerve in the supraspinatus fossa and its vulnerability in muscle advancement. J Shoulder Elbow Surg 2003;12(3):256–9.
46. Hoellrich RG, Gasser SI, Morrison DS, et al. Electromyographic evaluation after primary repair of massive rotator cuff tears. J Shoulder Elbow Surg 2005;14(3):269–72.
47. Kuhn JE, Plancher KD, Hawkins RJ. Scapular winging. J Am Acad Orthop Surg 1995;3(6):319–25.
48. van Eijk J, van Alfen N. Neuralgic amyotrophy. AJR Am J Roentgenol 2011;196(6):W858 [author reply: W859].
49. Westerheide KJ, Dopirak RM, Karzel RP, et al. Suprascapular nerve palsy secondary to spinoglenoid cysts: results of arthroscopic treatment. Arthroscopy 2006;22(7):721–7.

Index

Note: Page numbers of article titles are in **boldface** type.

Magn Reson Imaging Clin N Am 20 (2012) 393–396
doi:10.1016/S1064-9689(12)00026-8

mri.theclinics.com

Moving?

Make sure your subscription moves with you!

To notify us of your new address, find your **Clinics Account Number** (located on your mailing label above your name), and contact customer service at:

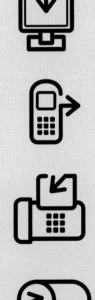

Email: journalscustomerservice-usa@elsevier.com

800-654-2452 (subscribers in the U.S. & Canada)
314-447-8871 (subscribers outside of the U.S. & Canada)

Fax number: 314-447-8029

Elsevier Health Sciences Division
Subscription Customer Service
3251 Riverport Lane
Maryland Heights, MO 63043

*To ensure uninterrupted delivery of your subscription, please notify us at least 4 weeks in advance of move.